Pelvic Pain

Editor

KELLY M. SCOTT

PHYSICAL MEDICINE AND REHABILITATION CLINICS OF NORTH AMERICA

www.pmr.theclinics.com

Consulting Editor
SANTOS F. MARTINEZ

August 2017 • Volume 28 • Number 3

ELSEVIER

1600 John F. Kennedy Boulevard ● Suite 1800 ● Philadelphia, Pennsylvania, 19103-2899

http://www.theclinics.com

**PHYSICAL MEDICINE AND REHABILITATION CLINICS OF NORTH AMERICA Volume 28, Number 3
August 2017 ISSN 1047-9651, ISBN 978-0-323-53253-2**

Editor: Lauren Boyle
Developmental Editor: Meredith Madeira

© **2017 Elsevier Inc. All rights reserved.**

This periodical and the individual contributions contained in it are protected under copyright by Elsevier, and the following terms and conditions apply to their use:

Photocopying
Single photocopies of single articles may be made for personal use as allowed by national copyright laws. Permission of the Publisher and payment of a fee is required for all other photocopying, including multiple or systematic copying, copying for advertising or promotional purposes, resale, and all forms of document delivery. Special rates are available for educational institutions that wish to make photocopies for non-profit educational classroom use. For information on how to seek permission visit www.elsevier.com/permissions or call: (+44) 1865 843830 (UK)/(+1) 215 239 3804 (USA).

Derivative Works
Subscribers may reproduce tables of contents or prepare lists of articles including abstracts for internal circulation within their institutions. Permission of the Publisher is required for resale or distribution outside the institution. Permission of the Publisher is required for all other derivative works, including compilations and translations (please consult www.elsevier.com/permissions).

Electronic Storage or Usage
Permission of the Publisher is required to store or use electronically any material contained in this periodical, including any article or part of an article (please consult www.elsevier.com/permissions). Except as outlined above, no part of this publication may be reproduced, stored in a retrieval system or transmitted in any form or by any means, electronic, mechanical, photocopying, recording or otherwise, without prior written permission of the Publisher.

Notice
No responsibility is assumed by the Publisher for any injury and/or damage to persons or property as a matter of products liability, negligence or otherwise, or from any use or operation of any methods, products, instructions or ideas contained in the material herein. Because of rapid advances in the medical sciences, in particular, independent verification of diagnoses and drug dosages should be made.

Although all advertising material is expected to conform to ethical (medical) standards, inclusion in this publication does not constitute a guarantee or endorsement of the quality or value of such product or of the claims made of it by its manufacturer.

Reprints. For copies of 100 or more of articles in this publication, please contact the Commercial Reprints Department, Elsevier Inc., 360 Park Avenue South, New York, NY 10010-1710. Tel.: 212-633-3874; Fax: 212-633-3820; E-mail: reprints@elsevier.com.

Physical Medicine and Rehabilitation Clinics of North America (ISSN 1047-9651) is published quarterly by Elsevier Inc., 360 Park Avenue South, New York, NY 10010-1710. Months of issue are February, May, August, and November. Business and Editorial Offices: 1600 John F. Kennedy Blvd., Suite 1800, Philadelphia, PA 19103-2899. Customer Service Office: 3251 Riverport Lane, Maryland Heights, MO 63043. Periodicals postage paid at New York, NY and additional mailing offices. Subscription price per year is $288.00 (US individuals), $560.00 (US institutions), $100.00 (US students), $210.00 (Canadian individuals), $737.00 (Canadian institutions), $210.00 (Canadian students), $210.00 (foreign individuals), $737.00 (foreign institutions), and $210.00 (foreign students). Foreign air speed delivery is included in all *Clinics* subscription prices. All prices are subject to change without notice. **POSTMASTER:** Send address changes to *Physical Medicine and Rehabilitation Clinics of North America*, Customer Service Office: Elsevier Health Sciences Division, Subscription Customer Service, 3251 Riverport Lane, Maryland Heights, MO 63043. **Customer Service: 1-800-654-2452 (US). From outside of the United States, call 314-447-8871. Fax: 314-447-8029. E-mail: JournalsCustomer Service-usa@elsevier.com (for print support); JournalsOnlineSupport-usa@elsevier.com (for online support).**

Physical Medicine and Rehabilitation Clinics of North America is indexed in *Excerpta Medica, MEDLINE/ PubMed (Index Medicus), Cinahl,* and *Cumulative Index to Nursing and Allied Health Literature.*

Contributors

CONSULTING EDITOR

SANTOS F. MARTINEZ, MD, MS
American Academy of Physical Medicine and Rehabilitation, Campbell Clinic
Orthopaedics, Department of Orthopaedics, University of Tennessee, Memphis,
Tennessee

EDITOR

KELLY M. SCOTT, MD
Medical Director, Comprehensive Pelvic Rehabilitation Program, Associate Professor,
Physical Medicine and Rehabilitation, University of Texas Southwestern Medical Center,
Dallas, Texas

AUTHORS

STACEY BENNIS, MD
Resident Physician, Northwestern-Feinberg School of Medicine Physical Medicine
and Rehabilitation, Chicago, Illinois

JACLYN H. BONDER, MD
Assistant Professor, Department of Rehabilitation Medicine, New York Presbyterian
Hospital, Weill Cornell Medical College, New York, New York

MICHELLE H. BRADLEY, PT, DPT, WCS, CLT-LANA
Physical Therapy, Outpatient PM&R, Physical Medicine and Rehabilitation Clinic,
University of Texas Southwestern Medical Center of Dallas, Dallas, Texas

C. ANNA BRINKER, PT, MHS
Physical Therapy, Outpatient PM&R, Physical Medicine and Rehabilitation Clinic,
University of Texas Southwestern Medical Center of Dallas, Dallas, Texas

BENJAMIN M. BRUCKER, MD
Assistant Professor, Division of Female Pelvic Medicine and Reconstructive Surgery,
Neurourology and Voiding Dysfunction, Medical Director, Tisch Hospital; Associate
Program Director Residency Program, Departments of Urology and Obstetrics and
Gynecology, NYU Langone Medical Center, New York, New York

JOHN CHANG, MBBS
Department of Urology, St George Hospital, Kogarah, New South Wales, Australia

AVNEESH CHHABRA, MD
Associate Professor, Department of Radiology and Department of Orthopedic Surgery,
University of Texas Southwestern Medical Center, Dallas, Texas

MICHELLE CHI, MD
PGY 3, Department of Rehabilitation Medicine, New York Presbyterian Hospital,
New York, New York

SARAH M. EICKMEYER, MD
Assistant Professor, Medical Director of Inpatient Rehabilitation Services, Residency Program Director, Department of Rehabilitation Medicine, University of Kansas, Kansas City, Kansas

NICHOLAS ELKINS, DO
Physical Medicine and Rehabilitation, University of Texas Southwestern Medical Center, Dallas, Texas

KIMBERLY L. FERRANTE, MD
Assistant Professor, Division of Female Pelvic Medicine and Reconstructive Surgery, Department of Obstetrics and Gynecology, Department of Urology, Associate OB/GYN Residency Program Director, New York University School of Medicine, New York, New York

COLLEEN M. FITZGERALD, MD, MS
Medical Director, Chronic Pelvic Pain Program, Loyola University Chicago, Stritch School of Medicine, Maywood, Illinois

PATRICK M. FOYE, MD
Professor and Interim Chair, Physical Medicine and Rehabilitation, Director, Coccyx Pain Center, Rutgers New Jersey Medical School, Newark, New Jersey

JASON HUNT, MD
Physical Medicine and Rehabilitation, University of Texas Southwestern Medical Center, Dallas, Texas

SARAH HWANG, MD
Assistant Professor of Clinical Physical Medicine and Rehabilitation, University of Missouri, Columbia, Missouri

AMBEREEN KHAN, MD
Assistant Professor, Department of Radiology, University of Texas Southwestern Medical Center, Dallas, Texas

GAURAV KHATRI, MD
Assistant Professor, Department of Radiology, University of Texas Southwestern Medical Center, Dallas, Texas

PHUONG U. LE, DO
Pain Medicine Fellow, Department of Physical Medicine and Rehabilitation, West Los Angeles Veterans Affairs Medical Center, University of California at Los Angeles, Los Angeles, California

DOMINIC LEE, MBBS, FRACS (Urology)
Department of Urology, St George Hospital, Kogarah, New South Wales, Australia

DOMINIQUE R. MALACARNE, MD
Division of Female Pelvic Medicine and Reconstructive Surgery, Department of Urology, Department of Obstetrics and Gynecology, NYU Langone Medical Center, New York, New York

ERIKA L. MOODY, MD, MBS
Clinical Fellow, Department of Anesthesiology, UT Health San Antonio, San Antonio, Texas

AMEET S. NAGPAL, MD, MS, MEd
Clinical Assistant Professor, Department of Anesthesiology, UT Health San Antonio, San Antonio, Texas

JASON PAN, MD
Chief Resident, Department of Physical Medicine and Rehabilitation, University of Pennsylvania, Philadelphia, Pennsylvania

GARGI RAVAL, MD
Assistant Professor, Department of Physical Medicine and Rehabilitation, Dallas VA Medical Center, University of Texas Southwestern Medical Center, Dallas, Texas

ASHLEY RAWLINS, PT, DPT
Physical Therapy, Outpatient PM&R, Physical Medicine and Rehabilitation Clinic, University of Texas Southwestern Medical Center of Dallas, Dallas, Texas

LEIA RISPOLI, MD
PGY 3, Department of Rehabilitation Medicine, New York Presbyterian Hospital, New York, New York

KELLY M. SCOTT, MD
Medical Director, Comprehensive Pelvic Rehabilitation Program, Associate Professor, Physical Medicine and Rehabilitation, University of Texas Southwestern Medical Center, Dallas, Texas

KATE E. TEMME, MD, CAQSM
Co-Director, Penn Center for the Female Athlete, Assistant Professor, Departments of Physical Medicine and Rehabilitation, and Orthopaedics, University of Pennsylvania, Philadelphia, Pennsylvania

PHILIPPE E. ZIMMERN, MD
Department of Urology, University of Texas Southwestern Medical Center, Dallas, Texas

Contents

Although the cause of chronic pelvic pain (CPP) is multifactorial, a substantial number of cases have musculoskeletal and neuromuscular causes. Multiple stakeholders, including physicians with varying degrees of pain training ranging from primary care physicians, obstetricians, gynecologists, urologists, neurologists, gastroenterologists, psychologists, physical therapists, and physiatrists, are involved in the care of these patients. Physiatrists play a pivotal role in the treatment of patients with CPP because their training focuses on improving quality of life through a holistic approach to patient management and on the musculoskeletal and neuromuscular systems.

Understanding the anatomic relationship of the pelvic floor muscles with the pelvic girdle, spine, and hips aids the rehabilitation provider in diagnosis, management, and appropriate referrals. The bony anatomy of the pelvic girdle consists of 3 bones and 3 joints. The pelvic floor muscles are comprised mainly of the levator ani muscles with somatic innervation from the lumbosacral plexus. The bony and muscular pelvis is highly interconnected to the hip and gluteal musculature, which together provide support to the internal organs and core muscles. Pelvic floor physiology is centered on bladder and bowel control, sexual functioning, and pregnancy.

The history and physical examination are important keys to diagnosis and treatment of patients with chronic pelvic pain. The comprehensive history should include questioning regarding patient's pain complaint and a thorough history and review of any body system that may be involved, including neuromusculoskeletal, obstetric, gynecologic, gastrointestinal, urologic, dermatologic, infectious, oncologic, and psychiatric. The physical examination should also follow a focused systems-based approach and includes examination of gastrointestinal, dermatologic, neurologic, and musculoskeletal (including lumbosacral spine, sacroiliac joints, pelvis, and hips) systems, and the pelvic floor (internal and external examination, including neuromuscular anatomy).

Chronic pelvic pain can result from various intra- and extra-pelvic etiologies. Although patient history and physical examination may narrow the differential diagnosis, frequently, the different etiologies have overlapping presentations. Imaging examinations such as US and/or MR imaging may help delineate the cause of pain, particularly when related to intra-pelvic organs, pelvic floor dysfunction or prolapse, synthetic material such as pelvic mesh or slings, and in some cases of neuropathic pain. Etiologies of neuropathic pain can also be assessed with non-imaging tests such as nerve conduction studies, electromyography, and testing of sacral reflexes.

Myofascial pelvic pain refers to pain in the pelvic floor muscles, the pelvic floor connective tissue, and the surrounding fascia. The cause is often multifactorial and requires treatment that encompasses multiple modalities. This type of pain is often associated with other abdominopelvic disorders, so providers in these specialties need to be aware of these connections. A comprehensive musculoskeletal examination, including evaluation of the pelvic floor muscles, and history are key to diagnosing myofascial pelvic pain. Treatments include physical therapy, muscle relaxers, oral neuromodulators, cognitive-behavioral therapy, and pelvic floor muscle injections.

Visceral and somatic causes of pelvic pain are often inter-related, and a musculoskeletal examination should always be considered for the successful diagnosis and treatment of pelvic pain. For the diverse etiologies of hip pain, there are many unique considerations for the diagnosis and treatment of these various disorders. Pelvic pain is often multidimensional due to the overlap between lumbo-hip-pelvic diagnoses and may require a multidisciplinary approach to evaluation and management.

Coccyx (tailbone) pain substantially decreases the quality of life for patients who suffer with this condition. Classic symptoms include midline pain located below the sacrum and above the anus. Symptoms are worse while sitting or during transitions from sitting to standing. Physical examination typically reveals focal tenderness during palpation of the coccyx. Diagnostic tests include radiographs. Advanced studies may include MRI, computerized tomography scans, or nuclear medicine bone scans.

Treatments may include the use of cushions, medications by mouth, topical medications, local pain management injections, pelvic floor physical therapy, and (in rare cases) surgical removal of the coccyx (coccygectomy).

PHYSICAL MEDICINE AND REHABILITATION CLINICS OF NORTH AMERICA

RELATED INTEREST

Obstetrics & Gynecology Clinics, September 2014 (Vol. 41, Issue 3)
Pelvic Pain in Women
Mary T. McLennan, Andrew Steele, Fah Che Leong, *Editors*

VISIT THE CLINICS ONLINE!
Access your subscription at:
www.theclinics.com

Foreword

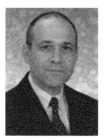

Santos F. Martinez, MD, MS
Consulting Editor

It is with great anticipation that this issue on pelvic pain becomes available to our readers. The format is artfully and effectively presented by Dr Scott and colleagues and will serve as a landmark reference compendium on the topic. Although there has been an awareness of this group of disorders, it frequently escapes our traditional training curriculum as there are few who dedicate themselves to this niche. There is a significant shortage of qualified specialists to manage this patient population, and as Dr Scott alluded to, the Physiatrist certainly has the potential to refine his/her skills to become the subspecialist to take on the task. This compendium can serve as a primer for our residents in training and those in private practice alike. Our extensive anatomic training is complemented by a review in pelvic anatomy/physiology with guidance in clinical assessment and further inclusion of interventional techniques. This issue fills a void in our armamentarium and provides the physiatrist with practical tools to manage this population to help restore function and optimize our patients' quality of life. It is our hope that more PMR residency programs will include this review in their basic curriculum.

Santos F. Martinez, MD, MS
American Academy of Physical Medicine
and Rehabilitation
Campbell Clinic Orthopaedics
Department of Orthopaedics
University of Tennessee
Memphis, TN 38104, USA

E-mail address:
smartinez@campbellclinic.com

Phys Med Rehabil Clin N Am 28 (2017) xiii
http://dx.doi.org/10.1016/j.pmr.2017.05.001
1047-9651/17/© 2017 Published by Elsevier Inc.

Preface

Pelvic Pain

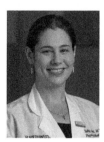

Kelly M. Scott, MD
Editor

It is my distinct pleasure to present this *Physical Medicine and Rehabilitation Clinics of North America* issue focused on pelvic pain. Pelvic pain is an extremely common phenomenon, particularly in women, and patients with pelvic pain suffer greatly—not only due to their pain but also because of the associated problems they experience with bladder, bowel, and sexual functioning. Physiatrists are encountering pelvic pain patients with increasing frequency, whether in pain management practices, in occupational health settings, in spine centers, or even within the context of general rehabilitation medicine. And, believe it or not, this is a GOOD THING! Pelvic pain patients need us, because we are the doctors who understand muscles, nerves, and joints, structures that are largely ignored by most of the surgical specialists who typically see patients with pelvic complaints. As this issue will delineate, there are many musculoskeletal and neurologic causes of pelvic pain that we can diagnose and treat successfully using our physiatric principles. Patients who previously have been shuttled from one surgeon to the next, receiving at best multiple rounds of antibiotics and at worst surgeries to remove healthy organs, can finally find relief from their suffering when the actual cause of their pain is discovered and managed appropriately.

The 12 articles in this issue are meant to give a strong foundational education in the treatment of musculoskeletal and neurologic pelvic pain. First, Phuong U. Le and Colleen M. Fitzgerald provide a general overview of the topic, including epidemiology, risk factors, clinical presentation, and formulating a differential diagnosis. Then, Sarah M. Eickmeyer details the anatomy and physiology of the pelvic floor, and Stacey Bennis and Sarah Hwang describe the office evaluation of pelvic pain with a focus on history-taking and physical examination (including a detailed description of how to conduct a pelvic floor neuromuscular evaluation). Diagnostic studies for pelvic pain are covered by Gaurav Khatri, Ambereen Khan, Gargi Raval, and Avneesh Chhabra with a focus on both radiologic imaging studies and electrodiagnosis. Pelvic floor myofascial pain is one of the most common causes of chronic pelvic pain, and Jaclyn H. Bonder, Michelle Chi, and Leia Rispoli describe pelvic floor dysfunction and its

Phys Med Rehabil Clin N Am 28 (2017) xv–xvi
http://dx.doi.org/10.1016/j.pmr.2017.03.013
1047-9651/17/© 2017 Published by Elsevier Inc.

associated syndromes. As many who practice musculoskeletal medicine know, there are many musculoskeletal causes of pelvic pain apart from the pelvic floor muscles, and Kate Elizabeth Temme and Jason Pan delve into these topics in their article. Patrick Foye's article focuses on coccydynia, a common condition seen in many pain and spine practices, but which is truly also a pelvic musculoskeletal disorder. Little is known about neurogenic causes of pelvic pain, but Nicholas Elkins, Jason Hunt, and Kelly Scott attempt to shed light on these excruciatingly painful conditions such as pudendal neuralgia. Dominique R. Malacarne, Kimberly L. Ferrante, and Benjamin M. Brucker give an overview of gynecologic and urologic causes of pelvic pain, so that we as physiatrists can be familiar with these entities and know when to refer to our surgical colleagues when a patient does not have musculoskeletal or neurologic pathology in the pelvis. Pelvic floor physical therapy is rapidly emerging as one of the best treatment methods for chronic pelvic pain, and the article by Michelle Bradley, Ashley Rawlins, and Cynthia Brinker provides the physical therapy perspective on what techniques are important for successful treatment. D. Lee, J. Chang, and P. Zimmern describe the evaluation and management of iatrogenic pelvic pain after synthetic mesh placement—a scenario that has unfortunately become far too common among our chronic pelvic pain patients. The issue ends with Ameet S. Nagpal and Erica L. Moody detailing interventional pain management techniques for the treatment of pelvic pain.

I would like to extend my sincere thanks to the expert authors, who contributed their time and talents to this issue, and I would like to dedicate this work to the countless patients who suffer and to the devoted practitioners and therapists who try to help them. It is my hope that this issue will enable more physiatrists to join our ranks and provide healing to these patients who truly need it.

Kelly M. Scott, MD
Physical Medicine and Rehabilitation
University of Texas Southwestern Medical Center
5323 Harry Hines Boulevard
Dallas, TX 75390-9055, USA

E-mail address:
kelly.scott@utsouthwestern.edu

Pelvic Pain: An Overview

Phuong U. Le, DO[a],*, Colleen M. Fitzgerald, MD, MS[b]

KEYWORDS

- Chronic pelvic pain • Pelvic pain of myofascial origin • Downtraining pelvic floor

KEY POINTS

- Although the cause of chronic pelvic pain (CPP) is multifactorial, a substantial number of cases have musculoskeletal and neuromuscular causes.
- Multiple stakeholders, including physicians with varying degrees of pain training ranging from primary care physicians, obstetricians, gynecologists, urologists, neurologists, gastroenterologists, psychologists, physical therapists, and physiatrists, are involved in the care of these patients.
- Unfortunately, little cross-collaboration occurs among specialty providers, and the patient often consults with these varying specialists in sequential order because few interdisciplinary centers exist.
- Physiatrists play a pivotal role in the treatment of patients with CPP because their training focuses on improving quality of life through a holistic approach to patient management and on the musculoskeletal and neuromuscular systems.

Pelvic pain is defined as pain localizing to the pelvis, the anterior abdominal wall at or below the umbilicus, the lumbosacral back, or the buttocks.[1] Acute pelvic pain has a sudden onset that requires prompt diagnosis and expeditious treatment. Chronic pelvic pain (CPP) is constant or recurring and arbitrarily defined as lasting for more than 6 months and frequently carries significant physical, functional, and psychological burdens that negatively affect quality of life (QoL). Consequently, the management of patients with CPP is drastically different from that of acute pelvic pain and can be very challenging. CPP is a multifactorial condition with overlapping causes driven by visceral, somatic, as well as complex pelvic neural circuitry.[2] More than 70 different diagnoses[3] are associated with CPP, with most patients often suffering from coexisting bowel, bladder, and sexual dysfunction. Multiple stakeholders, including physicians with varying degrees of pain training ranging from primary care physicians, obstetricians, gynecologists, urologists, neurologists, gastroenterologists, psychologists, physical therapists, and physiatrists, are involved in the care of these patients.

The authors have nothing to disclose.
[a] Department of Physical Medicine and Rehabilitation, West Los Angeles Veterans Affairs Medical Center, University of California at Los Angeles, 11301 Wilshire Boulevard, Los Angeles, CA 90073, USA; [b] Chronic Pelvic Pain Program, Loyola University Chicago, Stritch School of Medicine, 2160 S First Avenue, Maywood, IL 60153, USA
* Corresponding author.
E-mail address: le.u.phuong@gmail.com

Unfortunately, little cross-collaboration occurs among specialty providers. The patient often consults with these varying specialists in sequential order because few interdisciplinary centers exist. Physiatrists play a pivotal role in the treatment of patients with CPP because their training focuses on improving QoL through a holistic approach to patient management and on the musculoskeletal and neuromuscular systems.

EPIDEMIOLOGY

Although CPP affects women of all ages, epidemiologic studies of CPP have been hampered by a lack of a unifying definition, unclear cause and pathophysiology, and the absence of a definitive diagnostic marker. Overall, the prevalence of CPP in women ranged between 5.7% and 26.6% worldwide.[4] More than 15% of women experience CPP for over a period of 1 year,[5] with the average duration of symptoms of 2.5 years.[6] Lifetime prevalence may reach 33% in women. There is no significant correlation with mean gravidity and parity, rates of elective abortion, race, or mean educational level.[7] Annually, approximately 400,000 laparoscopies are performed to evaluate CPP with 40% of patients having negative results.[1] The prevalence by CPP subtype varies with endometriosis in 11% of reproductive age women, interstitial cystitis or painful bladder syndrome ranging from 1.2 to 4.5 per 100,000[8] to as high as 1 in 4.5 women,[9] vulvodynia from 8.3%[10] to 16%,[11] and pelvic floor myofascial pain from 9% to 24%.[12] Pelvic floor myofascial pain often coexists in patients with these subtypes of CPP. For example, more than 50% of patients with endometriosis also have pelvic floor myofascial pain.[13] CPP also afflicts men, with a worldwide prevalence of 2% to 16% in those less than 50 years old.[5]

DISABILITY

Patients with CPP have a significantly poorer QoL. The Short Form 36 Health Survey Questionnaire (SF-36) is the most frequently used subjective measurement of QoL in CPP studies.[14] SF-36 scores are inversely proportional to the degree of pelvic pain. In other words, higher pain scores correlate with lower QoL. Physical function, bodily pain, general health, vitality, social function, and mental health scores are lower among women with CPP.[15] Urinary symptoms, including frequency, nocturia, and dysuria, also negatively impact both men and women with CPP. In addition, sexual dysfunction secondary to pain and discomfort related to intercourse is common to both genders. However, overall, women with CPP are less sexually active than men.[16] Bowel dysfunction such as irritable bowel syndrome is also prevalent[17–20] and can significantly decrease QoL. Women with a history of physical and sexual trauma have a significantly higher rate of CPP and experience more posttraumatic stress,[21] which can further impair their mental health QoL.[22] These women experience a higher incidence of sleep disturbances as well as limitations of mobility.[23,24]

Risk Factors for Chronic Pelvic Pain

Multiple factors can predispose a patient to the development of CPP. A list of risk factors that have been identified follows[25]:

- Trauma/microtrauma
  - Timing may be remote or recent
  - In many cases, the specific trauma or inciting event may not be identified
- Vaginal or urinary tract infections
- Pregnancy and childbirth (vaginal or operative delivery)
- Musculoskeletal problems affecting the back, hips, and legs or pelvic girdle

- Pelvic or vaginal surgery or procedure
- Chronic constipation
- Chronic anxiety or depression can worsen pain or trigger a flare
- History of sexual abuse[26]

Acute-on-Chronic and Red Flags

Patients with CPP may suffer from acute medical conditions involving the pelvic structures. Therefore, it is important that the treating physicians not overlook the clinical manifestations of acute pain while treating patients with an established diagnosis of CPP. For patients on existing opioid medications, providers may downplay the patient's acute pain as a sign of drug seeking. If there is a change in the characteristics of the pain, a thorough investigation is warranted. New-onset fever or chills, recent weight loss, new postcoital bleeding, changes in bowel habits, gross hematuria, and any bright red blood per rectum or melena warrant immediate investigation. Acute-on-chronic pelvic pain can result from a variety of infectious and inflammatory conditions across specialties, including urologic (kidney stones, urinary tract infection), neurologic (multiple sclerosis), colorectal (gastroenteritis), gynecologic (sexually transmitted infection, pelvic inflammatory disease, ovarian cyst), musculoskeletal (acute herniated disc, synovitis). Malignancy must always also be ruled out with any change in symptom presentation no matter what the age range of the patient.

Differential Diagnoses

CPP is a multifactorial condition with possible sources, including visceral organs, soft tissues, muscles, nerves, and osseous structures. It is important to distinguish subtypes or more specific diagnoses within the overarching umbrella of CPP, especially pelvic girdle pain. PGP is musculoskeletal pain that localizes in the region of the sacroiliac joint and/or the pubic symphysis.[2]

Common causes of CPP are listed by organ system in **Table 1**. Specific neuromuscular causes of CPP are listed in **Table 2**.

EVALUATION

The evaluation for CPP of neuromuscular origin by a physiatrist is different from and cannot substitute for the pelvic or rectal examination performed by a gynecologist, a primary care physician, or other specialists. The gynecologic examination includes the evaluation of the external genitalia, speculum examination, and bimanual

Table 1
Common causes of chronic pelvic pain and comorbid diagnoses

Urologic	Gynecologic	Gastrointestinal	Psychological
Interstitial cystitis/ bladder pain syndrome	Endometriosis	Proctalgia fugax	Depression
	Vulvodynia	Anorectal pain syndrome	Physical or sexual abuse
Urethral pain syndrome	Adenomyosis	Irritable bowel syndrome	Sleep disturbance
Penile pain syndrome	Pelvic adhesions	Chronic appendicitis	Psychological stress
Prostate pain syndrome	Ovarian cysts	Inflammatory bowel disease	Substance abuse
Scrotal pain syndrome	Residual ovary syndrome	Hemorrhoids	
Chronic urinary tract infection	Posthysterectomy pain	Functional bowel disorder	
Chronic prostatitis	Pelvic congestion syndrome		
	Fibroids		

Table 2
Neuromuscular causes of chronic pelvic pain

Category	Diagnoses
Muscular/fascia	• Pelvic floor myofascial pain/levator ani syndrome/tension myalgia • Myofascial pain syndromes of associated extrinsic muscles (iliopsoas, adductor, piriformis) • Dyssynergia of the PFMs • Vaginismus/dyspareunia • Iatrogenic (synthetic mesh infection, exposure through vaginal mucosa, contraction and band formation)
Skeletal/joint	• Pelvic insufficiency/stress fracture • Sacroiliac joint dysfunction/servilities • Pelvic obliquity or derangement, pelvic asymmetry • Pubic symphysitis/osteitis pubis/pubic symphysis separation • Coccydynia • Lumbar degenerative disc disease/spondylosis or listhesis (with referral to posterior pelvis [L4-L5-S1]) • Hip osteoarthritis/hip fracture/acetabular labral tears/chondrosis/developmental hip dysplasia/femoral acetabular impingement/avascular necrosis of the femoral head • Bony metastasis
Neurologic	• Radiculopathy • Plexopathy • Peripheral neuropathy–pudendal neuropathy • Sacral postherpetic neuralgia
Viscerosomatic (presumed)	• Endometriosis • Irritable bowel syndrome • Bladder pain syndrome • Dysmenorrhea • Chronic prostatitis (in men)

examination[27] to evaluate cervical malignancy, vaginal infection, and sexually transmitted disease, whereas the focus of the neuromuscular examination is the evaluation of the overall external postural alignment as well as the internal and external myofascial, neurologic assessment.

Patients with CPP often have "overactive" pelvic floor muscles (PFMs) on physical examination.[28] Overactive PFMs are hypertonic and shortened, often in spasm and tender to palpate. Hence, PFM training for CPP primarily focuses on "downtraining" the pelvic floor by teaching patients to relax and lengthen the PFM. Downtraining can consist of myofascial release, scar/connective tissue mobilization, diaphragmatic breathing, mental imagery, paradoxic relaxation, perineal bulges (also called "reverse Kegels"), stretches, vaginal or anal dilation, rectal balloon catheter training, desensitization, skin rolling, visceral mobilization, and dry needling.

ASSOCIATED CONDITIONS THAT ACCOMPANY PELVIC PAIN

The uterus, cervix, adnexa, and bladder share the same visceral innervation as the lower ileum, sigmoid colon, and rectum. Signals travel via the sympathetic nerves to spinal cord segments T10 through L1. Because of this shared pathway, distinguishing between pain of gynecologic, urologic, and gastrointestinal origin is often difficult.[29] It is not surprising then that symptoms associated with CPP include bowel, bladder, and sexual dysfunction. Symptoms that are commonly associated with CPP include suprapubic pain, urinary urgency with or without incontinence, constipation, dyspareunia, and postcoital pain. Psychiatric comorbidities include depression, sleep disturbance, and psychological stress.

SUMMARY

Not only does CPP pose enormous suffering on the individual patient but also diagnostic and therapeutic endeavors are costly for society. Although the cause of CPP is multifactorial, a substantial number of cases have musculoskeletal and neuromuscular causes. Therefore, an emphasis must be placed on the importance of the evaluation of patients from a musculoskeletal and neuromuscular perspective. The authors recently investigated trends in clinicaltrials.gov to assess the current number and characteristics of randomized controlled trials addressing female CPP of myofascial origin. Their review revealed a dearth of clinical trials investigating this condition (Le Phuong and colleagues, unpublished data, 2015-2016). Thus, clinicians are forced to assemble a ragtag anthology of expert opinions and evidence from studies of other pelvic pain disorders. From the authors' investigation, it is also evident that there is a lack of a uniform terminology to address this condition perhaps due to the involvement of multiple stakeholders caring for these patients. In order to allow for better cross-talk among subspecialties, the development of a common terminology is of utmost importance because the condition is broad, challenging, and multifaceted and requires an interdisciplinary management approach. In addition, it is imperative that original research and clinical trials focused on pelvic girdle and pelvic floor myofascial pain be pursued.

REFERENCES

1. Howard FM. The role of laparoscopy in chronic pelvic pain: promise and pitfalls. Obstet Gynecol Surv 1993;48(6):357–87.
2. Hoffman D. Understanding multisymptom presentations in chronic pelvic pain: the inter-relationships between the viscera and myofascial pelvic floor dysfunction. Curr Pain Headache Rep 2011;15(5):343–6.
3. Hahn L. Chronic pelvic pain in women. A condition difficult to diagnose–more than 70 different diagnoses can be considered. Lakartidningen 2001;98(15): 1780–5 [in Swedish].
4. Ahangari A. Prevalence of chronic pelvic pain among women: an updated review. Pain Physician 2014;17(2):E141–7.
5. Krieger JN, Nyberg L Jr, Nickel JC. NIH consensus definition and classification of prostatitis. JAMA 1999;282(3):236–7.
6. Reiter RC, Gambone JC. Demographic and historic variables in women with idiopathic chronic pelvic pain. Obstet Gynecol 1990;75(3 Pt 1):428–32.
7. Mathias SD, Kuppermann M, Liberman RF, et al. Chronic pelvic pain: prevalence, health-related quality of life, and economic correlates. Obstet Gynecol 1996; 87(3):321–7.
8. Ito T, Miki M, Yamada T. Interstitial cystitis in Japan. BJU Int 2000;86(6):634–7.
9. Parsons CL, Dell J, Stanford EJ, et al. Increased prevalence of interstitial cystitis: previously unrecognized urologic and gynecologic cases identified using a new symptom questionnaire and intravesical potassium sensitivity. Urology 2002; 60(4):573–8.
10. Reed BD, Harlow SD, Sen A, et al. Prevalence and demographic characteristics of vulvodynia in a population-based sample. Am J Obstet Gynecol 2012;206(2): 170.e1-9.

11. Harlow BL, Stewart EG. A population-based assessment of chronic unexplained vulvar pain: have we underestimated the prevalence of vulvodynia? J Am Med Womens Assoc (1972) 2003;58(2):82–8.

12. Adams K, Gregory WT, Osmundsen B, et al. Levator myalgia: why bother? Int Urogynecol J 2013;24(10):1687–93.

13. Dos Bispo AP, Ploger C, Loureiro AF, et al. Assessment of pelvic floor muscles in women with deep endometriosis. Arch Gynecol Obstet 2016;294(3):519–23.

14. Neelakantan D, Omojole F, Clark TJ, et al. Quality of life instruments in studies of chronic pelvic pain: a systematic review. J Obstet Gynaecol 2004;24(8):851–8.

15. Haggerty CL, Schulz R, Ness RB. Lower quality of life among women with chronic pelvic pain after pelvic inflammatory disease. Obstet Gynecol 2003;102(5 Pt 1): 934–9.

16. Quaghebeur J, Wyndaele JJ. Prevalence of lower urinary tract symptoms and level of quality of life in men and women with chronic pelvic pain. Scand J Urol 2015;49(3):242–9.

17. Liao CH, Lin HC, Huang CY. Chronic prostatitis/chronic pelvic pain syndrome is associated with irritable bowel syndrome: a population-based study. Scientific Rep 2016;6:26939.

18. Choung RS, Herrick LM, Locke GR 3rd, et al. Irritable bowel syndrome and chronic pelvic pain: a population-based study. J Clin Gastroenterol 2010; 44(10):696–701.

19. Matheis A, Martens U, Kruse J, et al. Irritable bowel syndrome and chronic pelvic pain: a singular or two different clinical syndrome? World J Gastroenterol 2007; 13(25):3446–55.

20. Hooker AB, van Moorst BR, van Haarst EP, et al. Chronic pelvic pain: evaluation of the epidemiology, baseline demographics, and clinical variables via a prospective and multidisciplinary approach. Clin Exp Obstet Gynecol 2013;40(4):492–8.

21. Meltzer-Brody S, Leserman J, Zolnoun D, et al. Trauma and posttraumatic stress disorder in women with chronic pelvic pain. Obstet Gynecol 2007;109(4):902–8.

22. Smith KB, Tripp D, Pukall C, et al. Predictors of sexual and relationship functioning in couples with chronic prostatitis/chronic pelvic pain syndrome. J Sex Med 2007;4(3):734–44.

23. Grace V, Zondervan K. Chronic pelvic pain in women in New Zealand: comparative well-being, comorbidity, and impact on work and other activities. Health Care Women Int 2006;27(7):585–99.

24. Vivian D, Barnard A. Prevalence and correlates of three types of pelvic pain in a nationally representative sample of Australian women. The Med J Aust 2009; 190(1):47–8 [author reply: 48].

25. Moynihan LK, Elkadry EA, Myofascial Pelvic Pain Syndrome, First Consult January 2014.

26. Paras ML, Murad MH, Chen LP, et al. Sexual abuse and lifetime diagnosis of somatic disorders: a systematic review and meta-analysis. JAMA 2009;302(5): 550–61.

27. American College of Obstericians and Gynecologists: ACOG Committee Opinion No. 534. A Well Woman Visit. August 2012.

28. Butrick CW. Pathophysiology of pelvic floor hypertonic disorders. Obstet Gynecol Clin North Am 2009;36(3):699–705.

29. Baggish MS. Advanced Pelvic Anatomy. Atlas of Pelvic Anatomy and Gynecologic Surgery. 4th edition. Chapter 2. Elsevier; 2016.

Anatomy and Physiology of the Pelvic Floor

Sarah M. Eickmeyer, MD

KEYWORDS

• Pelvic floor muscles • Levator ani • Pelvic girdle • Sacroiliac joint • Pubic symphysis

KEY POINTS

- The bony anatomy of the pelvic girdle consists of 3 bones—the 2 innominate bones and the sacrum, and 3 joints—the sacroiliac joints and the pubic symphysis.
- The pelvic floor muscles are comprised mainly of the levator ani muscles with somatic innervation from the lumbosacral plexus.
- The bony and muscular pelvis is highly interconnected to the hip and gluteal musculature, which together provide support to the internal organs and core muscles.
- Pelvic floor physiology is centered on bladder and bowel control, sexual functioning, and pregnancy.

INTRODUCTION

Understanding the anatomic relationship of the pelvic floor muscles with the pelvic girdle, spine, and hips aids the rehabilitation provider in diagnosis, management, and appropriate referrals. This article reviews the anatomy of the pelvic girdle, the pelvic floor musculature, and its innervation, and highlights the normal physiology of the pelvic floor.

ANATOMY OF THE PELVIC FLOOR

The pelvic floor is composed of muscles, ligaments, and fascia that act as a sling to support the bladder, reproductive organs, and rectum. This sling of soft tissue is enclosed by the bony scaffolding of the pelvis, formed by 2 innominate bones made from the ilium, ischium, and pubis, which articulate with the sacrum posteriorly and each other anteriorly (**Fig. 1**). Extending from the sacrum is the coccyx, which acts as an important ligamentous and tendinous anchor.

The stability of the articulating surfaces of the pelvis is thought to arise through mechanisms termed "force closure" and "form closure." Force closure is achieved

The author has nothing to disclose.
Department of Rehabilitation Medicine, University of Kansas, 3901 Rainbow Boulevard, Kansas City, KS 66160, USA
E-mail address: seickmeyer@kumc.edu

1047-9651/17/© 2017 Elsevier Inc. All rights reserved.
pmr.theclinics.com

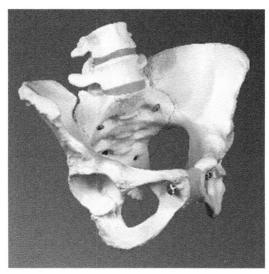

Fig. 1. The bony pelvic girdle consists of the 2 innominate bones and the sacrum, which are connected by 2 posterior sacroiliac joints and 1 anterior pubic symphysis joint.

through the interlocking of the ridges and grooves of the bony joint surfaces in the pelvis, whereas form closure is achieved through the compressive forces of the muscles, ligaments, and fascia, providing passive stability.[1,2]

In the posterior pelvic ring, there are 2 sacroiliac joints. The anterior sacroiliac ligaments, composed of the anterior longitudinal ligament, the anterior sacroiliac ligament, and the sacrospinous ligament, stabilize the joint by resisting upward movement of the sacrum and lateral movement of the ilium. The posterior sacroiliac ligaments are made up by the short and long dorsal sacroiliac ligaments, the supraspinous ligament, the iliolumbar ligament, and the sacrotuberous ligament. These ligaments function to resist downward and upward movement of the sacrum and medial motion of the ilium. Of note, the long dorsal sacroiliac ligament is believed to be a source of posterior pelvic pain owing to the forces transmitted from the sacroiliac joints and hip joint to the nociceptors and proprioceptors within the ligament.[3] Anteriorly, the pubic symphysis is a cartilaginous joint between the 2 pubic bones reinforced by superior, inferior, anterior, and posterior ligaments. Functionally, it resists tension, shearing, and compression, and is subject to great mechanical stress as it widens during pregnancy.

The superficial pelvic floor muscles are the bulbospongiosus, ischiocavernosus, and superficial and deep transverse perineal muscles. The deep pelvic floor muscles that line the inner walls of the pelvis are the levator ani and coccygeus that, along with the endopelvic fascia, comprise the pelvic diaphragm (**Table 1**). The levator ani is composed of 3 muscles—the puborectalis, pubococcygeus, and iliococcygeus (**Fig. 2**). The pubococcygeus is located most anteriorly. It originates from both the posterior pubic bone and the anterior portion of the arcus tendineus; it inserts into the anococcygeus ligament and the coccyx. The iliococcygeus is the posterior part of the levator ani. It originates from the posterior part of the arcus tendineus and ischial spine and attaches along the anococcygeal raphe and coccyx. Last, the puborectalis is located below the pubococcygeus and forms a U-shaped sling around the rectum. Its sphincterlike action pulls the anorectal junction forward, contributing to continence.

Table 1
Pelvic floor musculature anatomic origins, insertions, innervation and function

Muscle	Origin	Insertion	Innervation	Function
Puborectalis	Pubic symphysis	Pubic symphysis		Raise the pelvic floor
Pubococcygeus	Posterior pubic bone and arcus tendineus	Anococcygeus ligament and coccyx	S3–5, direct innervation from sacral nerve roots	Maintains floor tone in upright position
Iliococcygeus	Ischial spine and arcus tendineus	Anococcygeal raphe and coccyx		Voluntary control of urination
Coccygeus	Ischial spine	Lower sacral and upper coccygeal bones		Support of fetal head
Piriformis	Anterior sacrum	Posterior-surface greater trochanter	S1-2 via Nerve to Piriformis	Lateral rotation, Abduction of thigh. Retroversion of pelvis
Obturator Internus	Pelvic surface of ilium, ischium, and obturator membrane	Posterior surface greater trochanter	L5, S1-2 via Nerve to Obturator internus	Lateral rotator of thigh

The coccygeus muscle is triangular in shape, reinforcing the posterior pelvic floor by arising from the ischial spine and inserting on the lower sacral–coccygeal bones and is contiguous with the sacrospinous ligament. The perineal body or central perineal tendon is located between the vagina and anus. This is a site where the pelvic muscles and sphincters converge to provide support to the pelvic floor. Rupture of this entity during childbirth can lead to pelvic organ prolapse.

Lining the lateral walls of the pelvis, the piriformis arises from the anterior sacrum, with the sacrotuberous ligament and attaches on the superior border of the greater

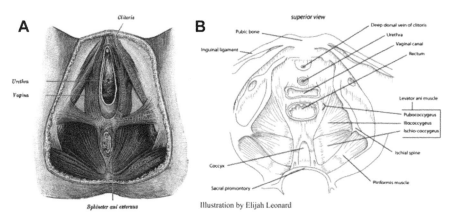

Fig. 2. The muscles of the (A) superficial pelvic floor and (B) deep pelvic floor. (*From* Prather H, Dugan S, Fitzgerald C, et al. Review of anatomy, evaluation, and treatment of musculoskeletal pelvic floor pain in women. PM R 2009;1:349; with permission.)

trochanter. When the sacrum is fixed, the piriformis laterally rotates an extended thigh, or abducts a flexed thigh. If the femurs are fixed, it can retrovert the pelvis. The obturator internus, also a lateral rotator of the thigh, arises from the pelvic surfaces of the ilium, ischium, and obturator membrane. It too attaches just distally to the piriformis on the greater trochanter.

The pelvic floor muscles receive innervation through somatic, visceral, and central pathways. Skin innervation of the lower trunk, perineum, and proximal thigh is mediated through the iliohypogastric, ilioinguinal, and genitofemoral nerves (L1-L3). Perhaps the most clinically relevant nerve to this article is the pudendal nerve and its branches (**Fig. 3**). Arising from the ventral branches of S2-S4 of the sacral plexus, the pudendal nerve passes between the piriformis and coccygeal muscle as it traverses through the greater sciatic foramen, over the spine of the ischium, and back into the pelvis through the lesser sciatic foramen. It courses along the lateral wall of the ischiorectal fossa where it is contained in a sheath of the obturator fascia termed the pudendal (or Alcock's) canal. There are 3 main terminal branches of the pudendal nerve—the inferior rectal nerve (which typically originates proximal to Alcock's canal), the perineal nerve, and the dorsal nerve of the penis/clitoris. The pudendal nerve innervates the penis/clitoris, the bulbospongiosus and ischiocavernosus muscles, the perineum, the anus, the external anal sphincter, and the urethral sphincter. This nerve contributes to external genital sensation, continence, orgasm, and ejaculation. Muscles of the levator ani are thought to have direct innervation from sacral nerve roots S3-S5.[4]

PHYSIOLOGY OF THE PELVIC FLOOR

The pelvic floor muscles function to support the pelvic organs by coordinated contraction and relaxation.[5] The pelvic floor provides active support through a constant state

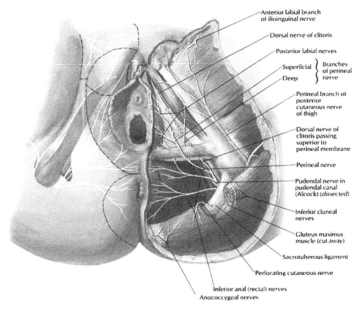

Fig. 3. Innervation of the pelvic floor. (Copyright © 2017. Used with permission of Elsevier. All rights reserved. www.netterimages.com.)

of muscular contraction and passive support from the surrounding connective tissue and fascia. With an increase in intraabdominal pressure, the pelvic floor muscles reflexively contract with upward movement and closure of the vagina and urethral and anal sphincters. This action is important for maintaining continence. Pelvic floor relaxation occurs only briefly and intermittently during the processes of normal micturition and defecation.

Micturition occurs when the bladder detrusor contracts and the urethral sphincter relaxes through involuntary autonomic nervous control, mainly under parasympathetic influences. During the same time, the pelvic floor muscles also voluntarily relaxes—chiefly the pubococcygeus of the levator ani muscle.[6] The coordination of these muscular actions is essential to maintain urinary continence and allow for micturition in a socially acceptable time and place.

Defecation occurs when the anal sphincter and puborectalis muscles simultaneously relax, thereby opening the rectoanal angle and allowing feces to pass. In addition, the abdominal muscles contract during a Valsalva action to increase abdominal pressure.[6] The relaxation of the anal sphincter is reflexive through the autonomic nervous system, mainly under parasympathetic control. The pelvic floor muscles and abdominal muscles are under voluntary control to allow defecation to occur in a socially acceptable time and place, similar to micturition.

Normal sexual function is coordinated by the pelvic floor muscles, genitalia, and autonomic nervous system. For females during the excitement phase, psychological and physical factors initiate arousal, generalized vasocongestion, and lubrication of the vaginal introitus from Bartholin's glands. During sexual orgasm, the pelvic floor muscles, anal sphincter, and uterus undergo repeated muscle contractions occurring at 0.8-second intervals; this action is coordinated via a spinal cord reflex from the pudendal nerve via S2-S4 sacral segments to the perineum and external genitalia.[7] In males, erection is under parasympathetic control, allowing the smooth muscle of the corpus cavernosa to relax and fill with blood, while the perineal striated pelvic floor muscles contracts to promote rigidity. Seminal emission is under sympathetic control as the ejaculate moves into the proximal urethra. Ejaculation is mainly a spinal cord reflex as the semen forcefully expulses from the urethra.[7] Thus, both female and male sexual response is under control of the autonomic nervous system, with the parasympathetic division responsible for the excitement phase and the sympathetic division responsible for the orgasm phase.

Many musculoskeletal changes occur during pregnancy to accommodate for the growing fetus and prepare the woman's body for childbirth.[8,9] In addition to the increase in body mass, the abdominal muscles lengthen, there is an increase in lumbar lordosis, an increase in the anterior pelvic tilt, an increase in the pelvic width, and the center of gravity shifts anteriorly as the fetus grows. Hormonal changes also increase joint laxity. All of these changes lead to an increased demand being placed on the hip extensors, hip abductors, ankle plantar flexors, and the pelvic floor muscles.

In 2005, the International Continence Society presented a standardized terminology for pelvic floor muscles function and dysfunction.[5] The pelvic floor muscles function by coordinated contraction and relaxation as a unit. Voluntary contraction is when the patient can contract the pelvic floor muscles on demand; voluntary relaxation is when the patient can relax the pelvic floor muscles on demand after a contraction. Involuntary contraction of the pelvic floor muscles occurs during an increase in intraabdominal pressure to prevent incontinence, such as during a cough. Involuntary relaxation occurs during a strain or Valsalva maneuver to allow for normal micturition or defecation.

Contraction and relaxation can be observed during the pelvic floor physical examination, as described elsewhere. Based on examination of pelvic floor muscles, the following conditions have been defined by the International Continence Society. Normal pelvic floor muscles refers to muscles that can voluntarily and involuntarily contact with normal strength and relax completely. Overactive pelvic floor muscles (also sometimes termed nonrelaxing pelvic floor muscles) do not relax and may paradoxically contract when relaxation is needed, such as during micturition or defecation. Underactive pelvic floor muscles (also called noncontracting pelvic floor muscles) cannot voluntarily contact when desired. Nonfunctioning pelvic floor muscles refer to no palpable pelvic floor muscle action and can be based on a noncontracting, nonrelaxing pelvic floor where the muscles are both weak and hypertonic. These categories can be helpful for generating a differential diagnosis for possible etiologies of pelvic floor dysfunction.

SUMMARY

A clear understanding of the bones, muscles, and nerves of the pelvic floor sets the stage for understanding normal and abnormal function of bowel and bladder continence, sexual functioning, and pregnancy-related issues.[10]

REFERENCES

1. Pool-Goudzwaard AL, Vleeming A, Stoeckart R, et al. Insufficient lumbopelvic stability: a clinical, anatomical and biomechanical approach to 'a-specific' low back pain. Man Ther 1998;3:12–20.
2. Vleeming A, Stoeckart R, Volkers AC, et al. Relation between form and function in the sacroiliac joint. Part I: clinical anatomical aspects. Spine 1990;15:130–2.
3. Vleeming A, Pool-Goudzwaard AL, Hammudoghlu D, et al. The function of the long dorsal sacroiliac ligament: its implication for understanding low back pain. Spine 1995;21:556–62.
4. Barber MD, Bremer RE, Thor KB, et al. Innervation of the female levator ani muscles. Am J Obstet Gynecol 2002;187(1):64–71.
5. Messelink B, Benson T, Berghmans B, et al. Standardization of terminology of pelvic floor muscle function and dysfunction: report from the pelvic floor clinical assessment group of the International Continence Society. Neurourol Urodyn 2005;24:374–80.
6. Rocca Rossetti S. Functional anatomy of pelvic floor. Arch Ital Urol Androl 2016; 88(1):28–37.
7. Boron WF, editor. Medical physiology. 1st edition. Philadelphia: Saunders; 2003.
8. Foti T, Davids JR, Bagley A. A biomechanical analysis of gait during pregnancy. J Bone Joint Surg Am 2000;82:625–32.
9. Gilleard W, Crosbie J, Smith R. Effect of pregnancy on trunk range of motion when sitting and standing. Acta Obstet Gynecol Scand 2002;81:1011–20.
10. Prather H, Dugan S, Fitzgerald C, et al. Review of anatomy, evaluation, and treatment of musculoskeletal pelvic floor pain in women. PM R 2009;1:346–58.

Office Evaluation of Pelvic Pain

Stacey Bennis, MD[a], Sarah Hwang, MD[b],*

KEYWORDS

- Chronic pelvic pain • Pelvic floor examination • Clinical evaluation of pelvic pain
- Musculoskeletal examination of pelvic pain

KEY POINTS

- A comprehensive history and physical examination will help guide treatment of patients with chronic pelvic pain.
- All patients with chronic pelvic pain should be questioned regarding a history of abuse.
- A thorough musculoskeletal examination should be performed on all patients with chronic pelvic pain, because many musculoskeletal disorders can contribute to chronic pelvic pain.
- The physiatric pelvic floor examination is a nongynecologic assessment of the superficial and deep pelvic floor muscles, ligaments, and nerves.
- It should be explained that this examination is an extension of the neurologic and musculoskeletal assessment.

INTRODUCTION

Chronic pelvic pain (CPP) is a common and debilitating disease defined as noncyclic pelvic pain that persists for more than 6 months.[1,2] The prevalence of CPP has been estimated around 5.7% to 26.6% based on a 2014 systematic review of 7 CPP studies.[1,2] However, the exact incidence and prevalence of disability and overall medical cost owing to CPP is unknown.[3] The etiology can be complex and multifactorial. Anatomically, CPP can involve structures in the anatomic pelvis, anterior abdominal wall below the level of the umbilicus, pelvic girdle, lumbosacral spine, and buttocks. Furthermore, CPP may be visceral, somatic, neuropathic, or referred. Given this breadth of anatomic involvement, the pain generator in CPP is often elusive to diagnose. Potential etiologies of CPP include gynecologic, urologic, gastrointestinal, musculoskeletal, neurologic, or psychosomatic/central sensitization disorders.[3] CPP is, thus, an umbrella term encompassing a variety of diagnoses and disorders that

The authors have nothing to disclose.
[a] Northwestern University Feinberg School of Medicine/McGaw Medical Center, 565 W. Quincy Street, Unit #517, Chicago IL 60661, USA; [b] University of Missouri, One Hospital Drive, DC046.00, Columbia, MO 65212, USA
* Corresponding author.
E-mail address: hwangsa@health.missouri.edu

are not mutually exclusive and may overlap, making appropriate diagnosis and management challenging for even the most experienced of clinicians.[4] A multidisciplinary approach to diagnosis and management involving obstetrician/gynecologists, urologists/urogynecologists, gastroenterologists, internists, oncologists, physiatrists, and pelvic floor physical therapists is important to provide a thorough evaluation. Even with a multidisciplinary approach, conservative medical and surgical therapies may fail to provide relief. Given the potential for therapy failure, functional impairment, high comorbidity of mood disorders, the subjective reaction to the disorder, and the possibility of premorbid abuse, there is often a strong psychosomatic component to CPP.[5] Psychological evaluation with a psychologist or psychiatrist may be a beneficial part of the multidisciplinary approach as well. Physiatrists are uniquely well-suited to play a significant role in the evaluation of CPP owing to the specialty's expertise in the diagnosis of complex musculoskeletal issues, ability to conservatively manage bowel and bladder dysfunction, understanding of chronic pain management, and natural focus on restoring functional ability and improving quality of life.

The initial clinical evaluation of CPP should include a thorough history and physical examination. The comprehensive clinical history should include a history of present illness of the pain complaint, including any medications or interventions, as well as a thorough history and review of any body system that may be involved (including neuromusculoskeletal, obstetric, gynecologic, gastrointestinal, urologic, dermatologic, infectious, oncologic, and psychiatric). The physical examination should also follow a focused systems-based approach and ideally includes examination of gastrointestinal, dermatologic, neurologic, and musculoskeletal (including lumbosacral spine, sacroiliac [SI] joints, pelvis, and hips) systems, and the pelvic floor (internal and external examination including neuromuscular anatomy). Given the breadth of this history and examination, it should be tailored to the individual patient's complaints and presenting signs or symptoms.

THE CLINICAL HISTORY

The workup of the patient with chronic pelvic pain entails a thorough medical history, which includes the history of present illness, medical history, surgical/procedural history, obstetric/gynecologic history, social history, psychiatric history, current and prior medications, pertinent family history, and a full review of systems. As with any patient, it is important to discuss any allergies. Additionally, in the female population of childbearing age, it is important to determine a menstrual and pregnancy history, including if the patient is currently pregnant, trying to get pregnant, or currently breastfeeding, because this can impact further workup and management.

An history of present illness of the pain complaint can follow the "OPPQRSTA" approach:

- Onset/duration of pain, and any inciting events or injuries;
- Palliative factors;
- Provoking factors;
- Quality of pain;
- Region (location) of pain;
- Severity of pain;
- Temporal factors (ie, when is the pain worst); and
- Associated symptoms (ie, numbness, tingling, radiation).

An assessment of any previously trialed over-the-counter or prescription medications (oral, topical, vaginal suppository, or rectal suppository), modalities (heat, ice, ultrasound, biofeedback, chiropractic, acupuncture, therapies), and interventional procedures (including injections or procedures such as cystoscopy, colonoscopy, and sigmoidoscopy) and surgeries (exploratory laparoscopy, hysterectomy, or other surgical procedures) should be obtained.

The past medical history, past surgical history, and review of systems can be easily subdivided into their related body systems to further delineate possible sources for pain. Because of the sensitive nature of many of these questions, it is recommended to start with more general questions for each system to establish patient–clinician rapport before proceeding with more sensitive questions. It may be beneficial to explain to the patient that these questions are asked of all patients with pelvic pain to help determine the etiology of pain. **Box 1** includes a suggested outline of questions, which can be adapted and modified depending on the patient's presenting complaint. It is important to remember that this list is not exhaustive and may not apply

---

Box 1
Review of systems questions for patients presenting with chronic pelvic pain

Neuromusculoskeletal

- Do you have low back pain?

- Do you have hip pain?

- Do you have pain in your pelvis?

- Do you have pain that radiates into your buttocks, legs, or feet?

- Are there any positions that make your pain worse?

- Is your pain worse with sitting, standing, or walking?

- Is your pain worse with coughing, sneezing, or bending over?

- Is your pain worse with transitional movements (getting in/out of a chair, getting in/out of a car, getting in/out of bed)?

- Do you have any weakness in your legs? Is it due to pain?

- Do you have any history of tripping frequently or falling?

- Do you need to use an assistive device such as a cane or walker for ambulation?

- Do you have any numbness or tingling? If so, where?

- Can you feel the tissue paper when you wipe after urinating or having a BM?

- Can you feel when you have a BM and when you urinate?

Obstetric

- Gravida/para status
  - How many times have you been pregnant?
  - How many children have you delivered?
  - Have you had any ectopic pregnancies, miscarriages, or abortions? Any procedures?

- For each pregnancy
  - Did you have pain during your pregnancy?
  - Did you have a vaginal delivery or cesarean section (C-section)?
  - What was the birth weight of your child?
  - How long were you in labor?
  - How long did you push/how long was your active labor?
  - Did your delivery require vacuum or forceps assistance?
  - Did you have perineal tearing or an episiotomy? Do you know what grade?
  - Were there any complications with the labor or delivery?
  - Did you have any bowel or bladder changes after your delivery?

Gynecologic

- Do you have any history of gynecologic surgeries? D&C? Biopsies? LEEP? Tubal ligation? C-section? Hysterectomy? Salpingoopherectomy? Vaginal Sling? Mesh?
- Are gynecologic examinations painful for you?
- Have you ever been diagnosed with endometriosis? How was it diagnosed?
- Have you ever been diagnosed with chronic yeast infections?
- For premenopausal patients
  - When was your last menstrual period? Are your periods regular?
  - Are you taking hormonal contraceptives?
  - Is there any chance you could be pregnant?
  - Do you wear tampons? Is it painful to wear tampons?
- Menopausal/postmenopausal patient
  - When was your last menstrual period? Do you ever have any vaginal bleeding?
  - Did your pain start before or after menopause?
  - Have you been or are you currently on any hormonal replacement therapy?
  - Have you ever been diagnosed with vaginal dryness or lichen sclerosis?
  - Have you ever been diagnosed with pelvic organ prolapse? Do you use a pessary?
- Sexual history
  - Are you sexually active? Do you have 1 partner or multiple partners? Is/are your partner(s) male or female or both?
  - Do you have pain with intercourse?
    - What is painful? Initial penetration? Deep penetration?
  - Do you have pain after intercourse?
    - How long does it last?
  - Is it painful when you orgasm?

Gastrointestinal

- Do you have any history of intraabdominal surgeries? Hernia surgery? Appendectomy? Cholecystectomy? Other?
- Do you ever have constipation or diarrhea? Are your stools hard or soft?
- Have you ever been diagnosed with irritable bowel syndrome?
- How often do you have a BM?
- Do you have pain before, during, or after a BM?
- Do you have to strain to empty your bowels?
- Do you ever have fecal urgency?
- Do you ever have fecal incontinence or leakage?
- Do you take any stool softeners or bowel medications?

Urologic

- Do you have a history of any urologic disorders? Any prior urologic surgeries?
- General incontinence symptoms
  - Do you every experience urinary incontinence or leaking? How often?
  - Do you have to wear an incontinence pad? If so, how frequently do you have to change the pad?
  - What do you drink throughout the day? How much coffee? Tea? Soda? Juice? Water?
- Stress urinary symptoms
  - Do you experience urinary incontinence or leaking with coughing and sneezing? With standing from a chair? With exercise?
- Urgency–frequency urinary symptoms
  - How often do you have to go to the bathroom to urinate?
  - Do you ever have difficulty making it to the toilet?

- ○ Do you ever have urinary incontinence or leaking when you have the urge to empty your bladder?
- Nocturia symptoms
  - ○ How many times per night do you wake up to use the bathroom?
  - ○ Do you ever have incontinence or leakage at night while sleeping?
- Retention symptoms
  - ○ Do you ever feel that you incompletely empty your bladder?
  - ○ Do you ever feel like you are straining to empty your bladder?
- UTI symptoms
  - ○ Do you have burning or pain with urination?
  - ○ Do you have blood in your urine?
  - ○ Do you have a history of UTIs? If so, did you have positive cultures? How frequently have you been treated for UTIs?
- Urinary symptoms associated with sexual intercourse
  - ○ Do you ever have urinary incontinence or leakage with sexual intercourse?
- Do you take any medications or supplements for your bladder?

Dermatologic

- Have you noticed any rashes or lesions in the pelvic region?
- Have you noticed dryness of the skin in the pelvic region?
- Have you noticed pruritus (itchy skin) in the pelvic region?

Infectious

- Have you had any recent fevers or chills?
- Have you had any recent weight loss?
- Have you ever been diagnosed with any sexually transmitted diseases?

Oncologic

- Have you had any recent unintentional weight loss?
- Do you have any personal history of breast, ovarian, uterine, or colon cancer?
- Do you have any family history of breast, ovarian, uterine, or colon cancer?

Psychiatric

- What are your hobbies? What do you enjoy doing in your spare time?
- How many hours do you sleep on average? What time do you go to bed? What time do you wake up? Do you take any sleep aids?
- Do you drink caffeinated beverages? How many per day?
- Do you use tobacco? How many cigarettes per day? For how long?
- Do you use alcohol? How many drinks per week? For how long?
- Do you use any recreational drugs? Which drugs? How often? For how long?
- Are you married? Single? Divorced? Widowed?
- Do you feel that you have a strong support system?
- Do you currently have any stressors in your life?
- Do you feel safe at home and at work?
- Have you ever been the victim of emotional abuse?
- Have you ever been the victim of verbal abuse?
- Have you ever been the victim of physical abuse?
- Have you ever been the victim of sexual abuse?

- Have you ever been diagnosed with depression or anxiety?
- Do you follow with a psychiatrist, psychologist, or social worker?
- Have you ever been hospitalized for a psychiatric illness?
- Have you ever had thoughts of harming yourself?
- Have you ever been diagnosed with an eating disorder?
- Have you ever been the victim of abuse? Physical? Sexual? Emotional? Verbal?

Abbreviations: BM, bowel movement; D&C, dilatation and curettage; LEEP, loop electrosurgical excision procedure; UTI, urinary tract infection.

to every patient. These questions can be included on an intake form to guide the clinical history. However, it is important to note that, when an intake form is used, patients may not complete the forms, may omit answers, may not feel comfortable answering the questions, or may not understand the questions being asked. Therefore, once patient–clinician rapport is established, it is imperative to approach these questions in person, and with the care and sensitivity required to ensure the most accurate history is obtained. It may help to explain to patients that a thorough and accurate history (including all of the above questions) will improve the chances of identifying the etiology of the patient's CPP and thus improve the chances or providing appropriate care. **Box 2** describes several clinical pearls that can be gathered from the history obtained from the patient.

THE CLINICAL PHYSICAL EXAMINATION

Similar to the clinical history, the physical examination can be split up by body and organ system. For the purposes of this article, the physical examination described focuses on the physiatric approach to pelvic pain. In patients presenting with symptoms based on clinical history that are more consistent with a urologic, gynecologic, gastrointestinal, dermatologic, infectious, or oncologic process, a referral to an appropriate specialist may be warranted. Given the frequent overlap of symptoms, a physiatric examination is still recommended for any patient presenting to a physiatrist with CPP to assess for any neuromuscular disorders contributing to their pain. The following physical examination is proposed and can be modified and focused based on the patient's presenting complaint.

Box 2
Clinical pearls from the history

1. Pain with sitting, pain with sexual intercourse, pain with gynecologic speculum examination, prior episiotomy/vaginal tearing with delivery, urinary urgency-frequency, urinary tract infection symptoms (in the absence of positive cultures), urinary retention, and constipation may all be signs of myofascial pelvic pain or pelvic floor function disorders.

2. Back pain that is worse with coughing, sneezing, laughing, or bending over is suggestive of a discogenic process.

3. Pelvic girdle pain (including at the pubic symphysis or sacroiliac joints) is suggestive of a pubic symphysis or sacroiliac joint disorder.

4. A history of abuse or premorbid mood disorder is associated with the development of chronic pelvic pain.

ABDOMINAL EXAMINATION
Inspection

The examiner assesses for any obvious distention, masses, hernias, or scars.

Auscultation

The examiner listens to all 4 quadrants for hypoactive, hyperactive, or normoactive bowel sounds.

Palpation

Superficial and deep palpation is performed to assess for any focal tenderness, trigger points, scar tissue, or masses. The examiner then palpates the intraabdominal muscles and their insertions. Palpation of the iliacus muscle and iliopsoas muscle is also performed.

Special Tests

The examiner assesses for diastasis rectus abdominus. Diastasis rectus abdominis (DRA) or "rectus diastasis" is a separation of the 2 muscle bellies of the rectus abdominis at the linea alba.[6] Although the exact clinical implications of DRA are unknown, it has been proposed that DRA may change posture, which may lead to lumbosacral or pelvic pain. DRA is measured by palpation at 4.5 cm above and 4.5 cm below the umbilicus in both the "standardized supine" position with arms crossed over the chest and in an abdominal crunch position to the level of the shoulder blades being elevated off the examination table. DRA is classified as greater than 2 fingerbreadths widening (mild is 2–3 fingerbreadths, moderate is 3–4 fingerbreadths, and severe is >4 fingerbreadths).[6]

NEUROLOGIC EXAMINATION

Strength examination is performed for the upper and lower extremities and should include the following:

- Upper extremities: shoulder abduction, elbow flexion, elbow extension, wrist extension, finger flexion, hand grip
- Lower extremities
  - Seated: hip flexion, hip abduction, hip adduction, knee flexion, knee extension, ankle dorsiflexion, ankle plantarflexion, ankle inversion, ankle eversion, great toe extension
  - Sidelying: hip abduction for gluteus medius and gluteus maximus
  - Prone: hip extension, resisted knee flexion
  - Standing: single leg raise to assess for Trendelenburg (a sign of gluteus weakness)

Sensory examination to light touch and pinprick is performed in the upper and lower extremities, including the C3 to -T2 dermatomes for the upper extremities and the L2 to S2 dermatomes for the lower extremities.

Reflexes are tested, including the biceps, triceps, brachioradialis, patellar, medial hamstrings, and Achilles tendons in the bilateral upper and lower extremities. Evaluation for ankle clonus is performed and primitive reflexes are assessed, including Hoffman's in the upper extremities and Babinski in the lower extremities.

Gait assessment is conducted, observing the patient during casual walking, toe walking, heel walking, and tandem gait. The examiner should note any gait abnormalities, including antalgic gait, Trendelenburg gait, hip hiking, steppage gait, foot internal/external rotation in gait, and step length asymmetry.

Finally, a functional assessment is performed and may include single leg calf raises and double and single leg squats.

MUSCULOSKELETAL EXAMINATION
Inspection

The muscles are inspected for any muscular hypertrophy or atrophy and the examiner assesses for abnormalities of alignment or leg length discrepancy. During inspection, the examiner notes any abnormalities of the feet, ankles, knees, hips, pelvis, and lumbo-sacral spine. If there is concern for joint hypermobility, an assessment is performed using the Beighton criteria and Brighton score (**Box 3**).[7] The Beighton score for joint hypermobility can help to provide a picture of joint laxity in patients, which may predispose them to injury or early osteoarthritis. In patients who meet criteria concerning for a connective tissue disorder, referral to a rheumatologist should be pursued.

Palpation

The muscles insertions and muscles bellies of the pelvic girdle are palpated, including gluteus maximus, gluteus medius, piriformis, iliotibial band, tensor fascia lata, iliopsoas tendon, iliacus muscle, quadriceps, adductors, and hamstrings. The examiner palpates the long dorsal ligament of the spine and the lumbosacral, pelvic girdle, and hip bony landmarks (as described below). The ilioinguinal nerve is palpated anteriorly (inferior and medial to the anterior superior iliac spine) and sciatic nerve posteriorly.

LUMBOSACRAL SPINE

The lumbosacral examination helps to differentiate lumbosacral pain generators from pelvic pain generators.

Inspection

The spine is inspected for alignment, shift, and the presences of scoliosis.

Palpation

Palpation of the paraspinal muscles, spinous processes, and z-joints is performed in standing. The examiner also assesses for step-off deformities and shifts.

Range of Motion

The examiner assesses lumbar range of motion, including forward flexion, extension, lateral side bending, and rotation. Pain with range of motion is noted as well as any restrictions in range of motion.

Box 3
Beighton criteria

1. Passive dorsiflexion of the little fingers beyond 90° (1 point for each hand) – 2 points
2. Passive apposition of the thumbs to the flexor aspects of the forearm (1 point for each thumb) – 2 points
3. Hyperextension of the elbows beyond 10° (1 point for each elbow) – 2 points
4. Hyperextension of the knee beyond 10° (1 point for each knee) – 2 points
5. Forward flexion of the trunk with knee – 1 point

Data from Beighton P. Assessment of hypermobility. London: Springer-Verlag London Limited; 2012.

Special Tests

Axial facet loading test (to assess for facet arthropathy) is performed. The examiner performs straight leg raise and seated slump. The straight leg raise and seated slump tests place traction on the exiting spinal nerve roots and can indicate a symptomatic discogenic pain.[8] The straight leg raise is performed on 1 leg at a time with the patient supine. The leg is passively raised by the examiner to the end range or to the point of pain.[8] A positive test is reproduction of symptoms in the range of 30° to 70° of passive elevation. The straight leg raise mainly places stretch on the ipsilateral exiting L5 to S1 nerve roots. In contrast, the seated slump test places maximum stretch or traction on the neural foramen and exiting spinal nerve roots throughout the lumbar spine.[8,9] The seated slump test is a progressive series of maneuvers[8,9] in which the patient sits erect, looking straight ahead. The patient places hands on their lower back, palms facing out and then slumps forward allowing the thoracic and lumbar spines to collapse into flexion, while looking straight ahead. The patient is then instructed to fully flex the cervical spine by bringing their chin to their chest. The examiner then extends 1 knee and dorsiflexes the foot. If symptoms are provoked, the patient then extends the neck to assess for improvement in symptoms (this releases neural tension). The test is repeated on the other side. A positive seated slump test provokes reproduction of the patient's radicular symptoms.

PELVIC GIRDLE EXAMINATION

The pelvic girdle has stability through force closure (fascial and tendinous attachments of muscles within the pelvis) and form closure (bony congruency of joint surfaces). It is important to remember that disruption of either the form or force closure of the pelvis can lead to pelvic instability, which may contribute to CPP.

Inspection

The patient is assessed for pelvic obliquity or shift in standing. Leg length discrepancy is evaluated while patient is in supine position. Before testing leg length discrepancy, the patient should perform a supine pelvic tilt ("bridge") to reset the pelvis.

Palpation

The examiner palpates the bilateral sacral sulcus, the long dorsal ligament, bilateral posterior superior iliac spines (PSIS), bilateral iliac crests, bilateral anterior superior iliac spines, bilateral greater trochanteric regions, bilateral buttocks, bilateral ischial tuberosities, bilateral sciatic nerve distributions, and iliotibial bands.

Special Tests

There are several screening tests to assess for SI joint dysfunction including the standing flexion test (tests for iliosacral dysfunction), the seated flexion test (tests for SI dysfunction), the Gillet test, and the Stork test (thought to be the most sensitive test for SI joint dysfunction). Normally, there is no relative motion of the pelvis during load transfer. In the standing flexion test, the examiner places both thumbs on the bilateral PSIS and the patient flexes forward at the hips in a standing position, in a positive test the dysfunctional SI joint exhibits more cephalad motion.[10,11] In the seated flexion test, the patient sits in a chair with hips and knees flexed to 90°, feet flat on the floor, and flexes forward to reach hands toward the floor. In a positive test, the dysfunctional SI joint exhibits more cephalad motion.[10] In the Gillet test, 1 thumb is placed over the PSIS on the tested side and the other thumb is placed on the contralateral second sacral tubercle, the subject flexes the hip and knee on the tested side. A positive test is lack of posteroinferior movement of the iliac spine in relation to S2 on the tested side.[10] For the Stork test, 1 thumb is placed over the PSIS on the side providing single leg support, and the other thumb is placed in midline at S2. The patient flexes the hip and knee of the untested side. The PSIS of the supporting leg should stay level with the thumb at S2 (negative test); if the examine reveals cephalad motion, this indicates inappropriate load transfer through the SI joint (positive test). The test can also be reported as the direction of movement of the PSIS as compared with the sacrum (cephalad, caudad, or none).[11] In each of these 4 screening tests, the examiner places the dominant eye over midline to assess motion.

In the active straight leg raise test, the clinician prompts the patient to lift 1 leg with the knee extended about 2 inches off the examination table, and then the test is repeated on the other side.[12] A positive test can include pain, weakness, or a feeling of instability. The test can be repeated with manual compression or stabilization of the pelvis or using an SI joint belt to support the pelvis. If the patient has a reduction in pain or can complete the test more easily, then underlying pelvic joint dysfunction or joint hypermobility can be presumed.[12]

These tests are used to test for SI joint dysfunction. The tests described below are SI joint pain provocation tests.

SI joint distraction simultaneously tests the right and left SI joint by applying vertically oriented pressure to the bilateral anterior superior iliac spinous processes (directed posteriorly), thereby distracting the bilateral SI joint.[13]

The posterior pelvic pain provocation test (P4) is also known as the thigh thrust or anteroposterior compression test. This test assesses the ipsilateral SI joint by grounding the sacrum with 1 examiner's hand and applying a vertically oriented and posteriorly directed pressure with the other hand.[13]

The Gaenslen's maneuver tests the ipsilateral SI joint in posterior rotation and the contralateral SI joint in anterior rotation by applying a superior/posterior torsion force to the ipsilateral knee (with hip and knee in flexion) and a posteriorly directed force to the contralateral knee (which is flexed over the edge of the examination table).[13]

The compression test maneuver tests the right and left SI joint simultaneously by placing the patient in sidelying and applying a vertically directed force through the iliac crest to compress the bilateral SI joint toward the floor.[13]

The sacral thrust test simultaneously tests the right and left SI joint by placing the patient in prone and applying a vertically directed shearing force over the midline of the sacrum at its apex.[13]

The drop test assesses the ipsilateral SI joint by having the patient raise the ipsilateral heel off the floor to bear near full bodyweight, then dropping the heel to the floor to create a cranially directed shear force at the ipsilateral SI joint. The test is repeated on the contralateral side.[13]

The SI joint as the etiology of primary low back and/or lower extremity pain is estimated in about 15% of patients.[14,15] The gold standard for symptomatic SI joint pain is a fluoroscopically guided, contrast-enhanced, intraarticular anesthetic block.[15,16] No specific tests have been validated to correctly identify a symptomatic SI joint.[14] However, Laslett[13] has described that these tests are reliable if performed in a highly standardized manner with sufficient force to stress the SI joint. Of the 6 SI joint tests described, the best predictors for a positive intraarticular SI joint block (the gold standard for diagnosis of a symptomatic SI joint) is either 2 out of 4 positive tests (distraction, compression, thigh thrust, or sacral thrust) or 3 or more of the full set of 6 tests (distraction, thigh thrust, Gaenslen's, compression, sacral thrust, drop test).[16]

HIP EXAMINATION

Hip pain can be intraarticular, extraarticular, or referred from the gastrointestinal system, genitourinary system, lumbosacral spine, SI joint, pelvic girdle, pelvic floor neuromuscular structures, and pelvic organs.[17] Confounding the picture is that hip pain can refer not only to the anterior groin and lateral hip, but to the buttock, low back, and knee as well.[17] Because of these variables, it is important to consider hip pathology in patients who present with CPP. The following tests can help to distinguish between intraarticular and extraarticular hip disorders.

- Intraarticular hip tests
  - Passive hip range of motion: asymmetry or restriction, pain with range of motion
  - Provocative tests
- Anterior hip impingement test
- Internal rotation over pressure test
- Scour test
- Flexion, abduction, external rotation (FABER)/Patrick's test
- Stinchfield's test/resisted hip flexion test
- Posterior hip impingement tests
- Extraarticular hip tests
  - Palpation: greater trochanteric region, iliopsoas tendon and iliacus muscle, abdominal muscle insertions, adductor muscle origin, hamstring origin, conjoint tendon, inguinal ring/posterior inguinal canal, pubic tubercle
  - Muscle length tests
- Ober test: tests the tightness of the iliotibial band in sidelying
- Thomas test: assesses for hip contracture or psoas syndrome in supine with the contralateral hip and knee flexed

PELVIC FLOOR EXAMINATION

The physiatric pelvic floor examination is a nongynecologic assessment of the superficial and deep pelvic floor muscles, ligaments, and nerves. It should be explained to the patient that this examination is an extension of the neurologic and musculoskeletal assessment. As in other regions of the body, the pelvic floor examination involves inspection, palpation, sensory testing, reflex testing, strength testing, and special testing. The perineum and pelvic floor is described by a clock face diagram with the pubic bone at 12 o'clock and the perineal body/anus/coccyx at 6 o'clock, this is important for description of external findings as well as for identification of pelvic floor muscles on internal pelvic floor examination. In female patients, the examination should include both a vaginal and rectal pelvic floor examination to optimally identify and examine the pelvic floor anatomy and improve chances for localizing the pain generator. In male patients, the pelvic floor can be examined rectally. The visceral structures, including pelvic organs, are typically not assessed during the physiatric physical examination. The goals of the pelvic floor examination include localizing pain generators within the musculoskeletal and neurologic structures (such as trigger points) and determining the type and extent of pelvic floor muscle dysfunction. Pelvic floor muscles can be underactive (also described as weak or noncontracting), overactive (tight or nonrelaxing), or have qualities of both underactivity and overactivity. Coordination of pelvic floor motion is also assessed.

Before proceeding with the examination, the rationale for the examination should be thoroughly explained to the patient, including that it is not a gynecologic examination, and the patient's verbal consent should be obtained. It is important to note that the examiner should stop to advise the patient before proceeding with each step of the pelvic floor examination. As in a gynecologic examination, it is also recommended that the examiner touch the dorsum of the gloved hand against the patient's medial thigh before proceeding with external genital palpation and before proceeding with the internal pelvic floor examination to decrease the reflexive withdrawal response. The following outline describes the external and internal pelvic floor examination.

EXTERNAL PELVIC FLOOR NEUROMUSCULAR EXAMINATION
Inspection

The examination begins with inspection of the external genitalia to assess for rashes, lesions, cysts, scars, swelling, venous varicosities, hemorrhoids, skin color changes, clitoromegaly, or high-grade pelvic organ prolapse. The pelvic floor muscle function (including the perianal region) is assessed by having the patient perform a voluntary pelvic floor muscle ("Kegel") contraction (the pelvic floor moves ventrally and cranially with the contraction), assessing for voluntary relaxation after the contraction (the pelvic floor descends from the ventral position), having the patient perform an involuntary contraction by coughing (takes place preceding an increase in abdominal pressure), and involuntary relaxation via Valsalva maneuver (takes place when bearing down, as in defecation). Inspection for pelvic organ prolapse or incontinence can also be assessed when the patient performs a cough and Valsalva maneuver. **Box 4** describes some key points to remember when assessing pelvic floor muscle function.

Palpation

Next, the examiner palpates externally for tenderness over the superficial pelvic floor muscles in the "urogenital triangle" (ischiocavernosus, bulbospongiosus, superficial transverse perineal) and palpates for tenderness over the levator ani in the "anogenital triangle" (located near the ischial tuberosities bilaterally).

Sensation

Sensation is assessed by using a cotton swab applicator to assess light touch and a neurotip to assess pinprick in the S2 to S5 sacral dermatomes bilaterally. Light touch and pinprick sensation should also be checked in the iliohypogastric, ilioinguinal, genitofemoral, and pudendal cutaneous distributions of the groin, mons pubis, and labia. The "Q-tip" test is performed by lightly touching a cotton swab at the vulvar vestibule to assess for hyperalgesia/allodynia, a positive test elicits pain and may suggest a diagnosis of vulvodynia.

Box 4
Assessment of pelvic floor muscle function: key points

- The pelvic floor and perineal body lifts during contraction.
- The pelvic floor and perineal body descends during relaxation.
- Pelvic floor muscle impairments and dysfunction can include underactive pelvic floor, overactive pelvic floor, noncontracting pelvic floor, and nonrelaxing pelvic floor.

Reflexes

Anal wink should be assessed bilaterally to test the sacral reflex arc by drawing a sweeping arc with a cotton swab applicator just anterior to the ischial tuberosities.

INTERNAL PELVIC FLOOR NEUROMUSCULAR EXAMINATION

The internal pelvic floor vaginal examination is best performed on a flat table without the use of stirrups. As it is a manual and nongynecologic examination, a speculum is also not used. Gloves must be used (latex or nitrile for patients or providers with latex allergies). For the vaginal internal pelvic floor examination, the patient is placed in a supine position with the knees bent, and if comfortable, abducted slightly (a position often referred to as "hook-lying"). The rectal internal pelvic floor examination is most easily performed with the patient in the lateral decubitus position. As in the external examination, it is best to prompt the patient before starting the internal examination by discussing the steps that the examiner will take, as well as using light pressure from the dorsum of the gloved hand against the patient's medial thigh before proceeding with the internal examination. It is recommended that a 1-finger approach with lubricant gel be used for the examination, because it is proposed that this causes less distortion to the pelvic floor anatomy.[18] Furthermore, this method can be used to assess for strength of contraction, control of contraction, sustained contraction, and tone.[18] All of the muscles assessed on the internal pelvic neuromuscular examination should be assessed for length, tenderness (including trigger points and spasms), taught bands, and scar tissue. A thorough pelvic floor examination should include both per vaginum and per rectum assessments to optimize the evaluation of all of the deep pelvic floor anatomy.

INTERNAL PELVIC FLOOR NEUROMUSCULAR EXAMINATION—PER VAGINUM
Palpation

The superficial pelvic floor muscles (bulbospongiosus, ischiocavernosus, and superficial transverse perineus) and deep transverse perineal muscles can be assessed for focal or diffuse tenderness in a clockwise fashion at the vaginal introitus to the level of the distal interphalangeal joint of the examining finger. The rectum can be identified posteriorly at the 6 o'clock position. The levator ani should be palpated between the 3 o'clock and 5 o'clock position on the left and between the 7 o'clock and 9 o'clock position on the right. The levator ani should be palpated for any focal or diffuse tenderness. The obturator internus is located just above 3 o'clock on the left and 9 o'clock on the right, and separated from the levator ani by locating the arcus tendineus. The arcus tendinous feels similar to a guitar string and connects between the pubic bone and ischial spine bilaterally. It is a suspensory ligament formed by the levator ani, obturator, and pelvic fascia to form a strong support for the pelvic floor. It is an important landmark that helps to locate the obturator internus muscle. The obturator internus is palpated for focal or diffuse tenderness over the muscle belly. Having the patient externally rotate the ipsilateral thigh against resistance will help to localize the muscle, and will assess for contraction and contraction-associated pain of the obturator internus. The ischial spines can be palpated bilaterally. The examiner also palpates for any cystocele, rectocele, or pelvic organ prolapse.

Strength Testing

The examiner performs strength testing in all 4 quadrants. Contraction of the pelvic floor muscles results in squeezing and lifting around the examiner's finger. The

---

Box 5
Oxford scale

0/5: No contraction of the pelvic floor muscles.

1/5: A flicker or pulsation of the muscle is felt but there is no discernible lifting or tightening.

2/5: Weak contraction with no discernible lifting or tightening.

3/5: Moderate contraction with some lifting of the posterior wall and some tightening around the examiners finger. Contraction is visible.

4/5: Good contraction with elevation of the vaginal wall felt against resistance and drawing in of the perineum.

5/5: Strong resistance is felt, if 2 fingers are inserted, fingers will be approximated.

---

examiner first assesses the resting tone of the muscle. When a contraction is performed, the examiner is assessing multiple aspects of that contraction, including the coordination of contraction and relaxation, the symmetry of muscle tone, contraction, relaxation, and coordination and the quality of the contraction strength for each muscle identified. The quality of the contraction can be assessed using the Oxford Scale (**Box 5**), Modified Oxford Scale (**Box 6**) or the International Continence Society criteria (**Box 7**).[18,19] In the Oxford Scale, the muscle contraction is graded on a 0 of 5 to 5 of 5 scale, similar to grading muscle contractions in the extremities. The International Continence Society criteria uses the descriptions absent, weak, moderate/normal, and strong to describe the contraction. The endurance of the muscle contraction is assessed for each muscle identified and the patient should be prompted to "hold the contraction" for 10 seconds.[19] The examiner then assesses the fast contraction/relaxation for each muscle identified using the "quick-flick" test. The examiner prompts the patient to make 5 to 10 "fast, short, and strong contractions" and repeat "contract, relax, contract, relax." Quick-flick testing can be helpful in eliciting a nonrelaxing quality of the pelvic floor muscles.

Special Tests

Tinel's test is performed by tapping lightly over the pudendal nerve, which is located just inferior to the ischial spines bilaterally. A positive test provokes pain or paresthesias in the pelvic floor or perineum, which is suggestive of pudendal neuralgia.

Box 6
Modified Oxford scale

0/5: No contraction of the pelvic floor muscles.

1/5: A flicker or pulsation of the muscle is felt, but there is no discernible lifting or tightening.

2/5: Weak contraction with no discernible lifting or tightening.

3/5: Some lifting and tightening of the muscle around the examiner's finger.

4/5: Good contraction with lifting and tightening and patient is able to hold contraction for 5 seconds.

5/5: Strong contraction with lifting and tightening and patient is able to hold contraction for 10 seconds.

Box 7
International Continence Society
Absent
Weak
Moderate/normal
Strong

INTERNAL PELVIC FLOOR NEUROMUSCULAR EXAMINATION—PER RECTUM

In men, the examination of the muscles above can be performed per rectum. In females, the rectal examination is important to gain a full picture of the pelvic floor muscle function.

Palpation

The resting tone and contractile tone of the internal and external anal sphincter is assessed. The examiner should palpate for tenderness (including trigger points and spasms), taught bands, and scar tissue over the coccygeus, piriformis, and puborectalis muscles. These muscles can then be assessed for resting tone, contractility, endurance, and fast contraction/relaxation. The coccyx is then assessed for tenderness, deviation, and mobility. The coccyx can be mobilized with the examiners internal finger anterior to the coccyx and the external finger posterior to the coccyx. The examiner should also palpate the sacrococcygeal, sacrospinous, and sacrotuberous ligaments as well as the ischial spine and pudendal canal. It is important to ask the patient to perform a Valsalva while the examiner's finger inside the anal canal to assess for dyssynergia of the pelvic floor muscles (contraction with either ascent or descent), which may be a cause of outlet dysfunction-type constipation and defecatory straining or pain.

At the end of the examination, the patient should be provided with tissue or hygienic wipes. The examiner should dispose of gloves and soiled sheets, and wash their hands. It is recommended to allow the patient privacy to change back into their street clothes after completion of the examination. The examiner can then return to discuss the physical examination findings, assessment, and plan.

REFERENCES

1. Ahangari A. Prevalence of chronic pelvic pain among women: an updated review. Pain Physician 2014;14:E141–7.
2. Speer LM, Mushkbar S, Erbele T. Chronic pelvic pain in women. Am Fam Physician 2016;93(5):380–7.
3. Wesselmann U, Czakanski PP. Pelvic pain: a chronic visceral pain syndrome. Curr Pain Headache Rep 2001;5:13–9.
4. Abrams P, Baranowski A, Berger RE, et al. A new classification is needed for pelvic pain syndromes - are existing terminologies of spurious diagnostic authority bad for patients? J Urol 2006;175:1989–90.
5. Bodden-Heidrich R, Kuppers V, Beckmann MW, et al. Chronic pelvic pain syndrome (CPPS) and chronic vulvar pain syndrome (CVPS): Evaluation of psychosomatic aspects. J Psychosom Obstet Gynaecol 1999;20(3):145–51.
6. Bakken Sperstad J, Tennfjord MK, Hilde G, et al. Diastasis recti abdominis during pregnancy and 12 months after childbirth: prevalence, risk factors and report of lumbopelvic pain. Br J Sports Med 2016;0:1–6.

7. Beighton P. Assessment of hypermobility. London: Springer-Verlag London Limited; 2012.

8. Majlesi J, Togay H, Unalan H, et al. The sensitivity and specificity of the slump and the straight leg raising tests in patients with lumbar disc herniation. J Clin Rheumatol 2008;14(2):87–91.

9. Maitland GD. The slump test: examination and treatment. Aust J Physiother 1985; 31(6):215.

10. Dreyfuss P, Dreyer S, Griffin J, et al. Positive sacroiliac screening tests in asymptomatic adults. Spine 1994;19(10):1138–43.

11. Hungerford BA, Gilleard W, Moran ME, et al. Evaluation of the ability of physical therapists to palpate intrapelvic motion with the stork test on the support side. Phys Ther 2007;87(7):879–87.

12. Mens JM, Vlemming A, Snijders CJ, et al. The active straight leg raising test and mobility of the pelvic joints. Eur Spine J 1999;8:468–73.

13. Laslett M. Evidence-based diagnosis and treatment of the painful sacroiliac joint. J Man Manipulative Ther 2008;16(3):142–52.

14. Dreyfuss P, Dreyer SJ, Cole A, et al. Sacroiliac joint pain. J Am Acad Orthop Surg 2004;12(4):255–65.

15. Dreyfuss P, Michaelsen M, Pauza K, et al. The value of medical history and physical examination in diagnosing sacroiliac joint pain. Spine 1996;21(22):2594–602.

16. Laslett M, Aprill CN, McDonald B, et al. Diagnosis of sacroiliac joint pain: validity of individual provocation tests and composites of tests. Man Ther 2005;10: 207–18.

17. Prather H, Cheng A. Diagnosis and treatment of hip girdle pain in the athlete. PM R 2016;8:S45–60.

18. Laycock J, Jerwood D. Pelvic floor muscle assessment: the perfect scheme. Physiotherapy 2001;87(12):631–42.

19. Slieker-ten Hove MCP, Pool-Goudzwaard AL, Eijkemans MJC, et al. Face validity and reliability of the first digital assessment scheme of pelvic floor muscle function conform the new standardized terminology of the international continence society. Neurourol Urodyn 2009;28:295–300.

Diagnostic Evaluation of Chronic Pelvic Pain

 CrossMark

Gaurav Khatri, MD[a],*, Ambereen Khan, MD[a], Gargi Raval, MD[b],
Avneesh Chhabra, MD[a],[c]

KEYWORDS

- Pelvic pain • Pelvic mesh • Pelvic ultrasound • MR defecography • MR neurography
- Nerve conduction tests • Electromyography

KEY POINTS

- Chronic pelvic pain can result from intrapelvic causes related to genitourinary structures, pelvic floor weakness, previously placed synthetic material in the pelvis, and neuromuscular pain.
- Ultrasound and magnetic resonance imaging including specialized techniques, such as magnetic resonance (MR) defecography and MR neurography may be indicated for evaluation of pelvic pain depending on the suspected cause.
- Evaluation of neurogenic pelvic pain may include nerve conduction studies, testing of sacral reflexes, electromyography, and MR neurography.

INTRODUCTION

Chronic pelvic pain refers to pelvic pain that occurs continuously or intermittently for a duration of more than 6 months[1] and is estimated to affect 14.7% of reproductive-age women.[2] Chronic pelvic pain may stem from causes related to native pelvic organs, pelvic floor dysfunction and prolapse, synthetic material placed in the pelvis for treatment of prolapse or urinary incontinence, or neuromuscular causes. Imaging evaluation of patients presenting with chronic pelvic pain usually begins with pelvic ultrasound (US) or occasionally with computed tomography (CT), although magnetic resonance imaging (MRI), including magnetic resonance (MR) defecography or MR neurography may be indicated depending on the suspected condition. This review discusses the diagnostic workup and imaging modalities that may aid in diagnosis of the various causes of pelvic pain.

The authors have nothing to disclose.
[a] Department of Radiology, University of Texas Southwestern Medical Center, 5323 Harry Hines Boulevard, Dallas, TX 75390, USA; [b] Department of Physical Medicine and Rehabilitation, Dallas VA Medical Center, University of Texas Southwestern Medical Center, 5323 Harry Hines Boulevard, Dallas, TX 75390, USA; [c] Department of Orthopedics, University of Texas Southwestern Medical Center, 5323 Harry Hines Boulevard, Dallas, TX 75390, USA
* Corresponding author.
E-mail address: gaurav.khatri@utsouthwestern.edu

Phys Med Rehabil Clin N Am 28 (2017) 477–500
http://dx.doi.org/10.1016/j.pmr.2017.03.004
1047-9651/17/© 2017 Elsevier Inc. All rights reserved.

PELVIC ORGANS

The most common causes of chronic or recurrent pelvic pain are related to pelvic organs and include endometriosis, uterine adenomyosis, uterine fibroids, and infection of the gynecologic structures or urinary bladder. Less common causes include pelvic congestion syndrome, adnexal and/or peritoneal inclusion cysts and pelvic adhesions, urethral diverticula, and infected Gartner duct or Bartholin gland cysts. Primary or metastatic malignancies in the pelvis can also cause pain; however, this review focuses on benign causes of pelvic pain.

US evaluation of pelvic organs includes transabdominal and transvaginal techniques. Limitations of US imaging include dependence on operator skill, patient body habitus, and degree of patient tolerance to transvaginal scanning. In cases whereby transvaginal imaging is not possible, presence of bowel gas may obscure anatomy on transabdominal imaging. MRI is generally performed in the supine position using a dedicated phase-array pelvic surface coil and includes T1-weighted (T1w) and T2-weighted (T2w) sequences in multiple planes. Dynamic contrast-enhanced imaging and diffusion-weighted imaging (DWI), which is based on the principle of Brownian motion of water molecules, may add sensitivity and specificity in MR evaluation of the pelvis. Contraindications to MRI, such as certain metallic implants and pacemakers, and high cost may limit use of this modality.

Endometriosis

Endometriosis is defined as the presence of endometrial glands and stroma outside of the endometrial cavity[3] and typically occurs in women of reproductive age. In addition to chronic or recurrent pelvic pain, patients may present with dysmenorrhea, dyspareunia, infertility, and abnormal uterine bleeding.[3,4] Endometriosis is seen in up to 80% of patients with uterine adenomyosis.[5]

Three types of endometriosis implants have been described: ovarian endometriomas, superficial endometrial implants on the surface of organs or the peritoneum, and deep infiltrating endometriosis.[4] Sites of involvement commonly include the ovaries, uterine ligaments, pouch of Douglas, bowel, fallopian tubes, and the peritoneal lining of the pelvis.[6,7] Less commonly, endometriosis may involve the cervix, vagina, bladder, or abdominal wall scars.[6,7] When urinary organs, such as the bladder or ureter, are involved, patients may report additional symptoms such as dysuria, hematuria, or flank pain due to urinary obstruction.

A normal clinical examination does not rule out endometriosis. Laparoscopy is the gold standard for diagnosis but is invasive and expensive. Transvaginal US (TVUS) and MRI demonstrate high sensitivity and specificity for diagnosis of ovarian endometriomas. Deep infiltrating endometriosis may also be identified on TVUS and MRI; however, accuracy for this form of endometriosis is lower.[8] On US, an ovarian endometrioma appears cystic with homogenous low level echoes, sometimes with small echogenic foci representing hemosiderin deposits within the wall of the lesion.[9] Less commonly, an endometrioma may demonstrate thin or thick septations, irregular walls, a fluid-fluid level, or a retractile clot (**Fig. 1**).[7] On MRI, endometriomas are cystic lesions, however, unlike simple cysts, they demonstrate high signal intensity (SI) on T1w images. On T2w images, they typically exhibit lower SI (shading) and may demonstrate SI gradient, appearing most hypointense in the dependent portion because of the layering of internal hemorrhagic debris (**Fig. 2**).[7] Other hemorrhage-containing ovarian lesions, such as hemorrhagic cysts, cystic neoplasms, or dermoid cysts, may mimic endometriomas. The presence of multiple cysts that are hyperintense on T1w images increases the likelihood of endometriomas.[10] Implants of deep

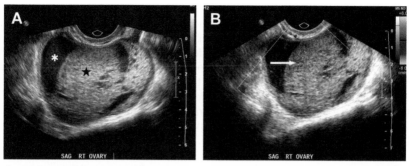

Fig. 1. A 29-year-old woman with recurrent pelvic pain found to have ovarian endometriomas at surgery. Sagittal gray-scale US image in the sagittal plane (*A*) demonstrates a complex lesion in the right ovary containing low-level internal echoes (*asterisk*). The increased echogenicity in the central portion of the lesion (*black star*) may represent retractile clot given the lack of vascularity on color doppler US image (*arrow* in *B*).

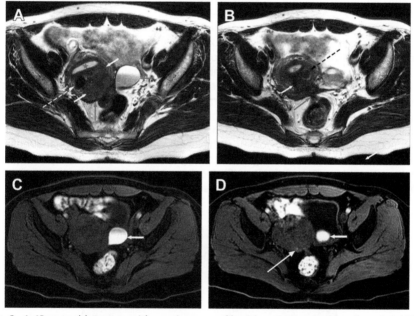

Fig. 2. A 43-year-old woman with ovarian mass, fibroid, and irregular bleeding. Axial T2w turbo spin echo (TSE) images through the pelvis demonstrate a well-circumscribed lesion arising from the left ovary (*short red arrows* in *A, B*) with layering low SI effect of hemorrhagic debris within the lesion. There is focal thickening of the junctional zone with poor margination (*short white arrows* in *A, B*), which contains tiny high SI foci on T2w images consistent with focal adenomyosis. Note the contiguity of the thickened junctional zone with the endometrium (*star* in *A, B*). In contrast, there are well-circumscribed small fibroids in the posterior uterus that are also low SI on T2w images (*dashed arrows* in *A, B*). Additionally, there is thick low SI tissue in the posterior rectovaginal space causing tethering of the anterior rectal wall (*long red arrows* in *A, B*) due to deep infiltrating endometriosis. The left ovarian endometrioma demonstrates high SI on precontrast T1w fat-suppressed (FS) images (*short arrows* in *C, D*) and did not enhance on postcontrast images (not shown). The plaque of deep endometriosis demonstrates tiny punctate foci of high SI on T1w FS images (*long arrow* in *D*).

endometriosis appear as hypointense round or stellate nodules on T2w images in expected locations discussed above. These nodules demonstrate foci of hyperintense signal on T1w images (see **Fig. 2**). Dilated fallopian tubes containing hemorrhagic material (hematosalpinx) should raise concern for pelvic endometriosis.[11] Adhesions are frequently described with endometriosis and may result in fixed retroflexion of the uterus, kinking or abnormal positioning of the bowel, tethering of bowel, abnormal positioning or fixation of the ovaries, and/or loculated fluid collections in the pelvis.[4,6,7] Endometriomas can undergo malignant transformation in an estimated 2.5% of cases,[11] more commonly in older patients, in larger or multiloculated endometriomas, and endometriomas with solid components.[12]

Adenomyosis

Adenomyosis represents migration of endometrial glands from the basal endometrial layer into the myometrium of the uterus, resulting in smooth muscle hyperplasia in the myometrium around the migrated glands.[7] It is typically seen in parous women ranging from 40 to 50 years old and is strongly associated with endometriosis. Prevalence of adenomyosis in patients with endometriosis may be as high as 91%.[5] About a third of patients diagnosed with adenomyosis are asymptomatic[13]; however, the most common presentations are dysmenorrhea, menorrhagia, and metrorrhagia. Dyspareunia is uncommon. The cause of dysmenorrhea in adenomyosis is unknown but is likely related to a variety of factors. One theory proposes that accumulated menstrual blood in foci of adenomyosis increases intramyometrial pressure resulting in pain.[13]

Adenomyosis may be diffuse with migrated endometrial tissue seen diffusely throughout the myometrium or focal where the migrated endometrial tissue forms circumscribed aggregates in the myometrium called adenomyomas.[7] MRI offers similar sensitivity but higher specificity than US for diagnosis of adenomyosis. US features of diffuse adenomyosis include linear subendometrial striations, subendometrial echogenic nodules, asymmetric myometrial thickness, subendometrial cysts, ill-defined endometrial-myometrial border, globular configuration of the uterus, and heterogeneous myometrium (**Fig. 3**).[14] On US, focal adenomyosis may appear as an ill-defined echogenic mass with infiltrating vessels on Doppler imaging. In contrast to

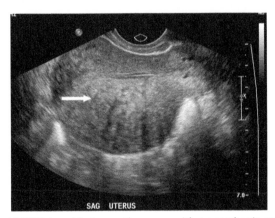

Fig. 3. A 33-year-old G1P1 (gravida 1 para 1) woman with menorrhagia and irregular cycles. Single gray-scale US image in the sagittal plane demonstrates an enlarged, globular uterus with asymmetric posterior myometrial thickening, poorly defined endometrial/myometrial border, and linear subendometrial striations (*white arrow*).

fibroids, focal adenomyomas do not cause mass effect and are relatively poorly marginated.[15]

MR features of diffuse adenomyosis include a thickened junctional zone (>12 mm) but without associated mass effect and poor definition of the endo-myometrial junction. Small hyperintense foci may be seen in the thickened junctional zone on both T2w and T1w images (**Fig. 4**).[15] Focal adenomyomas appear as ill-defined hypointense masses on T2w images with or without hyperintense foci internally on T2w and T1w images. Focal adenomyomas can mimic uterine fibroids; however, in contrast to fibroids, focal adenomyomas have poorly defined borders, do not cause mass effect on the endometrium, do not alter the uterine contour, and always demonstrate subendometrial components (see **Fig. 2**).

Uterine Fibroids

Uterine fibroids are benign tumors of the myometrium consisting of smooth muscle cells, fibrous and connective tissue, and collagen.[16] They are hormonally responsive tumors, typically seen in women of reproductive age, and can get quite large. As fibroids increase in size, they may outgrow their blood supply and undergo degeneration. Various types of degeneration, including hyaline, myxoid, hemorrhagic, and cystic degeneration, result in varied appearances on imaging. Fibroids may be intramural, subserosal, or submucosal in location. Patients may develop symptoms related to the size, number, and location of the fibroids. Chronic symptoms include uterine bleeding, infertility, pelvic pain and pressure, dysmenorrhea, dyspareunia, incontinence, and constipation.[16]

On US, nondegenerated fibroids appear as a well-circumscribed hypoechoic or isoechoic myometrial masses. Fibroid degeneration results in increasing heterogeneity of the mass with or without calcifications or cystic change.[9] On MR, nondegenerated fibroids are hypointense on T2w images, appear relatively well circumscribed, and demonstrate progressive enhancement (**Fig. 5**). Degenerated fibroids demonstrate heterogeneous SI with areas of hypoenhancement or nonenhancement and possible cystic or hemorrhagic change.[17]

Pelvic Congestion Syndrome

Pelvic congestion syndrome is a condition of pelvic pain typically seen in parous reproductive-age women resulting from dilated, incompetent pelvic veins. Although

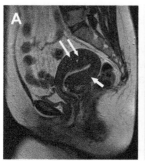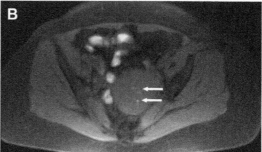

Fig. 4. A 42-year-old woman with intractable menorrhagia. Sagittal T2w TSE (A) and axial precontrast T1w FS (B) images through the pelvis demonstrate an enlarged uterus with loss of the endomyometrial border and diffuse thickening of the junctional zone (*short white arrow* in A) containing tiny high SI foci on both T2w and T1w images (*long white arrows* in A and B).

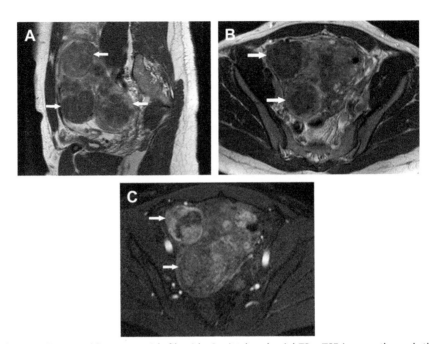

Fig. 5. A 33-year-old woman with fibroids. Sagittal and axial T2w TSE images through the pelvis (*A, B*) demonstrate multiple well-circumscribed, low SI myometrial masses (*short white arrows* in *A, B*) with distortion of the endometrium and uterine contour. Axial postcontrast T1w FS image through the pelvis (*C*) demonstrates heterogeneous enhancement of these masses (*short white arrows* in *C*).

diagnostic criteria are poorly defined, a combination of pelvic pain, dilated ovarian veins, and venous reflux is characteristic.[18] The pain associated with pelvic congestion is typically dull, achy, and pressurelike, is exacerbated by long periods of standing, and improved by recumbency. The pain may be unilateral or bilateral but is more frequently described as unilateral compared with other sources of pelvic pain.[18] The pain is typically on the side of the dilated pelvic veins,[1] more commonly on the left.[19] Additional findings that are highly suggestive of pelvic congestion include ovarian point tenderness and postcoital pain.[18] Physical examination may demonstrate vulvar or lower extremity varices.

Findings on Doppler US imaging include dilated pelvic veins adjacent to the ovary and uterus measuring greater than 4 mm (**Fig. 6**), slow blood flow (<3 cm/s) in the dilated pelvic veins, and reversal of flow in the ovarian vein. Additional supportive US findings include dilated uterine arcuate veins communicating with the pelvic veins, dilated ovarian veins, and/or cystic ovaries.[7,20]

MRI demonstrates dilated pelvic veins that appear as hypointense flow voids on T1w images and may be variable in SI on T2w images because of slow flow.[21] MR venography allows for optimal visualization of the varices that enhance after administration of contrast (**Fig. 7**). There may be retrograde filling of the ovarian veins on late-arterial-phase images. Time-resolved contrast-enhanced as well as noncontrast time-of-flight MRI techniques can be used to detect reversal of flow in the ovarian veins (toward the feet) (see **Fig. 7**).[22] MRI may demonstrate causal factors contributing to pelvic venous insufficiency, such as compression of the left renal vein (eg, by intra-

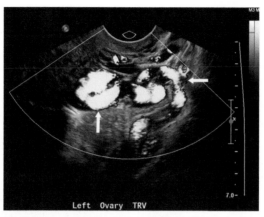

Fig. 6. A 54-year-old woman with pelvic pain. Single transverse color Doppler US image demonstrates dilated pelvic veins in the left adnexa (*white arrows*) adjacent to the left ovary (not shown).

abdominal masses or superior mesenteric artery), which in turn may result in retrograde flow in the left ovarian vein.[19,20]

Chronic Infection

Pelvic inflammatory disease (PID) is described as infection involving the uterus, fallo-pian tubes, or ovaries.[23] Chronic PID is thought to be multifactorial in cause. Associ-ated factors include inappropriate antibiotic management of acute pelvic infection, immune deficiency, septic abortion, infectious complications of child birth, and salpin-gitis. Chronic infection may manifest as tubo-ovarian abscesses (TOA), endometritis, oophoritis, or peritonitis. Patients may present with pelvic pain, low-grade fever, irreg-ular menses, and dysmenorrhea.[24]

Chronic PID presenting as a TOA may appear as a complex adnexal mass. US fea-tures are nonspecific and include an adnexal mass with heterogeneous echogenicity. US may also demonstrate hydrosalpinx, which appears as a tubular anechoic struc-ture with an echogenic wall and incomplete septations. Tubal wall thickening may be present in the setting of chronic salpingitis or pyosalpinx. US is limited in evaluation of chronic infection as the imaging features are nonspecific, and distinction between abscess and neoplasm is often difficult.[4,23]

Contrast-enhanced MRI has higher accuracy than US in differentiating TOA from ovarian cancer.[25] TOAs typically appear as heterogeneous thick-walled centrally non-enhancing structures with central hypointense signal on T1w images. On T2w images, TOAs demonstrate intermediate to high SI centrally with intermediate or low SI wall. Thick wall enhancement is typical.[23] DWI may be of additional value in differentiating TOAs from ovarian cancer,[26] particularly if contrast cannot be administered. Associ-ated features on MRI include infiltration of the adnexal fat, enlarged draining lymph nodes, and enhancing fascia or adhesions.[4,23]

Other Intrapelvic Causes of Pain

Peritoneal inclusion cysts may contribute to pelvic pain. They are formed by entrap-ment of physiologic pelvic fluid by adhesions and appear as septated, cystic lesions surrounding the ovaries. Peritoneal inclusion cysts can be identified on both US and MRI. Imaging features include large, irregular cystic masses with septations and

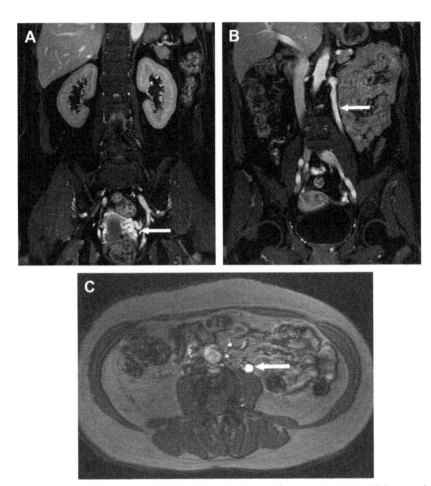

Fig. 7. A 56-year-old woman with left pelvic pain. Coronal postcontrast T1w FS images during the portal venous phase (*A, B*) demonstrate dilated left pelvic veins (*white arrow* in *A*) and enlarged left ovarian vein (*white arrow* in *B*). Axial 2-dimensional noncontrast time-of-flight image through the lower abdomen demonstrates retrograde flow toward the feet in the dilated left ovarian vein (*white arrow* in *C*).

margins that conform to the surrounding structures. The ovaries may be seen within or at the periphery of the cysts (**Fig. 8**).[9] Chronic or recurrent ovarian cysts may also be a source of pelvic pain.

Urethral diverticula result from infection of periurethral glands or cysts. Diverticula may cause symptoms of chronic pelvic pain, urinary urgency and frequency, posturination dribbling, urinary incontinence, and recurrent urinary tract infections. They are prone to calculi formation and infection and have a risk of malignant transformation. Urethral diverticula are best visualized on MRI and appear as nonenhancing structures surrounding the urethra. They are often located along the posterolateral wall of the midurethra.[7] Urethral diverticula may surround the lumen in a semiannular or horseshoe shape or, when large, may completely encircle the urethra. Chronic or recurrent urinary tract infections, cystitis, bladder outlet obstruction, and voiding dysfunction may also result in pain, typically in suprapubic location.

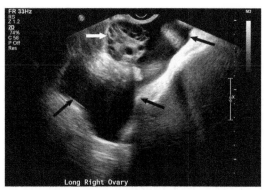

Fig. 8. A 21-year old woman with complex surgical history including bladder repair and urostomy placement, and long standing pelvic cyst status post multiple drainages, with pelvic pain. Single longitudinal gray-scale image through the right adnexa demonstrates a fluid collection conforming to boundaries of the peritoneum (*black arrows*) and surrounding the right ovary (*white arrow*).

Bartholin gland and Gartner duct cysts may become painful particularly when infected. Gartner duct cysts are remnants of Wolffian ducts located in the anterior vaginal wall above the level of the pubic symphysis. Obstruction of the Bartholin gland may result in formation of a Bartholin gland cyst in the posterior vulva at or just below the vaginal introitus, on either side of midline. Clinically, these may present as palpable masses. These cysts are more commonly evaluated with MRI than US, appear as avascular structures on both modalities, and are differentiated based on location. On MRI, these cysts may demonstrate hyperintense signal on T1w images if they contain hemorrhagic or proteinaceous debris.[7]

PELVIC FLOOR DYSFUNCTION

Pelvic floor dysfunction is a complex set of disorders including pelvic organ prolapse, urinary incontinence, obstructed urination, anal incontinence, and defecatory dysfunction. Patients frequently present with multi-compartment involvement of the pelvic floor,[27] and 17% to 44% of patients with pelvic floor dysfunction report pain.[28,29] Although the cause for pain in these patients is not clear, it may be associated with defecatory dysfunction.[28] Traditionally, fluoroscopic techniques, such as dynamic cystoproctography, have been used for evaluation of pelvic floor dysfunction. More recently, dynamic pelvic floor MRI has been emerged as an important tool for the evaluation of pelvic floor dysfunction.[30] It allows for high-resolution imaging of the pelvic anatomy as well as functional evaluation of the entire pelvic floor. Inclusion of defecation images during dynamic pelvic floor MR (MR defecography) is imperative for adequate assessment,[31,32] and necessitates instillation of contrast material into the rectum before imaging. MR defecography may be performed in the upright position with patients positioned in an open magnet; however, these types of magnets are not routinely available at most centers. At most institutions, MR defecography is performed with patients in the supine position within a closed magnet. Although supine positioning is not physiologic, studies have shown supine MR defecography to be a viable alternative to upright pelvic floor imaging.[33–37]

A comprehensive review of MR defecography technique and evaluation is beyond the scope of this review; however, because chronic pain in the setting of pelvic floor prolapse may be associated with defecatory dysfunction,[28] it is worth noting that various causes for defecatory dysfunction, such as rectocele, rectal intussusception, enterocele or peritoneocele, and pelvic floor dyssynergia, are well depicted on MR defecography. Peritoneoceles present with posterior vaginal bulges and, when large, may result in incomplete defecation due to mass effect on the rectum. Patients may also present with vaginal pressure, dyspareunia, low back pain,[38] and, in some cases, may report a sensation of dragging in the upright position that is relieved in the supine position because of stretching of bowel mesentery within the peritoneocele sac.[39] Similar to peritoneoceles, rectoceles may result in bulging of the posterior vaginal wall; however, the two entities are difficult to differentiate on physical examination. MRI is particularly helpful in this regard.[40] In the setting of pelvic floor dyssynergia, patients are unable to relax the puborectalis muscle and, in fact, may paradoxically contract the puborectalis muscle during attempts at defecation (**Fig. 9**). The lack of pelvic floor relaxation may impair the ability to defecate. Identification of this condition has important implications for management of defecatory dysfunction.

PELVIC FLOOR SYNTHETIC MATERIAL

In addition to functional evaluation of prolapse and defecatory dysfunction, US or MRI can be used to evaluate patients who present with pain after placement of urethral bulking agents, midurethral slings, or vaginal mesh. US for evaluation of the pelvic floor may be performed with transperineal or transvaginal technique. MR evaluation relies predominantly on high-resolution 2-dimensional (2D) and 3-dimensional (3D) T2w images. Patients with prior urethral bulking agent injection may present with recurrent incontinence secondary to resorption of injected agent over time or migration of bulking agent into the periurethral tissue. Periurethral migration of bulking agent may also cause an inflammatory reaction, which in turn may result in formation of a

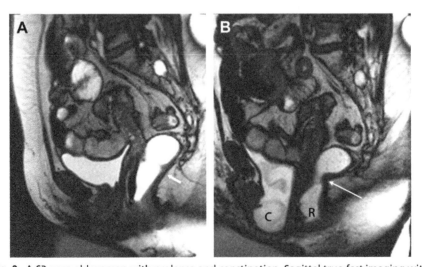

Fig. 9. A 63-year-old woman with prolapse and constipation. Sagittal true fast imaging with steady state precession (TrueFISP) images through the midline pelvis during rest (*A*) and defecation (*B*) demonstrate paradoxic contraction of the puborectalis muscle during defecation (*long white arrow, B*) with narrowing and posterior impression on the rectum (R). Short white arrow indicates levator plate at rest. C, cystocele during defecation.

subacute or chronic pseudoabscess. Patients may present with pain or dyspareunia, masslike sensation around the urethra, urinary tract infections, or other irritative voiding symptoms.[41] Urethral bulking agent may also extravasate into the lumen of the urethra and result in obstructive urinary symptoms. Finally, true abscess formation can also result in pain and signs of infection. Although imaging characteristics of various bulking agents may differ based on their chemical properties, they are generally well seen on US as isoechoic to hyperechoic material encircling the urethral lumen. US can be used to assess for nonuniform placement of bulking agent after the procedure and also changes in volume of bulking agent over time. Areas of extravasation may also be seen well. On MRI, certain urethral bulking agents appear hyperintense on T2w images, whereas others may be isointense or hypointense relative to the spongiform tissue. Bulking agents do not enhance and may mimic urethral diverticula, although may cause more mass effect on the urethral lumen than diverticula. Clinical history of prior bulking agent injection is important for differentiation. Certain formulations of urethral bulking agents may also calcify and can be seen on CT.

Midurethral slings are most commonly retropubic, transobturator, or single-incision slings. In contrast to the older bone-anchor slings, which were secured to the pubic bone with anchors, these newer slings are placed in a tension-free manner. The arms of the slings are allowed to scar down into soft or adipose tissue after placement. There are various proprietary types of slings; most are placed either via the transvaginal, suprapubic, or transobturator approach. Patients may present with symptoms, such as pain, dyspareunia, infection, or voiding dysfunction, due to erosion of sling material into the urethra or vagina. Imaging can be used to identify sling material and provide a road map for surgical exploration. Slings typically appear hyperechoic on US with posterior acoustic shadowing (**Fig. 10**) and hypointense on T2w MRI with a band or ribbonlike morphology (**Fig. 11**). Sling material in the suburethral space is difficult to delineate on MRI but is better seen on US, whereas evaluation in the retropubic space is better with MRI.[42] Consequently, erosion into the spongiform tissue may be depicted on US, whereas erosion of retropubic slings into the wall of the bladder may be more apparent on MRI. Scar tissue can mimic sling material on both modalities. Patients with transobturator slings may present with groin pain, whereas those with retropubic slings may report suprapubic pain more commonly. Although unclear, the cause for this pain may be related to scarring or nerve entrapment. Imaging of neuropathic pain is described later in this review.

Similar to urethral slings, various proprietary forms of vaginal mesh kits exist. These mesh kits may be placed along the anterior or posterior vaginal wall or both (see **Fig. 11**). Depending on the specific mesh placed and technique used, arms of the mesh may traverse the sacrospinous ligaments, levator muscles, ischiorectal fossae, or may extend into the obturator foramina. Mesh components along the vaginal wall may be difficult to differentiate from scarring; however, MRI often allows good visualization of peripheral extension of the mesh arms. US is limited in evaluation of these peripheral mesh components because of its smaller field of view. Patients may present with pain due to mesh contraction, scarring, or erosion. Mesh erosion rates are high, reported in up to 20% of cases.[43,44] Other complications include dyspareunia, infection, or urinary symptoms. Groin pain may be present in certain cases where mesh arms extend into the obturator foramen. In contrast to vaginal mesh kits, sacrocolpopexy mesh, which fixates the vaginal apex or cervix to the sacral promontory (**Fig. 12**), has lower rate of mesh erosion, ranging from 3% to 4%.[45] A unique potential complication of sacrocolpopexy mesh is sacral osteomyelitis of the sacrum, which can be seen on MRI. In general, normal mesh components appear thin and hypointense on T2w images. Focal or diffuse thickening

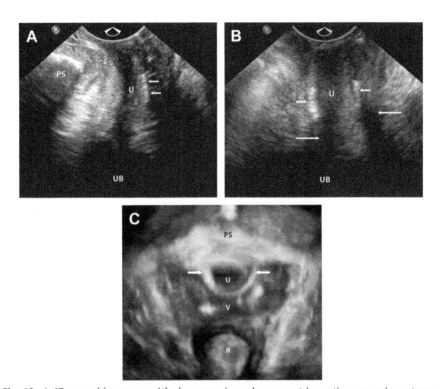

Fig. 10. A 47-year-old woman with dyspareunia and recurrent incontinence, prior retropubic sling placement. Transperineal sagittal (*A*) and coronal (*B*) gray-scale US images through the pelvic floor demonstrate midurethral sling (*short white arrows*) as linear echogenic material along the urethra (U). Note the posterior acoustic shadowing (*long white arrows* in *B*) due to attenuation of sound beam by synthetic material. Color volume rendered image in the axial plane demonstrates relationship of the sling (*short arrows* in *C*) to the U, vagina (V), and pubic symphysis (PS). R, rectum; UB, urinary bladder.

of these components may represent exuberant scarring, mesh erosion, or infection. Infected mesh or slings may also demonstrate high signal on T2w images, with or without associated collections.

NEUROGENIC PAIN

Pelvic pain may be neuropathic in origin. The major nerves implicated in pelvic pain disorders include the lumbosacral nerve roots, femoral, sciatic, superior and inferior gluteal, posterior femoral cutaneous, iliohypogastric, ilioinguinal, pudendal trunk and its branches, genitofemoral, lateral femoral cutaneous, superior and inferior cluneal nerves, and ganglion impar.[46] Neuropathy may be secondary to trauma, traction, prior surgery, tumors, or systemic causes, such as diabetes mellitus, radiation, and chemotherapy, or may be idiopathic.[47–49] Neuropathic symptoms include pain in the distribution of the affected nerve, paresthesia, and numbness. The location and distribution of pain and presence of associated signs, such as urinary or gastrointestinal symptoms or genital dysfunction, may suggest involvement of particular nerves (**Table 1**).

The clinical differential diagnosis of neuropathic pelvic pain includes hip pathology, hamstring tear, ischiofemoral impingement, and other intra-pelvic etiologies discussed earlier. Evaluation may consist of both imaging and non-imaging based tests.

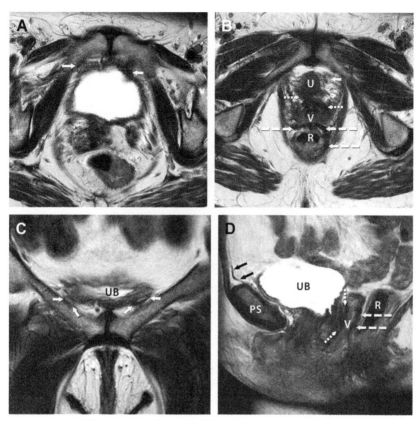

Fig. 11. A 72-year-old woman with hip pain, bilateral leg weakness after vaginal mesh surgery for prolapse. Axial T2w TSE images (*A, B*) through the pelvis demonstrate the arms of the retropubic urethral sling as low SI bands between the urinary bladder and pubic symphysis extending toward the urethra (*solid arrows* in *A, B*). Bandlike low SI material along the posterior vaginal wall and in close approximation to the left rectal wall (*long dashed white arrows* in *B*) and less well defined along the anterior vaginal wall (*short dashed white arrows* in *B*) is consistent with scar tissue versus vaginal mesh. Coronal (*C*) and sagittal (*D*) T2w TSE images through the pelvis demonstrate arms of the retropubic urethral sling as low SI bands in the retropubic space extending suprapubically (*solid arrows* in *C, D*). Low SI material along the anterior and posterior vaginal walls seen on sagittal image again consistent with vaginal mesh or scar tissue (*dashed white arrows* in *D*). PS, pubic symphysis; R, rectum; U, urethra; UB, urinary bladder; V, vagina.

Imaging of Neurogenic Pain: Magnetic Resonance Neurography

Imaging modalities for the diagnosis of neuropathy include US, CT, and MRI. US is operator dependent, however, can be used to detect superficial lesions, for instance, a canal of Nuck cyst compressing the genital branch of genitofemoral nerve. Occasionally, US may identify thickening of superficial nerves, such as the lateral femoral cutaneous nerve. US can also be used to guide injections around pudendal, genitofemoral, and lateral femoral cutaneous nerves.[50] CT is used to identify fractures, callous and space-occupying lesions, such as heterotopic ossification, that may compress the nerve. MRI offers the best soft tissue contrast for evaluation of pelvic viscera and nerves. Dedicated MR imaging of peripheral nerves, MR Neurography (MRN)

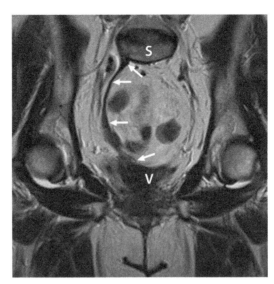

Fig. 12. A 58-year-old woman with pelvic pain, prior prolapse surgery, and pelvic mesh. Coronal T2 TSE image through the pelvis demonstrates sacrocolpopexy mesh as a thin linear low SI structure extending from the sacral promontory (S) to the vagina (V), with rightward curvature in the pelvis (*solid arrows*).

has been successfully used to demonstrate the nerves in various planes with superior conspicuity compared to conventional MRI.[51] MRN provides high-contrast and high-resolution imaging and uses a combination of 2D and 3D techniques. Thick-slab maximum-intensity projection (MIP) reconstructions generated from 3D MRN enhance the endoneurial fluid contrast while suppressing vascular flow signal and display the lumbosacral nerves and their branches in greater detail as compared with conventional MRI.[52] MRN findings in neuropathy include alterations in course, caliber, SI, and continuity of nerves, fascicles, and perineural fat planes (**Table 2**).[53,54]

Interpretation of MRN images requires an understanding of the normal appearances and possible variations of the pelvic nerves. The lumbosacral plexus nerves are symmetric in terms of SI and caliber bilaterally. The dorsal nerve root ganglia appear the most hyperintense on T2w images, and SI fades gradually in the distal nerve roots. The sciatic, femoral, and lateral femoral cutaneous nerves depict intermediate SI distal to the level of inguinal ligament.[55] These 3 major nerves as well as the superior gluteal, iliohypogastric, and ilioinguinal nerves are best seen on 3D images, whereas smaller nerves, such as the pudendal, genitofemoral, inferior gluteal, and posterior femoral cutaneous nerve, are best seen on axial 2D images[56] (**Fig. 13**). Anatomic variations in sciatic and femoral nerves, such as split nerves, intramuscular course, and distal branching patterns, can be seen in up to 20% of cases. The most common abnormal imaging finding on MRN is nerve hyperintensity that approaches the SI of the adjacent veins and is asymmetric to the contralateral normal side. This finding is evident on T2w fat-suppressed (FS) images and diffusion tensor imaging (DTI) (**Fig. 14**). DTI results in suppression of SI from adjacent veins in the neurovascular bundle and increases the conspicuity of SI alteration in the nerves.[57] Evaluation of T1w, T2w FS images, and DTI in tandem is important in evaluation for neuropathy. T1w images allow detection of perineural scarring and aid in characterization of space-occupying lesions in the vicinity of nerves (see **Fig. 14**).

Table 1
Nerve involvement and spatial distribution of symptoms

Nerve	Location and Distribution of Sensory Symptoms	Associated Signs
Lumbosacral nerve roots	Gluteal area, along distribution of affected nerve roots	
Femoral	Anterior pelvis, groin and thigh	Leg weakness
Sciatic	Posterior gluteal area, posterior thigh, posterior-lateral calf and top of foot	Leg weakness
Superior gluteal	Deep and superior gluteal area	Abductor muscle weakness
Inferior gluteal	Deep and inferior gluteal area	Hip extension weakness
Posterior femoral cutaneous	Inferior gluteal area and posterior thigh	
Iliohypogastric	Anterior and lateral lower abdominal wall	
Ilioinguinal	Groin and medial thigh	
Pudendal	Deep pelvis, anterior pelvis, genital area	
Pudendal branches	Rectal (inferior hemorrhoidal nerve), perineum (perineal branches), genitalia (dorsal nerve of clitoris or penis)	
Genitofemoral	Groin, scrotum and labia, and anterior thigh	
Lateral femoral cutaneous	Anterolateral pelvis and thigh	
Superior cluneal nerve	Posterior superior iliac spine and iliac crest	
Inferior cluneal nerve	Lateral gluteal crease and posterior perineum	
Ganglion impar	Coccyx and rectal area	

A multidisciplinary approach with clear communication of findings and correlation with clinical symptoms is essential in diagnosis and management of pelvic neuropathies. MRN findings also frequently direct the choice of diagnostic and therapeutic image-guided interventions using US, fluoroscopy, CT, or MRI, such as perineural anesthetic and steroid injections, intramuscular anesthetic and Botox injections, and hyaluronidase injections for adhesionolysis[58] (**Fig. 15**). With image guidance,

Table 2
Magnetic resonance neurography findings

Nerve Characteristic	Abnormal MRN Finding
Course	Alteration or abrupt deviation
Caliber	Focal or diffuse enlargement or attenuation
Signal intensity	Hyperintensity similar to adjacent veins or abrupt signal alterations along the course
Fascicles	Enlargement, disruption, atrophy, or abrupt signal alterations
Epineurium/perineurium	Thickening or discontinuity
Continuity	Neuroma in continuity or complete discontinuity
Perineural fat planes	Fibrosis, effaced perineural fat due to thickened fascia or ligament, mass lesion

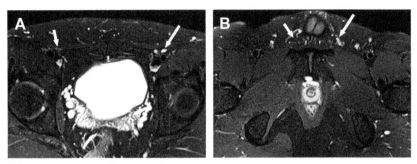

Fig. 13. Young male patient with left groin and scrotal pain. No prior inguinal surgery. Sequential axial MRN T2w spectral attenuated inversion recovery SPAIR images (*A, B*) show enlarged and high SI genital branch of the left genitofemoral nerve with prominent fascicles (*long arrows*), which was entrapped at the inguinal region. Note the normal isointense genitofemoral nerve on the right for comparison (*short arrows*).

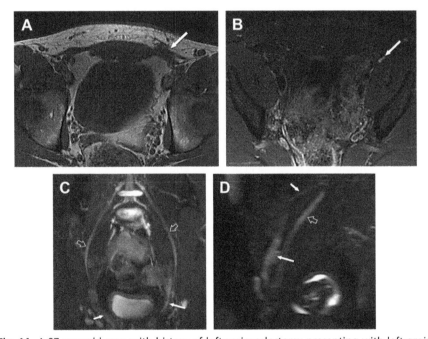

Fig. 14. A 27-year-old man with history of left varicocelectomy presenting with left groin, scrotal, and penile pain. Recent US of the scrotum was unremarkable. Axial T1w MRN image (*A*) shows left inguinal scarring (*arrow*). Axial T2w SPAIR image (*B*) shows enlarged and high SI left genitofemoral nerve (*arrow*). Coronal 3D T2w thick slab MIP image (*C*) shows normal symmetric femoral nerves (*open arrows*), enlarged and high SI left genitofemoral nerve (*long arrow*) as compared with normal right counterpart (*short arrow*). Oblique sagittal MIP image (*D*) shows the separation of abnormal left genitofemoral nerve (*long arrow*), normal femoral nerve (*open arrow*), and normal lateral femoral cutaneous nerve (*short arrow*).

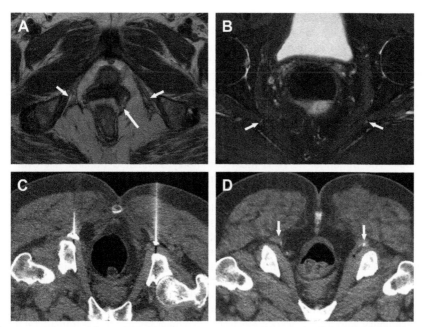

Fig. 15. A 71-year-old woman with metastatic ovarian cancer, prior hysterectomy and bilateral salpingo-oophorectomy, presenting with burning pain in the pelvis and vagina. Axial T2w MRN image (*A*) shows bilateral perivaginal and perineal scarring (*short arrows*) and distortion of the vagina (*long arrow*). Axial T2w SPAIR image (*B*) shows high SI bilateral pudendal nerves at the ischial spine (*arrows*). Axial images obtained during CT-guided pudendal perineural injections (*C, D*) show needle placements and injectates (*arrows* in *D*) composed of nonionic contrast, dexamethasone, and local anesthetic in the perineural space bilaterally and Alcock's canal on the right.

the face validity and technical success of these procedures is close to 100%. Although placebo effect can be seen with these injections in up to 20% to 30% of cases, a negative block under image guidance has substantial value in ruling out suspected pelvic neuropathy.[59]

Nonimaging Evaluation of Pelvic Pain

Electrodiagnostic testing can be used to aid in evaluation of neurogenic pelvic pain. A thorough history and physical examination should precede and guide the electrophysiologic evaluation. Diagnostic procedures to evaluate the more commonly implicated nerves in neurogenic pelvic pain include nerve conduction study techniques, sacral reflexes, and electromyography (EMG) of the external anal sphincter. In practice, testing may need to be expanded to exclude more proximal lumbosacral plexus and/or lumbosacral radicular lesions.

Nerve conduction studies

Nerve stimulation typically results in nerve depolarization and propagation of an action potential when the threshold is reached. Nerves can be stimulated with a surface stimulator or monopolar needle electrode. Nerve responses can be recorded directly from the stimulated nerve or from the innervated muscles. Typically, the responses studied in pelvic floor disorders are compound motor action potentials (CMAPs). CMAPs are obtained by stimulating a motor nerve proximal to the muscle it innervates and recording a response over the muscle. The CMAP represents a summated response of all the muscle fibers innervated by that nerve in the muscle. Parameters, such as latency, amplitude, duration, and conduction velocity, can be measured and compared with normal values or to the unaffected side. The onset or terminal latency reflects the time from stimulation of the nerve to the first CMAP positive deflection from baseline. The onset latency reflects the conduction of the fastest, large myelinated axons of the nerve.[60]

The pudendal, ilioinguinal, iliohypogastric, and genitofemoral nerves have been implicated in chronic pelvic pain. Electrophysiologic evaluation of these nerves is discussed. Pudendal nerve conduction studies were first described by Kiff and Swash[61] in 1984. The pudendal nerve is most commonly stimulated transrectally over the ischial spine, and CMAPs are recorded from the external anal sphincter (EAS) on both sides. The pudendal nerve is stimulated using a disposable St. Mark's electrode attached to a gloved hand. The bipolar stimulating electrode is located at the tip of the index finger, and the recording electrode is positioned at the base of the index finger over the EAS. Low-intensity stimulation at 10 to 30 mA is generally used, and the supramaximal response is recorded. The nerve is stimulated on both sides. The onset or terminal latency is measured. The expected mean latency to the EAS is 1.9 milliseconds,[62,63] but latencies up to 2.5 milliseconds have been reported in normal subjects.[64] The pudendal terminal motor latency (PTML) is more reliable than amplitude measurement.[65] In women, pudendal nerve conduction studies can also be performed transvaginally with the St. Mark's electrode, in similar fashion to the transrectal technique. The transvaginal technique may be better tolerated in women.[66] Normative data using this approach have been established in continent women.[64]

Electrophysiologic testing of the ilioinguinal, iliohypogastric, and genitofemoral nerves is technically difficult and not routinely performed, although specific techniques have been described. The ilioinguinal nerve can be stimulated with a needle just medial to the anterior superior iliac spine and a CMAP response recorded over the lower abdominal muscles. Expected mean motor latency reported is 4.0 milliseconds with a mean amplitude of 1.2 mV.[67] More than a 50% difference in amplitude relative to the unaffected side is considered significant.[68]

Ertekin and colleagues[69] described a motor nerve conduction technique to study the genitofemoral nerve by measuring the response in the cremaster muscle. The genitofemoral nerve is stimulated at the anterior superior iliac spine with bipolar surface electrodes with a duration of 0.1 to 0.3 milliseconds. Responses are recorded with a concentric needle electrode (CNE) inserted into the inguinal canal after palpation of structures within the canal. It is positioned in the midline approximately 1 cm above the penile root and also 2 to 3 cm lateral to the midline. Needle localization is confirmed by detection of motor unit activity by EMG before the nerve conduction study. Using this technique, Ertekin and colleagues[69] observed mean latencies of 6.4 ± 1.8 milliseconds depending on the length of the nerve. In studying genitofemoral nerve motor conduction time to the cremasteric muscle reflex as well as needle EMG of the cremasteric muscle, Bademkiran and colleagues[70] demonstrated motor involvement of the genitofemoral nerve in 47% of patients undergoing herniorrhaphy and in 23% of those treated nonsurgically. Genitofemoral motor nerve conduction studies may be helpful in evaluation of nerve injuries when compared with the unaffected side.

Sacral reflexes

Sacral reflexes have been used to evaluate patients with fecal incontinence, urinary incontinence, and impotence. In the evaluation of neurogenic pelvic pain, sacral reflex abnormalities may suggest a more proximal lesion. Electrodiagnostic evaluation of the bulbocavernosus reflex (BCR) in men and the clitoral anal reflex (CAR) in women are discussed. The BCR in males can be evaluated by stimulation of the dorsal nerve of the penis and recording at the bulbocavernosus muscle or EAS muscle. Ring electrodes placed over the shaft of the penis and glans can be used for bilateral stimulation. A recording needle electrode may be placed in the bulbocavernosus muscle or in the EAS muscle. A surface electrode located on an anal plug can also be placed in the rectum to record from the EAS. Alternatively, the reflex can also be recorded in the urethral sphincter.[71,72] The CAR in women is elicited by transcutaneous stimulation of the dorsal nerve of the clitoris on either side of the base. The reflex response is recorded with surface or needle electrode in similar fashion as described earlier.[62] Onset latencies range from 30 to 50 milliseconds.[73–75] The reflexes are inhibited during voiding and loss of this inhibition may be seen in suprasacral lesions.[76]

Needle electromyography

EMG studies electrical activity using surface or disposable needle electrodes from striated muscles. Voluntary electrical activity is studied as motor unit action potentials (MUAPs), which are a summation of several motor units. A motor unit is defined as an anterior horn cell, a motor neuron, and the muscle fibers it innervates. Characteristic changes in motor unit morphology and recruitment are noted in denervated and reinnervated muscle. Insertional activity, which is electrical activity recorded by the needle electrode as it passes through the muscle, and spontaneous activity, which is electrical activity that persists even after the needle electrode stops moving, suggests membrane instability in denervated muscle fibers. Unlike their limb counterparts, pelvic floor muscles are tonically active even at rest with the exception of electrical silence during voiding due to reflex inhibition of these muscles.[77,78] The continuous tone makes it difficult to evaluate spontaneous activity. The motor amplitudes are lower in amplitude and shorter in duration than in limb muscles.[77–79] Needle EMG of the EAS can be performed as part of the evaluation for suspected pudendal neuropathy. The EAS can be examined in women in the dorsal lithotomy position and in men in the lateral decubitus position after obtaining informed consent, draping patients appropriately and applying topical anesthetic cream. The EAS is preferably examined with a CNE,[80] which can be inserted 2 to 3 cm lateral to the anus and directed toward the midline until EMG activity is noted at a depth of 1 to 3 cm.[62] The EAS is examined at the 3- and 9-o'clock positions during a bilateral examination.[81] Podnar and Vodusek[82] have proposed a standardized and more quantitative EMG approach to EAS needle examination assessing all 4 quadrants of the muscle. Presence of denervation potentials, reduced interference pattern, increased presence of polyphasic MUAPs, and increased MUAP size and duration suggest a neurogenic sphincter lesion.[83]

Iliohypogastric and ilioinguinal neuropathies can also be assessed by needle EMG examination of abdominal wall muscles. The muscles should be examined bilaterally. Needle EMG abnormalities may include denervation potentials and signs of reinnervation. Knockaert and colleagues[84] demonstrated that the needle EMG abnormalities most commonly seen in iliohypogastric and ilioinguinal neuropathies were chronic motor unit changes, not active denervation. Unfortunately, EMG testing in iliohypogastric and ilioinguinal neuropathies is not sensitive or specific.

Utility of electrodiagnostic tests for pelvic pain

Pudendal and perineal nerve conduction studies have helped establish a connection between pudendal neuropathy, urinary stress incontinence, and fecal incontinence.[85–89] The role of electrodiagnostic testing in neurogenic pelvic pain is less clear.

In the evaluation of nerve entrapment syndromes for neurogenic pelvic pain, it is important to consider the limitations of neurophysiologic testing. Current electrophysiologic techniques cannot directly assess pain mechanisms but correlate more with structural changes, such as demyelination or axon loss, and primarily evaluate motor function of the nerves. In addition, these techniques cannot precisely localize the site of compression. For example, a prolonged PTML may be observed in a severe proximal lesion accompanied by Wallerian degeneration.[90]

Electrophysiologic testing alone of the pudendal, ilioinguinal, iliohypogastric, and genitofemoral nerves is not sensitive or specific[91]; however, future studies should focus on use of electrodiagnostic testing in conjunction with imaging studies and clinical examination and their role in confirming diagnoses, assessing severity, and potentially predicting outcomes with treatment.

SUMMARY

Chronic pelvic pain can result from various intrapelvic and extrapelvic causes. Although patient history and physical examination may narrow the differential diagnosis, frequently, the different causes have overlapping presentations. Imaging examinations, such as US and/or MRI, may help delineate the cause of pain, particularly when related to pelvic organs; pelvic floor dysfunction or prolapse; synthetic material, such as pelvic mesh or slings; and in some cases of neuropathic pain. Patients with neuropathic pain can also be evaluated with nonimaging tests, such as nerve conduction studies, EMG, and testing of sacral reflexes.

ACKNOWLEDGMENTS

The authors thank Glenn Katz for his invaluable contribution in preparing the figures for publication.

REFERENCES

1. Wozniak S. Chronic pelvic pain. Ann Agric Environ Med 2016;23(2):223–6.
2. Mathias SD, Kuppermann M, Liberman RF, et al. Chronic pelvic pain: prevalence, health-related quality of life, and economic correlates. Obstet Gynecol 1996; 87(3):321–7.
3. Howard FM. Endometriosis and mechanisms of pelvic pain. J Minimally Invasive Gynecol 2009;16(5):540–50.
4. Juhan V. Chronic pelvic pain: an imaging approach. Diagn Interv Imaging 2015; 96(10):997–1007.
5. Leyendecker G, Bilgicyildirim A, Inacker M, et al. Adenomyosis and endometriosis. Re-visiting their association and further insights into the mechanisms of auto-traumatisation. An MRI study. Arch Gynecol Obstet 2015;291(4):917–32.
6. Bazot M, Darai E, Hourani R, et al. Deep pelvic endometriosis: MR imaging for diagnosis and prediction of extension of disease. Radiology 2004;232(2):379–89.
7. Kuligowska E, Deeds L 3rd, Lu K 3rd. Pelvic pain: overlooked and underdiagnosed gynecologic conditions. Radiographics 2005;25(1):3–20.
8. Nisenblat V, Bossuyt PM, Farquhar C, et al. Imaging modalities for the non-invasive diagnosis of endometriosis. Cochrane Database Syst Rev 2016;(2):CD009591.
9. Amirbekian S, Hooley RJ. Ultrasound evaluation of pelvic pain. Radiol Clin North Am 2014;52(6):1215–35.

10. Togashi K, Nishimura K, Kimura I, et al. Endometrial cysts: diagnosis with MR imaging. Radiology 1991;180(1):73–8.
11. Siegelman ES, Oliver ER. MR imaging of endometriosis: ten imaging pearls. Radiographics 2012;32(6):1675–91.
12. Kadan Y, Fiascone S, McCourt C, et al. Predictive factors for the presence of malignant transformation of pelvic endometriosis. Eur J Obstet Gynecol Reprod Biol 2015;185:23–7.
13. Bergeron C, Amant F, Ferenczy A. Pathology and physiopathology of adenomyosis. Best practice & research. Clin Obstet Gynaecol 2006;20(4):511–21.
14. Atri M, Reinhold C, Mehio AR, et al. Adenomyosis: US features with histologic correlation in an in-vitro study. Radiology 2000;215(3):783–90.
15. Reinhold C, Tafazoli F, Mehio A, et al. Uterine adenomyosis: endovaginal US and MR imaging features with histopathologic correlation. Radiographics 1999; 19(Spec No):S147–60.
16. Doherty L, Mutlu L, Sinclair D, et al. Uterine fibroids: clinical manifestations and contemporary management. Reprod Sci 2014;21(9):1067–92.
17. Murase E, Siegelman ES, Outwater EK, et al. Uterine leiomyomas: histopathologic features, MR imaging findings, differential diagnosis, and treatment. Radiographics 1999;19(5):1179–97.
18. Champaneria R, Shah L, Moss J, et al. The relationship between pelvic vein incompetence and chronic pelvic pain in women: systematic reviews of diagnosis and treatment effectiveness. Health Technol Assess 2016;20(5):1–108.
19. Knuttinen MG, Xie K, Jani A, et al. Pelvic venous insufficiency: imaging diagnosis, treatment approaches, and therapeutic issues. Am J Roentgenol 2015;204(2): 448–58.
20. Ganeshan A, Upponi S, Hon LQ, et al. Chronic pelvic pain due to pelvic congestion syndrome: the role of diagnostic and interventional radiology. Cardiovasc Intervent Radiol 2007;30(6):1105–11.
21. Coakley FV, Varghese SL, Hricak H. CT and MRI of pelvic varices in women. J Comput Assist Tomogr 1999;23(3):429–34.
22. Pandey T, Shaikh R, Viswamitra S, et al. Use of time resolved magnetic resonance imaging in the diagnosis of pelvic congestion syndrome. J Magn Reson Imaging 2010;32(3):700–4.
23. Thomassin-Naggara I, Darai E, Bazot M. Gynecological pelvic infection: what is the role of imaging? Diagn Interv Imaging 2012;93(6):491–9.
24. Liang Y, Gong D. Acupuncture for chronic pelvic inflammatory disease: a qualitative study of patients' insistence on treatment. BMC Complement Altern Med 2014;14:345.
25. Tukeva TA, Aronen HJ, Karjalainen PT, et al. MR imaging in pelvic inflammatory disease: comparison with laparoscopy and US. Radiology 1999;210(1):209–16.
26. Wang T, Li W, Wu X, et al. Tubo-ovarian abscess (with/without pseudotumor area) mimicking ovarian malignancy: role of diffusion-weighted MR imaging with apparent diffusion coefficient values. PLoS One 2016;11(2):e0149318.
27. Maglinte DD, Kelvin FM, Fitzgerald K, et al. Association of compartment defects in pelvic floor dysfunction. Am J Roentgenol 1999;172(2):439–44.
28. Asfaw TS, Saks EK, Northington GM, et al. Is pelvic pain associated with defecatory symptoms in women with pelvic organ prolapse? Neurourol Urodyn 2011; 30(7):1305–8.
29. Ellerkmann RM, Cundiff GW, Melick CF, et al. Correlation of symptoms with location and severity of pelvic organ prolapse. Am J Obstet Gynecol 2001;185(6): 1332–7 [discussion: 1337–8].

30. Yang A, Mostwin JL, Rosenshein NB, et al. Pelvic floor descent in women: dynamic evaluation with fast MR imaging and cinematic display. Radiology 1991; 179(1):25–33.

31. Flusberg M, Sahni VA, Erturk SM, et al. Dynamic MR defecography: assessment of the usefulness of the defecation phase. Am J Roentgenol 2011;196(4): W394–9.

32. Kumar N, Khatri G, Xi Y, et al. Valsalva maneuvers versus defecation for MRI assessment of multi-compartment pelvic organ prolapse. Paper presented at American Roentgen Ray Society Annual Meeting 2014, San Diego (CA).

33. Bertschinger KM, Hetzer FH, Roos JE, et al. Dynamic MR imaging of the pelvic floor performed with patient sitting in an open-magnet unit versus with patient supine in a closed-magnet unit. Radiology 2002;223(2):501–8.

34. Gufler H, Ohde A, Grau G, et al. Colpocystoproctography in the upright and supine positions correlated with dynamic MRI of the pelvic floor. Eur J Radiol 2004; 51(1):41–7.

35. Kelvin FM, Maglinte DDT, Hale DS, et al. Female pelvic organ prolapse: a comparison of triphasic dynamic MR imaging and triphasic fluoroscopic cystocolpoproctography. Am J Roentgenol 2000;174(1):81–8.

36. Lienemann A, Anthuber C, Baron A, et al. Dynamic MR colpocystorectography assessing pelvic-floor descent. Eur Radiol 1997;7(8):1309–17.

37. Kumar N, Khatri G, Sims R, et al. Supine magnetic resonance defecography for evaluation of anterior compartment prolapse – correlation with standing voiding cystourethrogram. Paper presented at: American Roentgen Ray Society Annual Meeting 2013; Washington, DC.

38. Bitti GT, Argiolas GM, Ballicu N, et al. Pelvic floor failure: MR imaging evaluation of anatomic and functional abnormalities. Radiographics 2014;34(2):429–48.

39. Kelvin FM, Maglinte DD, Hornback JA, et al. Pelvic prolapse: assessment with evacuation proctography (defecography). Radiology 1992;184(2):547–51.

40. Tunn R, Paris S, Taupitz M, et al. MR imaging in posthysterectomy vaginal prolapse. Int Urogynecol J Pelvic Floor Dysfunct 2000;11(2):87–92.

41. Khatri G, Carmel ME, Bailey AA, et al. Postoperative imaging after surgical repair for pelvic floor dysfunction. Radiographics 2016;36(4):1233–56.

42. Schuettoff S, Beyersdorff D, Gauruder-Burmester A, et al. Visibility of the polypropylene tape after tension-free vaginal tape (TVT) procedure in women with stress urinary incontinence: comparison of introital ultrasound and magnetic resonance imaging in vitro and in vivo. Ultrasound Obstet Gynecol 2006;27(6):687–92.

43. Maher C, Feiner B, Baessler K, et al. Surgical management of pelvic organ prolapse in women. Cochrane Database Syst Rev 2013;(4):CD004014.

44. van Geelen JM, Dwyer PL. Where to for pelvic organ prolapse treatment after the FDA pronouncements? A systematic review of the recent literature. Int Urogynecol J 2013;24(5):707–18.

45. Nygaard IE, McCreery R, Brubaker L, et al. Abdominal sacrocolpopexy: a comprehensive review. Obstet Gynecol 2004;104(4):805–23.

46. Fritz J, Dellon AL, Williams EH, et al. 3-tesla high-field magnetic resonance neurography for guiding nerve blocks and its role in pain management. Magn Reson Imaging Clin N Am 2015;23(4):533–45.

47. Dellon AL, Coady D, Harris D. Pelvic pain of pudendal nerve origin: surgical outcomes and learning curve lessons. J Reconstr Microsurg 2015;31(4):283–90.

48. Lewis AM, Layzer R, Engstrom JW, et al. Magnetic resonance neurography in extraspinal sciatica. Arch Neurol 2006;63(10):1469–72.

49. Possover M, Forman A. Pelvic neuralgias by neuro-vascular entrapment: anatomical findings in a series of 97 consecutive patients treated by laparoscopic nerve decompression. Pain Physician 2015;18(6):E1139–43.
50. Onat SS, Ata AM, Ozcakar L. Ultrasound-guided diagnosis and treatment of meralgia paresthetica. Pain Physician 2016;19(4):E667–9.
51. Cho Sims G, Boothe E, Joodi R, et al. 3D MR neurography of the lumbosacral plexus: obtaining optimal images for selective longitudinal nerve depiction. Am J Neuroradiol 2016. [Epub ahead of print].
52. Chhabra A, Carrino J. Current MR neurography techniques and whole-body MR neurography. Semin Musculoskelet Radiol 2015;19(2):79–85.
53. Chhabra A, Del Grande F, Soldatos T, et al. Meralgia paresthetica: 3-Tesla magnetic resonance neurography. Skeletal Radiol 2013;42(6):803–8.
54. Chhabra A, Faridian-Aragh N. High-resolution 3-T MR neurography of femoral neuropathy. Am J Roentgenol 2012;198(1):3–10.
55. Soldatos T, Andreisek G, Thawait GK, et al. High-resolution 3-T MR neurography of the lumbosacral plexus. Radiographics 2013;33(4):967–87.
56. Chhabra A, McKenna CA, Wadhwa V, et al. 3T magnetic resonance neurography of pudendal nerve with cadaveric dissection correlation. World J Radiol 2016; 8(7):700–6.
57. Menezes CM, de Andrade LM, Herrero CF, et al. Diffusion-weighted magnetic resonance (DW-MR) neurography of the lumbar plexus in the preoperative planning of lateral access lumbar surgery. Eur Spine J 2015;24(4):817–26.
58. Fritz J, Chhabra A, Wang KC, et al. Magnetic resonance neurography-guided nerve blocks for the diagnosis and treatment of chronic pelvic pain syndrome. Neuroimaging Clin N Am 2014;24(1):211–34.
59. Wadhwa V, Scott KM, Rozen S, et al. CT-guided perineural injections for chronic pelvic pain. Radiographics 2016;36(5):1408–25.
60. Benson J. Electrodiagnosis in pelvic floor neuropathy. In: Benson J, editor. Investigation and management of female pelvic floor disorder. New York: Norton Medical Books; 1992. p. 157–65.
61. Kiff ES, Swash M. Slowed conduction in the pudendal nerves in idiopathic (neurogenic) faecal incontinence. Br J Surg 1984;71(8):614–6.
62. Roberts MM, Park TA. Pelvic floor function/dysfunction and electrodiagnostic evaluation. Phys Med Rehabil Clin N Am 1998;9(4):831–51, vii.
63. Snooks SJ, Swash M. Perineal nerve and transcutaneous spinal stimulation: new methods for investigation of the urethral striated sphincter musculature. Br J Urol 1984;56(4):406–9.
64. Olsen AL, Ross M, Stansfield RB, et al. Pelvic floor nerve conduction studies: establishing clinically relevant normative data. Am J Obstet Gynecol 2003;189(4): 1114–9.
65. Tetzschner T, Sorensen M, Rasmussen OO, et al. Reliability of pudendal nerve terminal motor latency. Int J Colorectal Dis 1997;12(5):280–4.
66. Tetzschner T, Sorensen M, Lose G, et al. Vaginal pudendal nerve stimulation: a new technique for assessment of pudendal nerve terminal motor latency. Acta Obstet Gynecol Scand 1997;76(4):294–9.
67. Ellis RJ, Geisse H, Holub BA, et al. Ilioinguinal nerve conduction. Muscle Nerve 1992;15:1171–208.
68. Oh SJ. Nerve conduction in focal neuropathies. 3rd edition. Philadelphia: LWW; 2002. p. 661.
69. Ertekin C, Bademkiran F, Yildiz N, et al. Central and peripheral motor conduction to cremasteric muscle. Muscle Nerve 2005;31(3):349–54.

70. Bademkiran F, Tataroglu C, Ozdedeli K, et al. Electrophysiological evaluation of the genitofemoral nerve in patients with inguinal hernia. Muscle Nerve 2005; 32(5):600–4.
71. Ertekin C, Reel F. Bulbocavernosus reflex in normal men and in patients with neurogenic bladder and/or impotence. J Neurol Sci 1976;28(1):1–15.
72. Opsomer RJ, Caramia MD, Zarola F, et al. Neurophysiological evaluation of central-peripheral sensory and motor pudendal fibres. Electroencephalogr Clin Neurophysiol 1989;74(4):260–70.
73. Beck R, Fowler CJ. Clinical neurophysiology in the investigation of genitourinary tract dysfunction. In: Rushton D, editor. Handbook of Neuro-urology. New York: Marcel Dekker; 1994. p. 151–80.
74. Benson J. Clinical application of electrodiagnostic studies of female pelvic floor neuropathy. Int Urogynecol 1990;J1:164–7.
75. Vodusek DB. Evoked potential testing. Urol Clin North Am 1996;23(3):427–46.
76. Sethi RK, Bauer SB, Dyro FM, et al. Modulation of the bulbocavernosus reflex during voiding: loss of inhibition in upper motor neuron lesions. Muscle Nerve 1989; 12(11):892–7.
77. Dibenedetto M, Yalla SV. Electrodiagnosis of striated urethral sphincter dysfunction. J Urol 1979;122(3):361–5.
78. Siroky MB. Electromyography of the perineal floor. Urol Clin North Am 1996;23(2): 299–307.
79. Blaivas JG, Labib KL, Bauer SB, et al. A new approach to electromyography of the external urethral sphincter. J Urol 1977;117(6):773–7.
80. King DG, Teague CT. Choice of electrode in electromyography of the external urethral and anal sphincters. J Urol 1980;124(1):75–7.
81. Kenton K. Pelvic floor neurophysiology: an AANEM workshop. Rochester (MN): AANEM; 2005.
82. Podnar S, Vodusek DB. Protocol for clinical neurophysiologic examination of the pelvic floor. Neurourol Urodyn 2001;20(6):669–82.
83. Lefaucheur JP. Neurophysiological testing in anorectal disorders. Muscle Nerve 2006;33(3):324–33.
84. Knockaert DC, Boonen AL, Bruyninckx FL, et al. Electromyographic findings in ilioinguinal-iliohypogastric nerve entrapment syndrome. Acta Clin Belg 1996; 51(3):156–60.
85. Snooks SJ, Badenoch DF, Tiptaft RC, et al. Perineal nerve damage in genuine stress urinary incontinence. An electrophysiological study. Br J Urol 1985;57(4):422–6.
86. Snooks SJ, Barnes PR, Swash M. Damage to the innervation of the voluntary anal and periurethral sphincter musculature in incontinence: an electrophysiological study. J Neurol Neurosurg Psychiatr 1984;47(12):1269–73.
87. Snooks SJ, Henry MM, Swash M. Faecal incontinence due to external anal sphincter division in childbirth is associated with damage to the innervation of the pelvic floor musculature: a double pathology. Br J Obstet Gynaecol 1985;92(8):824–8.
88. Snooks SJ, Swash M, Henry MM, et al. Risk factors in childbirth causing damage to the pelvic floor innervation. Int J Colorectal Dis 1986;1(1):20–4.
89. Snooks SJ, Swash M, Mathers SE, et al. Effect of vaginal delivery on the pelvic floor: a 5-year follow-up. Br J Surg 1990;77(12):1358–60.
90. Lefaucheur JP, Labat JJ, Amarenco G, et al. What is the place of electroneuromyographic studies in the diagnosis and management of pudendal neuralgia related to entrapment syndrome? Neurophysiol Clin 2007;37(4):223–8.
91. Labat JJ, Delavierre D, Sibert L, et al. Electrophysiological studies of chronic pelvic and perineal pain. Prog Urol 2010;20(12):905–10 [in French].

Myofascial Pelvic Pain and Related Disorders

Jaclyn H. Bonder, MD[a],*, Michelle Chi, MD[b], Leia Rispoli, MD[b]

KEYWORDS

- Pelvic pain • Myofascial pain • Trigger points • Vulvodynia • Physical therapy
- Bladder pain • Constipation

KEY POINTS

- Myofascial pelvic pain can present as trigger points, taut muscle bands, or generalized muscle pain and may refer to other regions of the pelvis.
- A comprehensive history and physical examination provide the most reliable diagnostic information for patients with suspected myofascial pelvic pain.
- Myofascial pelvic pain is often associated with disorders, such as vulvodynia, constipation, bladder pain syndrome, endometriosis, and anxiety.
- Treatments for myofascial pelvic pain can include physical therapy, oral medications, cognitive-behavioral therapy, and botulinum toxin injections.

DEFINITION AND EPIDEMIOLOGY

Myofascial pelvic pain (MFPP) refers to pain in the pelvic floor muscles (PFMs), the pelvic floor connective tissue, and the surrounding fascia. MFPP can be a syndrome of its own and cause pelvic pain or it can be associated with a host of other abdominopelvic pain disorders. It is characterized by muscular pain, taut bands, and trigger points that refer pain to specific regions when pressure is applied. Trigger points in the PFMs can refer to many areas, including the suprapubic region, the lower abdomen, the posterior and inner thighs, the buttocks, and the low back. Historically, it has been undertreated as a result of being undiagnosed by providers who usually evaluate and treat patients with pelvic pain because detailed PFM examination is not routinely taught in their residency training. In studies assessing training of obstetrics/gynecology residents on diagnosing urogynecologic disorders, there were no questions addressing their knowledge of MFPP disorders.[1,2] In addition, there are no accepted

Disclosure Statement: The authors have nothing to disclose.
[a] Department of Rehabilitation Medicine, New York Presbyterian Hospital, Weill Cornell Medical College, 525 East 68th Street, Baker Pavilion 16th Floor, New York, NY 10065, USA; [b] PGY 3, Department of Rehabilitation Medicine, New York Presbyterian Hospital, 525 East 68th Street, Baker Pavilion 16th Floor, New York, NY 10065, USA
* Corresponding author.
E-mail address: jab9155@med.cornell.edu

laboratory or imaging tests that establish the diagnosis. In recent years, it is being recognized by practitioners because of studies that have consistently demonstrated its existence as part of other pelvic pain disorders.

A recent study that screened patients with chronic pelvic pain (CPP) for myofascial pelvic floor pain or pelvic floor trigger points via interview and physical examination found that 13.2% had pain that was related to the PFMs.[3] The prevalence of PFM tenderness in those with other CPP disorders is much higher though. Prevalence of levator ani pain in a CPP clinic over a 7-year period has been found to be 22%.[4] In another study of women in a CPP clinic, PFM tenderness was an isolated finding in 15% of these patients but was associated with other CPP disorders in 58.3% of patients versus 4.2% of healthy volunteers. Of the women in the CPP group, 89.0% had tenderness of the levator ani muscle, 50.8% had tenderness of the piriformis muscle, and 31.7% had tenderness of the internal obturator muscle.[5]

ANATOMY

The PFMs are composed of 2 major layers, the superficial PFMs, which are part of the urogenital (UG) diaphragm, and the deep PFMs (also called the pelvic diaphragm). The superficial muscles include the bulbospongiosus, ischiocavernosus, and superficial and deep transverse perineal muscles. In addition, the external urethral sphincter sits within the UG diaphragm. The UG diaphragm also contains fascial layers, which are situated on the muscles and act to form the deep and superficial perineal space. The superficial perineal fascia is the most inferior layer, sitting between the skin and the bulbospongiosus, ischiocavernosus, and superficial perineal muscles. The perineal membrane encompasses the deep transverse perineal muscle on its inferior and superior aspects. Beyond this rests the inferior pelvic fascia behind which the levator ani muscles sit. The muscles that compose the pelvic diaphragm and act to support the abdominopelvic cavity and viscera by closing the inferior aperture of the pelvis are the levator ani muscle and coccygeus muscle. The levator ani muscle is made of 3 individual muscles: the puborectalis, pubococcygeus, and the iliococcygeus. The muscles are bordered superiorly by the superior pelvic fascia. The coccygeus muscle is also a deep PFM located posteriorly, arising from the ischial spine and moving medially to the midline sacrococcygeal joint. Also located posteriorly is the piriformis muscle, originating from the sacrum and inserting onto the greater trochanter. Lastly, the obturator internus sits laterally above the arcus tendinous, attaching to the pelvic surface of the obturator foramen and exiting the pelvis around the ischial tuberosity to insert on the greater trochanter. Each of the PFMs can contribute to pelvic pain, as a primary source, as a referred source, or as component of a more widespread pelvic pain disorder.

HISTORY

A comprehensive history must be taken from patients with MFPP, with a particular focus on medical and surgical history involving the abdominopelvic organs and region. Patients must also be screened for a past history of physical, sexual, and emotional abuse given the high instance of MFPP in this population. A typical set of paramount questions regarding pain are asked, such as alleviating and aggravating factors, quality, severity, associated symptoms, and areas it radiates to. Pain may be constant or intermittent, at rest or with activity, and is usually described as sore, achy, heavy, and deep. Pain at the introitus with intercourse is often described as burning or sharp. It is also crucial to take an in-depth review of systems regarding urinary, bowel, and sexual dysfunction as patients with MFPP often have comorbid disorders of these organ systems. Patients often report dyspareunia, constipation, dyschezia, bladder pain, and vulvar pain. Knowledge of a history of anxiety and/or depression is also key as these patients are at high risk for these psychiatric issues, whether as a result of their pain condition or if it predates their pain. For women, an obstetric history should be obtained highlighting the type of delivery, vaginal tearing, and length of labor, as these can point to injury of the PFMs or nerves. To help physicians diagnose the cause of the pain and whether there are potentially structural issues contributing, patients should be screened for pain in the joints of the pelvic girdle, such as the lumbosacral junction, sacroiliac joints, hip joints, and pubic symphysis. Because of referral patterns of trigger points in the pelvic floor, patients with MFPP may have a history of being treated for any one of these joints with a poor or partial response.

PHYSICAL EXAMINATION

Palpation of the superficial and deep PFMs can assess for myofascial pain, trigger points, and other taut bands of muscle. Internal pelvic floor examination is probably the most valuable diagnostic resource for identifying pelvic floor myofascial pain; however, it has not been extensively studied. One group recently published a PFM hyperalgesia scoring system in which they palpated the levator ani, the obturator internus, bulbospongiosus, ischiocavernosus, and the transverse perineal muscles with minimal pressure. They rated PFM tenderness on a mild, moderate, and severe scale in both symptomatic and asymptomatic individuals. They found good interrater and intrarater reliability and that this was a simple way to screen for myofascial pain before and after treatment.[6]

On the pelvic floor examination, if tenderness is elicited with palpation of the levator ani and obturator internus muscles, a diagnosis of MFPP can be made. The pelvic clock is often used to describe the PFM locations, which allows providers to know if symptoms have improved after treatment. The levator ani is palpated from 3 to 5 o'clock and 7 to 9 o'clock on the left and right, respectively. The obturator internus is located just above 3 and 9 o'clock and can often be felt by first palpating for the arcus tendinous and then moving the finger just above it. It can then be further identified by having patients externally rotate the hip so that the muscle bulges into the examiner's fingertip. It is also possible to assess for piriformis pain on musculoskeletal vaginal pelvic floor examination. Rectal examination allows for assessment of the coccygeus, piriformis, and puborectalis muscles. Tender muscles can also be described as diffusely overactive or underactive or as hypotonic or hypertonic. Strength evaluation of the muscles is also important because weakness, dyssynergia, or improper contraction in the setting of MFPP points to possible nerve injury. In patients with a history of pelvic floor surgery or injury, it should be noted if scar tissue formation is present and restricting movement of the muscles.

For patients with known or suspected MFPP, a complete neurologic and musculoskeletal examination of the lumbar spine, pelvis, and hip is indicated because the state of the PFMs can be affected by disorders of these areas and vice versa. Testing of these regions should include range-of-motion evaluation, manual muscle testing, inspection for proper alignment, and assessment for sensory deficits. See **Box 1** for potential findings.

DIAGNOSIS AND DIAGNOSTIC TESTING

Diagnosis of MFPP is largely based on history and physical examination. There have been attempts to diagnose myofascial trigger points (MTrPs) via ultrasound or dry needling, but none of them have been accepted for routine use or specifically explored

> **Box 1**
> **Summary of potential physical examination findings**
>
> - Bone and joint pain
> - Muscle tightness
> - Muscle spasm
> - Muscle weakness
> - Trigger points
> - Radicular pain
> - Pelvic instability or obliquity
> - Neuropathic pain
> - Referred pain: lumbar spine, gluteal region, hips

for the pelvic floor. On ultrasound, MTrPs have been shown to appear as focal, hypoechoic regions with reduced vibration amplitude on vibration sonoelastography, indicating a localized, stiff nodule.[7,8] Although magnetic resonance elasticity has also been studied and shown that taut muscle bands have increased stiffness as compared with normal tissue, this is not regularly used to diagnose trigger points.[9,10]

Myofascial pain syndrome in the PFMs has been diagnosed through electromyography and measuring the turn-amplitude analysis. Itza and colleagues[11] showed that it is a reliable test to diagnose MFPP whereby the sensitivity was 83% and the specificity was 100%. This test is still not accepted in practice though, and more studies are needed.

TREATMENT

MFPP can exist independently, but it also frequently coexists with a variety of other medical conditions in the urologic, gynecologic, gastroenterological, musculoskeletal, neurologic, and psychological domains. Consequently, successful treatment encompasses treating multiple systems and is tailored to the individual. Therefore, not only does identification of MFPP require comprehensive clinical history taking but an effective treatment plan also necessitates a multidisciplinary team (**Box 2**) approach that involves treating concomitant medical pathologies.

> **Box 2**
> **Multidisciplinary team for pelvic pain**
>
> - Gastroenterology
> - Gynecology
> - Physical therapy
> - Physiatry
> - Psychiatry
> - Psychology
> - Neurology
> - Urologist
> - Urogynecologist/female pelvic medicine and reconstructive surgery

These providers should develop a treatment strategy combining physical therapy techniques along with patient education, pain management, and behavioral modification.[12] Several approaches have been introduced in the literature, including the use of nonsteroidal antiinflammatory drugs (NSAIDs), antidepressants, muscle relaxants, and neuromodulators. Interventions are targeted toward treating active pelvic floor MTrPs, which can develop from several mechanical, physical, organ system, and psychological stressors and are thought to be the primary pain generators.[13] In more refractory cases, various injections may also be used in conjunction with conservative management.[14,15] The various treatment interventions are outlined next.

Physical Therapy

Pelvic floor physical therapy (PFPT) encompasses a variety of techniques used to treat MFPP and pelvic floor dysfunction. Together, physicians and pelvic floor physical therapists develop an individualized treatment program based on a thorough assessment of the patients' symptoms and examination. This intake by a highly trained pelvic floor physical therapist begins with taking a full detailed history, musculoskeletal examination including external and internal pelvic examination, and, if warranted, rectal examination.[16] Musculoskeletal examination of patients with MFPP incorporates evaluation of patient posture, gait, range of motion of the spine and lower extremities, as well as the pelvic floor examination described earlier.

Treatment tools may include education, behavioral modifications, neuromuscular reeducation, PFM strengthening and relaxation techniques, biofeedback, and palliative methods. Manual techniques, such as massage, stretching, and soft tissue and bony mobilization, as well as electrical stimulation and ultrasound are also important treatments used by trained pelvic floor physical therapists.[17] Therapists will also address structural dysfunctions, provide home exercise programs and self-management techniques, and, if necessary, use cognitive-behavioral therapy skills to help patients cope with responses that may have developed because of chronic pain.[17] Education to patients by pelvic floor physical therapists is often done with a mirror, to assist in learning about their anatomy and visualize the problem regions.[16] Frequency of treatment may vary; however, typically patients are seen 1 hour per week; duration will depend on how long patients have been symptomatic as well as their response to therapy.

The goal of therapeutic exercise is to strengthen weak muscles, stretch tight muscles, improve mobility and flexibility, and decrease pain.[16] The therapist will work internally to manually release painful trigger points and restrictions in connective tissue related to the vagina and/or rectum. Soft tissue mobilization techniques, as well as passive and active range-of-motion exercises, are used to lengthen short muscle groups of the pelvis and pelvic floor. Patients may also be treated with scar tissue manipulation, which involves pulling strokes of skin and subcutaneous tissue to improve circulation to surrounding viscera and tissue. Once muscle groups are released and lengthened, strengthening exercises may begin. Effectiveness depends on synergistic coordination of certain muscle groups to recruit as well as relax appropriately. Exercises may include pelvic floor inhibition, with progression to active pelvic floor lengthening, while teaching patient self-myofascial and connective tissue manipulation. Additional techniques may involve pelvic floor biofeedback, which has shown about 50% effectiveness in reducing pelvic pain and electrical stimulation, which has also been reported to successfully improve pelvic pain.[18,19]

In addition to a home exercise program to reinforce the effects of PFPT, physical therapists may also recommend lifestyle and behavioral changes for patients. These changes may include certain activities to modify or eliminate, pain management strategies, avoidance of irritants, as well as use of vaginal dilators. Specifically, activities to avoid may include Kegel exercises, vaginal coitus, prolonged sitting, and wearing elastic underwear and tight jeans.[17]

Conservative Treatment

Conservative treatment is aimed toward relaxing the pelvic floor musculature and surrounding regions. The following treatments should be combined with physical therapy when appropriate:

- Topical heat/cold: It can be used as an adjunct to other conservative therapies to address muscular spasms. Examples include warm baths, particularly oatmeal baths, which can also prevent vaginal dryness. The recommended frequency is 2 times per day for greater than 15 minutes. In contrast, for women with comorbid vulvodynia, applying a cold pack may be preferable.[15]
- Behavior modification: It includes biofeedback (transvaginal or transrectal), avoidance of Kegel maneuvers or excessive straining with defecation.[20]
- Bowel/bladder management: Constipation is common in both CPP and MFPP as a result of increased pelvic floor tone and activity. Thus, an optimal bowel and bladder program is recommended to prevent worsening hypertonicity and subsequent development of MTrPs.[15]

Medications

Commonly used first-line treatments for MFPP include analgesics, such as acetaminophen and NSAIDs.[20] Opioids have also been used when other treatments modalities have failed. Low-dose skeletal muscle relaxants, such as diazepam, methocarbamol, cyclobenzaprine, and baclofen, have also been found to be effective in alleviating symptoms when combined with other therapies.[15,20] Vaginal diazepam or baclofen suppositories are another adjunctive treatment option that may be promising for patients with MFPP. A retrospective study by Rogalski and colleagues[21] investigated the use of vaginal diazepam suppositories for high-tone pelvic floor dysfunction and pain. A chart review was performed on patients who had received diazepam suppositories in conjunction with pelvic physical therapy and trigger point injections. The results showed significant improvement in pelvic floor muscular tone in multiple phases (resting, squeezing, relaxation), reduced sexual pain rated by the Female Sexual Function Index, and reduced pain as assessed on the visual analog scale (VAS) for pain.

Neuromodulators, particularly gabapentin, have also been found to be useful in treating pelvic pain. One prospective randomized study by Sator-Katzenschlager and colleagues[22] compared the efficacy of gabapentin, amitriptyline, and the combination of both in women with CPP. The patients were randomized to receive gabapentin, amitriptyline, or a combination of both, with doses titrated to their maximum equivalent daily doses. At the 6-, 12-, and 24-month follow-up, pain relief was significantly improved in the gabapentin and combination group compared with the amitriptyline group.[22] However, tricyclic antidepressants, such as amitriptyline, can be used for treating MFPP and have also been found to be effective in reducing depressive symptoms, increasing pain tolerance, and restoring abnormal sleeping patterns.[20]

Injections

Several studies have evaluated the use of various trigger point injections as adjuvants to pharmacotherapy, physical therapy, and behavioral therapy for treating MTrPs. The

PFMs that are most commonly injected include the levator ani (iliococcygeus, pubococcygeus, puborectalis), coccygeus, obturator internus, and superficial and deep transverse perineii.[15] Injections of extrapelvic MTrPs, such as the iliopsoas, hip adductors, and rectus abdominis, have also been shown to be effective in treating MFPP.

Local anesthetic myofascial trigger points injection
Local anesthetic MTrP injections are one method described in literature for treating refractory MFPP. The role of anesthetic has been suggested to involve the inactivation of active MTrPs and resultant reduction of pain through the following proposed theories:

- Mechanical disturbance of muscle fibers and associated nerves
- Disruption of the positive pain feedback loop
- Decreased concentration of nociceptive substances
- Endorphin release[15]

Local anesthetic injections have been reported to be preferable to dry needling because of its reduction in postinjection soreness as well as their analgesic effects. Three basic approaches have been described, transvaginal, paravaginal/subgluteal, and transperineal, using various needle trajectories. The transvaginal approach allows for closer proximity of the injection site to the trigger point resulting in easier access to the deeper PFM groups (ie, obturator internus). When the needle is inserted into the muscle, a local twitch response may also be elicited, resulting in pain at the site or at a referred site. The most common anesthetics used are 2.0% lidocaine, 0.5% bupivacaine, and 0.5% ropivacaine.[15] It is important to note that anesthetics containing epinephrine should be avoided because of the increased risk for local ischemia and production of MTrPs. Steroid injections into MTrPs should also be avoided because of the increased muscle wasting with subsequent injections as well as increased risk for muscle dimpling.

When injecting anesthetic, roughly no more than 0.25 to 0.5 mL per trigger point should be injected. Typically, no more than 3.5 mL to 5.0 mL of solution is injected on each side of the pelvic floor. It may take up to 3 injections before achieving a favorable effect. Adverse effects may include intravascular injection, infection, and hematoma. Contraindications to injections include local or systemic infection, anticoagulant therapy, bleeding disorder, allergy to anesthetic agents, and acute muscle trauma.[15]

Botulinum toxin-A
For MFPP that is unresponsive to more conservative treatments, such as physical therapy and medications, botulinum toxin-A (BTX-A) injections may be sought as an alternative treatment option. Several studies have examined the utility of BTX-A for treating MTrPs in MFPP and other similar conditions with promising results.[15,23] The theory behind the use of BTX-A for treating pelvic floor MTrPs is such that BTX-A blocks acetylcholine release at the neuromuscular junction, leading to decreased resting tone and contraction strength.[15] With regard to BTX-A dosing and injection technique, there is currently no standardized guideline; however, several approaches have been described in the literature with varying effects. Injection location is also often individualized based on clinical examination.

BTX-A was shown to be effective in the treatment of pain associated with levator ani spasm in a study conducted by Jarvis and colleagues.[24] In this pilot study, 12 women with a greater than a 2-year history of CPP were recruited. The bilateral puborectalis and pubococcygeus muscles were selected for injection and located by digital muscle palpation. A total of 10 units of BTX-A were injected at each site, totaling 40 units. Three different dilutions were used: 10 IU/mL, 20 IU/mL, and 100 IU/mL. The results showed significant decrease in pain for dyspareunia and dysmenorrhea as assessed by the VAS. PFM manometry also showed a significant reduction in resting pressures.

A later randomized-controlled study evaluated the effects of BTX-A injections into PFMs compared with saline. Participants were randomized to receive either 80 units of BTX-A at 20 units/mL or saline injections. Under sedation, the study drug was injected into 2 sites bilaterally in the puborectalis and pubococcygeus muscles in 1-mL aliquots. Similar to the pilot study, the BTX-A group reported significantly decreased nonmenstrual pelvic pain, dyspareunia, and pelvic floor pressures compared with saline controls.[25]

When administering BTX-A, it is important to note that injections should not be given sooner than every 3 months. BTX-A should also be used more judiciously in those with neuromuscular junction disorders, such as myasthenia gravis, and those taking anticholinergic agents or muscle relaxants. Some of the side effects that may be reported include pain at the injection site, malaise, flulike symptoms, bladder and bowel incontinence, and rare but serious life-threatening toxic effects when there is distant spread.[15]

Dry needling

Dry needling is an alternative method of MTrP therapy. Its therapeutic effects are based on the premise that when a painful, tender localized area is penetrated repetitively with a fine needle, an analgesic effect is produced. Studies have shown that dry needling may exert therapeutic effects by acting at sites distant from the active MTrP.[15] There are also several associated adverse effects that are important to note, including postneedling soreness, hematoma formation, hemorrhage at the needling site, and syncopal episodes.[15]

Neuromodulation Therapy

Sacral neuromodulation is another treatment option that has been studied to show promising results in patients with pelvic floor pain by altering PFM activity.[20,26] A prospective study by Siegel and colleagues[26] explored the utility of sacral nerve stimulation in 10 patients with CPP refractory to conservative treatment. Following a positive response to percutaneous test stimulation, a neuro-prosthetic sacral nerve stimulation device was implanted with electrode stimulation of the S3 and S4 sacral nerve roots. Pain was assessed at baseline and at 1-, 3-, 6-, and 19-month follow-up intervals. The results showed that at least 80% of patients experienced a decrease in the number of hours of pain and severity of pain at long-term follow-up. Thus, sacral neuromodulation may be considered as an alternative treatment option for patients with MFPP refractory to more conservative measures.

ASSOCIATED DISORDERS

Patients with MFPP frequently present with additional urologic, gynecologic, gastrointestinal, musculoskeletal, and/or psychological complaints. These symptoms should be recognized, addressed, and treated. Clinicians should be aware of the commonly associated disorders with MFPP, and they should be considered when collecting a detailed history.[12]

Gynecologic

Gynecologic disorders that are often linked to MFPP include vulvodynia, dyspareunia, and endometriosis. Vulvodynia is vulvar pain of greater than 3 months' duration, generally without any visualized abnormality. It can be divided into provoked or unprovoked and also described as localized or generalized. Localized, provoked vulvodynia presents precisely as described. Patients experience pain in one specific area of the vulva (ie, vaginal vestibule or clitoris) with various forms of contact, tampon, speculum, and/or sexual relations.[27] Generalized vulvodynia, on the other hand, is usually unprovoked vulvar pain. This pain may or may not be exacerbated by sexual activity or reproduced on physical examination. Treatments include topical anesthetics, tricyclic antidepressants, pelvic floor therapy, pudendal nerve block when warranted, or, in severe protracted cases, vestibulectomy.

It is common for patients with vulvodynia to have accompanying sexual dysfunction and PFM dysfunction.[28] Hypertonic muscle dysfunction with tenderness of the PFMs, high resting tension, muscle irritability, and weakness is usually present with vulvodynia.[29] In women with provoked vestibulodynia, a combination of the following pelvic floor muscular findings exist: elevated resting tone, taut bands and/or active trigger points, elevated tone of both obturator internus muscles, increased tension in one or both tendinous arches of the pelvic fascia and/or the levator ani, and increased tone or visceral spasm in the urethra, bladder, uterus, or rectum.[30] In 2015, the Evidence-Based Vulvodynia Assessment Project showed that 90% of women with vulvodynia had muscular abnormalities in the pelvic floor.[31] Vulvodynia and MFPP have been linked together under the broad category of *CPP syndromes* in the medical literature[32] and may present similarly, with overlapping symptoms. However, recognizing the presence of both conditions may broaden the options for treatment approaches. The correlation of MFPP with vulvodynia is best proved by the improvement in pain that these patients have after PFPT. Several studies have highlighted the effects of PFPT for women with vulvodynia. In 2002, Bergeron and colleagues[27] performed a retrospective study, evaluating patients with provoked vestibulodynia after 6 to 8 sessions of PFPT programs. Approximately 71% of women with provoked vulvodynia (PVD) reported moderate to complete improvement in pain when followed up. In 2008, Dionisi and colleagues[33] cited 110 of 145 patients with improvement in pain after 10 weekly sessions of PFPT. And finally, in 2016 the *Journal of Sexual Medicine* published updated evidence-based recommendations for the treatment of vulvodynia and concluded PFPT is recommended for the management of vulvodynia (grade B).[34]

Dyspareunia, defined as painful vaginal penetration, is often observed in women with MFPP. Pain can develop due to UG atrophy, perineal scarring from prior surgery or childbirth, vulvodynia, hypertonic pelvic floor musculature, or other more serious medical conditions, such as endometriosis.[28] Vaginismus, the most common cause of entry dyspareunia, affects more than 1% of all women. Vaginismus presents as persistent involuntary contraction of the pelvic floor musculature.[35] Butrick[35] describes a perpetual cycle involving a patient's conditioned response. Dyspareunia is frequently initiated by an unpleasant experience, causing the fear or anxiety of pain with the next attempt. This fear, in turn, leads to involuntary hypertonic pelvic floor musculature, or vaginismus, resulting in entry dyspareunia, with a persistent cycle to follow.

Endometriosis affects roughly 10% of women of reproductive age. It is defined as a chronic inflammatory condition that occurs when endometrial tissue implants outside of the uterine lining.[36] Endometriosis also affects 50% of women with pelvic pain.[37] Endometriosis can cause a range of symptoms, including dysmenorrhea, dyspareunia, lower abdominal pain, and infertility.[38] However, the direct association with endometriosis and MFPP has yet to be supported in literature. A recent study performed by Stratton and colleagues[39] in 2015 concluded that sensitization and MTrPs were common in women with pain regardless of whether or not they had endometriosis at surgery. But those with any history of endometriosis were most likely to have sensitization. Stratton and colleagues[39] also speak to the importance of nongynecologic factors contributing to pelvic pain, especially in the CPP population.

Urologic

The most common urinary tract dysfunction found in patients with MFPP is interstitial cystitis (IC) or painful bladder syndrome. Patients with IC typically present with bladder pain, urgency, frequency, dysuria, nocturia, and/or pelvic pain.[35] In one prospective trial, it was found that 84% of patients with CPP had symptoms consistent with IC.[40] Another study estimated 50% to 87% of patients with IC also present with pelvic floor hypertonic dysfunction.[41] Urinary frequency, urgency, and pain may also be referred sensations with a skeletal rather than smooth muscle cause. Spasm of the intermediate layer muscles of the pelvic floor, sphincter urethrae, and compressor urethrae may create the sensation of urgency, whereas MTrPs in the levator muscles, obturator internus, and even rectus abdominis may also create urgency as a referred sensation.[42] Treatments for IC include stress reduction, diet modification, pelvic floor therapy, and medications, such as amitriptyline, histamine blockers and pentosan polysulfate, or bladder instillation therapy.[28]

Chronic prostatitis, also known as CPP syndrome in men, is classified as infectious or noninfectious, symptoms that are acute or chronic, and with or without the presence of CPP. About 90% to 95% of these patients are without evidence of infection and with CPP.[43] Patients typically present with associated urinary symptoms or sexual dysfunction; however, the pathophysiology explaining the source of chronic pain is not well understood.[43] Various treatments have been proposed, yet not widely accepted; these include alpha blocker, antiinflammatory, PFPT aimed at myofascial release, and urology referral if any abnormal findings.

Gastrointestinal

Chronic constipation is commonly experienced problem, especially among women with pelvic floor disorders.[44] Minimal literature exists evaluating constipation and management with women with pelvic floor dysfunction. One cross-sectional study described chronic constipation symptoms in the pelvic floor dysfunction population as including multiple distressing and uncomfortable symptoms. These patients responded well to self-management strategies, such as laxatives, manual facilitation, and enema; however, a more thorough assessment within this population was warranted.[44] Irritable bowel syndrome (IBS) affects about 10% of the population and about one-third of women with pelvic pain.[45–47] IBS is defined as functional gastrointestinal disorder characterized by abdominal pain, cramping, bloating, constipation, and diarrhea, frequently exacerbated by menstruation.[45] Most patients either have IBS with constipation or IBS with diarrhea. The literature on diagnosis and treatment of IBS is vast; however, current treatments available include cognitive-behavioral therapy, hypnotherapy, antispasmodics, antidepressants, dietary manipulation, fiber, and 5-hydroxytryptamine 3 receptor antagonists.[28] In both chronic constipation and IBS with constipation, it is important to also recognize and address the potential role of pelvic floor muscular dysfunction. Hypertonic or painful levator ani muscles may refer pain to the abdomen and contribute to abdominal pains that may initially be suggestive of a gastrointestinal disease process.[43] Women with MFPP may complain of constipation; pain before, during, or after defecation; as well as sensations of incomplete evacuation of bowel or bladder. These complaints may be due to a shortened puborectalis muscle, which slings around the rectum, and may create an anorectal angle that is too acute making bowel evacuation difficult or painful.[12] Constipation may also be due to the inability of the puborectalis muscle to relax during defecation.

Musculoskeletal Disorders

Pelvic floor MTrPs can develop as a result of a primary dysfunction intrinsic to the pelvic floor or as a functional adaptation to other musculoskeletal imbalances and disorders associated with the hip, spine, or pelvis.[48] MTrPs become activated from underlying chronic muscle fatigue, overuse injuries, impaired posture, or altered body mechanics, which may result from a primary musculoskeletal pathology or occur secondarily from organ pathology.[15] Therefore, it is important to treat the other underlying musculoskeletal causes that play a role in the development of MFPP and MTrPs.[15]

Skeletal causes of MFPP include hip and sacroiliac joint dysfunction, lumbar spine pathology, pubic symphysis disorders, and coccydynia. Conditions such as osteoarthritis, acetabular labral tears, femoral acetabular impingement, lumbar spondylosis, and coccyx misalignment have been implicated in the development of MFPP.[49] Muscular causes include levator ani and piriformis syndromes, which may result in the setting of trauma, such as child birth. More commonly, pain in the PFMs is widely attributed to the functional demands of these muscles and occurs through overuse injuries, repetitive strains/sprains, and postural dysfunction.[13,14,48] When these problems are not addressed, CPP can result in the formation of MTrPs as a result of abnormal muscle activation patterns of the PFMs. Another studied theory is that an underlying musculoskeletal disorder or impairment can cause muscle pain and injury, resulting in muscular strains. Muscle strains then lead to reduced circulation and localized hypoxia/ischemia, which can subsequently result in the development of MTrPs.[12]

The location of pain in some patients may not be localized to the pelvic floor. Patients with MFPP may commonly describe symptoms of low back pain; gluteal, groin, and leg pain; as well as radiation to the sacrum. Radiation to the hip and posterior thigh is also characteristic of a neuropathy or radiculopathy, which should be evaluated and treated appropriately. Patients with underlying musculoskeletal conditions contributing to MFPP may also describe pain with prolonged sitting, standing, and/or physical activity.[48]

The association of fibromyalgia and MFPP has also been examined in literature. One study evaluated the differences in body-wide musculoskeletal tender points in women with different types of CPP, specifically bladder pain syndrome (BPS) and MFPP. The following tender points were palpated: pelvic floor, abdomen, groin, inner thigh, and all 18 fibromyalgia tender points as described by the American College of Rheumatology.[49] Pelvic floor tender points included bilateral levator ani and obturator internus muscles and a single midline perineal assessment. The findings showed that patients with MFPP were found to have higher pelvic floor and fibromyalgia tender points compared with those with BPS alone. Therefore, this study demonstrated a strong positive correlation between pelvic floor and fibromyalgia tender points for patients with MFPP.[50]

Psychosocial Disorders

When obtaining a clinical history for women experiencing MFPP, a thorough history of past trauma, such as pelvic trauma or history of physical abuse or sexual abuse, is also warranted. Literature has also found that psychological stressors are closely correlated with MFPP. Both mental and emotional stress have been demonstrated to activate underlying MTrPs.[12] In addition, anxiety and depression have been linked to MFPP and CPP on numerous occasions. A cross-sectional study conducted by Coelho and colleagues[50] evaluated conditions frequently associated with CPP. The study examined 284 women with CPP, and the results showed a significant association between CPP and depression as measured by the Patient Health Questionnaire with an odds ratio of 2.33. Similarly, a systematic review by Latthe and colleagues[51] also evaluated factors predisposing women to CPP and found that anxiety and depression were positively associated with dyspareunia with an odds ratio of 3.23 and 7.77, respectively.[52] In 2010, a study in Brazil examined the prevalence of pelvic muscle tenderness in women with CPP. They found that among those with CPP, women who also had pelvic muscle tenderness had higher Beck Depression Index scores as well as higher rates of dyspareunia and constipation than those without pelvic muscle tenderness.[5] Given the support of literature, it is reasonable to conclude that the treatment of MFPP associated with other psychosocial conditions warrants psychological services for cognitive-behavioral interventions, which may include relaxation techniques.[14]

SUMMARY/DISCUSSION

MFPP of the PFMs is a frequent cause CPP in women and men. It often coexists with other disorders of the abdomen and pelvis as well as problems of the joints, muscles, and ligaments of the pelvic girdle. Treatment needs to be multidisciplinary so that each syndrome, dysfunction, and related injury is addressed. Physical therapy, oral pain medications, behavioral changes, and cognitive-behavioral therapy are the mainstays of management for these patients. Research in this field is still evolving. More studies are needed to help providers diagnose MFPP and determine the best course of treatment.

REFERENCES

1. Casiano ER, Wendel GD Jr, Congleton MJ, et al. Urogynecology training and practice patterns after residency. J Surg Educ 2012;69(1):77–83.
2. Schimpf MO, Feldman DM, O'Sullivan DM, et al. Resident education and training in urogynecology and pelvic reconstructive surgery: a survey. Int Urogynecol J Pelvic Floor Dysfunct 2007;18(6):613–7.
3. Bedaiwy MA, Patterson B, Mahajan S. Prevalence of myofascial chronic pelvic pain and the effectiveness of pelvic floor physical therapy. J Reprod Med 2013;58(11–12):504–10.
4. Tu FF, As-Sanie S, Steege JF. Prevalence of pelvic musculoskeletal disorders in a female chronic pelvic pain clinic. J Reprod Med 2006;51(3):185–9.
5. Montenegro ML, Mateus-Vasconcelos EC, Rosa e Silva JC, et al. Importance of pelvic muscle tenderness evaluation in women with chronic pelvic pain. Pain Med 2010;11(2):224–8.
6. Bhide AA, Puccini F, Bray R, et al. The pelvic floor muscle hyperalgesia (PFMH) scoring system: a new classification tool to assess women with chronic pelvic pain: multicentre pilot study of validity and reliability. Eur J Obstet Gynecol Reprod Biol 2015;193:111–3.
7. Sikdar S, Shah JP, Gebreab T, et al. Novel applications of ultrasound technology to visualize and characterize myofascial trigger points and surrounding soft tissue. Arch Phys Med Rehabil 2009;90(11):1829–38.
8. Turo D, Otto P, Shah JP, et al. Ultrasonic characterization of the upper trapezius muscle in patients with chronic neck pain. Ultrason Imaging 2013;35(2):173–87.
9. Chen Q, Wang HJ, Gay RE, et al. Quantification of myofascial taut bands. Arch Phys Med Rehabil 2016;97(1):67–73.
10. Chen Q, Basford J, An KN. Ability of magnetic resonance elastography to assess taut bands. Clin Biomech (Bristol, Avon) 2008;23(5):623–9.

11. Itza F, Zarza D, Salinas J, et al. Turn-amplitude analysis as a diagnostic test for myofascial syndrome in patients with chronic pelvic pain. Pain Res Manag 2015;20(2):96–100.

12. Pastore EA, Katzman WB. Recognizing myofascial pelvic pain in the female patient with chronic pelvic pain. J Obstet Gynecol Neonatal Nurs 2012;41(5): 680–91.

13. Kotarinos R. Myofascial pelvic pain. Curr Pain Headache Rep 2012;16(5):433–8.

14. Spitznagle TM, Robinson CM. Myofascial pelvic pain. Obstet Gynecol Clin North Am 2014;41(3):409–32.

15. Moldwin RM, Fariello JY. Myofascial trigger points of the pelvic floor: associations with urological pain syndromes and treatment strategies including injection therapy. Curr Urol Rep 2013;14(5):409–17.

16. Rosenbaum TY, Owens A. The role of pelvic floor physical therapy in the treatment of pelvic and genital pain-related sexual dysfunction (CME). J Sex Med 2008;5(3):513–23.

17. FitzGerald MP, Kotarinos R. Rehabilitation of the short pelvic floor. II: treatment of the patient with the short pelvic floor. Int Urogynecol J Pelvic Floor Dysfunct 2003; 14(4):269–75.

18. Glazer HI, Rodke G, Swencionis C, et al. Treatment of vulvar vestibulitis syndrome with electromyographic biofeedback of pelvic floor musculature. J Reprod Med 1995;40:283–90.

19. Nappi RE, Ferdeghini F, Abbiati I, et al. Electrical stimulation (ES) in the management of sexual pain disorders. J Sex Marital Ther 2003;29(1 Suppl):103–10.

20. Srinivasan AK, Kaye JD, Moldwin R. Myofascial dysfunction associated with chronic pelvic floor pain: management strategies. Curr Pain Headache Rep 2007;11(5):359–64.

21. Rogalski MJ, Kellogg-Spadt S, Hoffmann AR, et al. Retrospective chart review of vaginal diazepam suppository use in high-tone pelvic floor dysfunction. Int Urogynecol J 2010;21(7):895–9.

22. Sator-Katzenschlager SM, Scharbert G, Kress HG, et al. Chronic pelvic pain treated with gabapentin and amitriptyline: a randomized controlled pilot study. Wien Klin Wochenschr 2005;117(21–22):761–8.

23. Avendaño-Coy J, Gómez-Soriano J, Valencia M, et al. Botulinum toxin type A and myofascial pain syndrome: a retrospective study of 301 patients. J Back Musculoskelet Rehabil 2014;27(4):485–92.

24. Jarvis SK, Abbott JA, Lenart MB, et al. Pilot study of botulinum toxin type A in the treatment of chronic pelvic pain associated with spasm of the levator ani muscles. Aust N Z J Obstet Gynaecol 2004;44:46–50.

25. Abbott JA, Jarvis SK, Lyons SD, et al. Botulinum toxin type A for chronic pain and pelvic floor spasm in women: a randomized controlled trial. Obstet Gynecol 2006; 108:915–23.

26. Siegel S, Paszkiewicz E, Kirkpatrick C, et al. Sacral nerve stimulation in patients with chronic intractable pelvic pain. J Urol 2001;166(5):1742–5.

27. Bergeron S, Brown C, Lord MJ, et al. Physical therapy for vulvar vestibulitis syndrome: a retrospective study. J Sex Marital Ther 2002;28:183.

28. Abercrombie PD. Caring for women with chronic pelvic pain. J Obstet Gynecol Neonatal Nurs 2012;41(5):666–7.

29. Edwards L. Vulvodynia. Clin Obstet Gynecol 2015;58(1):143–52.

30. Hartmann D, Sarton J. Chronic pelvic floor dysfunction. Best Pract Res Clin Obstet Gynaecol 2014;28(7):977–90.

31. Lamvu G, Nguyen RH, Burrows LJ, et al. The evidence-based vulvodynia assessment project. A national registry for the study of vulvodynia. J Reprod Med 2015; 60(5–6):223–35.

32. Newman DK. Pelvic disorders in women: chronic pelvic pain and vulvodynia. Ostomy Wound Manage 2000;46(12):48–54.

33. Dionisi B, Anglana F, Inghirami P, et al. Use of transcutaneous electrical stimulation and biofeedback for the treatment of vulvodynia (vulvar vestibular syndrome): result of 3 years of experience. Minerva Ginecol 2008;60(6):485–91 [in Italian].

34. Goldstein AT, Pukall CF, Brown C, et al. Vulvodynia: assessment and treatment. J Sex Med 2016;13(4):572–90.

35. Butrick CW. Pelvic floor hypertonic disorders: identification and management. Obstet Gynecol Clin North Am 2009;36(3):707–22.

36. Viganò P, Parazzini F, Somigliana E, et al. Endometriosis: epidemiology and aetiological factors. Best Pract Res Clin Obstet Gynaecol 2004;18(2):177–200.

37. Fauconnier A, Chapron C. Endometriosis and pelvic pain: epidemiological evidence of the relationship and implications. Hum Reprod Update 2005;11(6): 595–606.

38. Guidice LC. Clinical practice. Endometriosis. N Engl J Med 2010;362(25): 2389–98.

39. Stratton P, Khachikyan I, Sinaii N, et al. Association of chronic pelvic pain and endometriosis with signs of sensitization and myofascial pain. Obstet Gynecol 2015;125(3):719–28.

40. Parsons CL, Dell J, Stanford EJ, et al. The prevalence of interstitial cystitis in gynecologic patients with pelvic pain, as detected by intravesical potassium sensitivity. Am J Obstet Gynecol 2002;187(5):1395–400.

41. Peters KM, Carrico DJ, Kalinowski SE, et al. Prevalence of pelvic floor dysfunction in patients with interstitial cystitis. Urology 2007;70(1):16–8.

42. Simons DG, Travell JG, Simons LS. 2nd edition. Travell and Simon' myofascial pain and dysfunction: the trigger point manual, vol. 2. London: Williams and Wilkins; 1999.

43. Lin G, Reed-Maldonado AB, Lin M, et al. Effects and mechanisms of low-intensity pulsed ultrasound for chronic prostatitis and chronic pelvic pain syndrome. Int J Mol Sci 2016;17(7):1057.

44. Fuller E, Welch JL, Backer JH, et al. Symptom experiences of chronically constipated women with pelvic floor disorders. Clin Nurse Spec 2005;19(1):34–40 [quiz: 41–2].

45. Choung RS, Herrick LM, Locke GR 3rd, et al. Irritable bowel syndrome and chronic pelvic pain: a population-based study. J Clin Gastroenterol 2010; 44(10):696–701.

46. Williams RE, Hartmann KE, Sandler RS, et al. Prevalence and characteristics of irritable bowel syndrome among women with chronic pelvic pain. Obstet Gynecol 2004;104(3):452–8.

47. Tsynman DN, Thor S, Kroser JA. Treatment of irritable bowel syndrome in women. Gastroenterol Clin North Am 2011;40(2):265–90.

48. Gyang A, Hartman M, Lamvu G. Musculoskeletal causes of chronic pelvic pain: what a gynecologist should know. Obstet Gynecol 2013;121(3):645–50.

49. Sanses TV, Chelimsky G, McCabe NP, et al. The pelvis and beyond: musculoskeletal tender points in women with chronic pelvic pain. Clin J Pain 2016;32(8): 659–65.

50. Coelho LS, Brito LM, Chein MB, et al. Prevalence and conditions associated with chronic pelvic pain in women from São Luís, Brazil. Braz J Med Biol Res 2014; 47(9):818–25.
51. Latthe P, Mignini L, Gray R, et al. Factors predisposing women to chronic pelvic pain: systematic review. BMJ 2006;332(7544):749–55.
52. Adelowo A, Hacker MR, Shapiro A, et al. Botulinum toxin type A (BOTOX) for refractory myofascial pelvic pain. Female Pelvic Med Reconstr Surg 2013;19(5): 288–92.

Musculoskeletal Approach to Pelvic Pain

Kate E. Temme, MD[a,b,*], Jason Pan, MD[a]

KEYWORDS

- Musculoskeletal • Pelvic pain • Sacroiliac joint • Pubic symphysis
- Bone stress injury • Hip pain • Greater trochanteric pain syndrome

KEY POINTS

- Visceral and somatic causes of pelvic pain are often inter-related, and a musculoskeletal examination should always be considered for the successful diagnosis and treatment of pelvic pain.
- For the diverse etiologies of hip pain, there are many unique considerations for the diagnosis and treatment of these various disorders.
- Pelvic pain is often multidimensional due to the overlap between lumbo-hip-pelvic diagnoses and may require a multidisciplinary approach to evaluation and management.

INTRODUCTION

Etiologies of pelvic pain are vast, and differentiation between visceral and somatic sources of pelvic pain can be complex. Accurate diagnosis and successful treatment of musculoskeletal pelvic pain require an understanding of the possible effect of visceral pathology on somatic pain as well as an appreciation of the lumbo-hip-pelvic-pelvic floor interconnection to musculoskeletal pelvic pain. For these reasons, pelvic pain is often multidimensional and may require a multidisciplinary approach to evaluation and management.

Visceral pelvic pain may be related to urologic, gynecologic, obstetric, and gastroenterologic processes, which can have secondary musculoskeletal effects through the viscerosomatic reflex. Interstitial cystitis and irritable bowel syndrome have been associated with pelvic floor dysfunction, through increased pelvic floor muscular resting state and associated pain.[1] Endometriosis has been implicated in cyclic sciatic radiculopathy,[2,3] and pregnancy may cause pelvic girdle pain (PGP) through the

The authors have nothing to disclose.
[a] Department of Physical Medicine and Rehabilitation, University of Pennsylvania, 1800 Lombard Street, 1st Floor, Philadelphia, PA 19146, USA; [b] Department of Orthopaedics, University of Pennsylvania, 1800 Lombard Street, 1st Floor, Philadelphia, PA 19146, USA
* Corresponding author. Department of Physical Medicine and Rehabilitation, University of Pennsylvania, 1800 Lombard Street, 1st Floor, Philadelphia, PA 19146.
E-mail address: kate.temme@uphs.upenn.edu

hormonal, weight, and center of gravity change effects on pelvic joint stability and function. Given the complex overlap between visceral and somatic pelvic pain, the American College of Obstetricians and Gynecologists recommends musculoskeletal causes of pain be evaluated before laparoscopy or hysterectomy for chronic pelvic pain.[4]

This article focuses on the evaluation of musculoskeletal pelvic pain[4] as well as the relationship between disorders of the bony pelvis to hip and lumbar pathology. European guidelines have proposed that musculoskeletal pelvic pain be termed, PGP, for exclusion of gynecologic and/or urologic disorders while maintaining consistency of terminology[4] (**Box 1**).

SACROILIAC JOINT PAIN

Sacroiliac joint (SIJ) pain results when the joint is placed under stress and is often diagnosed in the setting of posterior pelvic pain. Pain can be a result, however, of intra-articular SIJ pain, ligamentous pain, associated muscular pain, or a combination of these factors.

Anatomy

The SIJ, a true synovial joint in the inferior portion, is surrounded by a capsule anteriorly and posteriorly and is reinforced by the anterior and posterior sacroiliac ligaments (**Fig. 1**). The dorsal longitudinal SIJ ligament crosses the SIJ to attach to the dorsal sacrum and ilium.[5] It contains nociceptors and proprioceptors and has been implicated in posterior pelvic pain because it absorbs forces from the SIJ and hip. Broad lumbar and sacral innervation contributes to the varied clinical presentations of SIJ pain.

- SIJ stability: relies on both form and force closure[6,7]
    - Form closure refers to passive stability achieved by the interlocking mechanism of articular grooves and ridges of the SIJ, which is more pronounced in men.
    - Force closure is achieved by intrinsic and extrinsic SIJ ligament tension, in addition to pelvic, hip, and lumbar muscular contraction, which further stabilizes the SIJ.

Clinical Presentation

Given the vast innervation to the SIJ, symptoms are diverse and may vary over time. SIJ pain may present with unilateral, bilateral or alternating symptoms.

Box 1
European guidelines for pelvic girdle pain

Occurs most frequently in relation to pregnancy, trauma and/or arthritis.

Pain is located between the posterior iliac crest and gluteal fold, particularly in the SIJ region.

Pain may occur in conjunction with or separately in the pubic symphysis.

Pain may radiate to the posterior thigh.

Standing, walking, and sitting tolerance is diminished.

Pain or functional limitations with PGP must be reproducible by specific physical examination tests.

Lumbar causes must be ruled out prior to diagnosis of PGP.

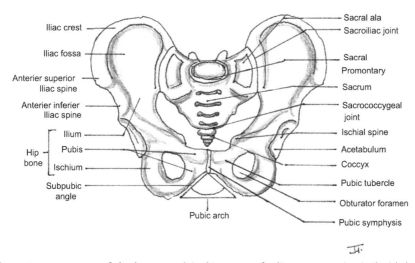

Fig. 1. Bony anatomy of the human pelvis. (*Courtesy of* Julie Temme, Miami, Florida.)

- Location: most commonly reported below the waistline, in the region of the posterior superior iliac spine.[8,9]
- Radiation: to the groin/pubic symphysis or lower extremity, especially the posterior thigh, but may radiate below the knee.
- Provocation: prolonged sitting, standing, and supine positions may incite symptoms. Transitional movements, asymmetric loading of the SIJ, including single-legged activities/sports, may provoke pain during which clicking, popping, or numbness may be reported. SIJ pain may result from trauma, pregnancy, or lumbar fusion or as a secondary adaption to another dysfunction (ie, altered gait due to an ankle sprain).

Diagnostic Evaluation

Physical examination

The diagnosis of SIJ pain through physical examination can be challenging. Alternative diagnoses, including hip and lumbar symptomatology, should be excluded. Posterior superior iliac spine region palpation may be painful. Flexibility of the hamstrings, rectus femoris, iliopsoas, and piriformis/obturator internus should be evaluated and core strength assessed (possibly including pelvic floor). SIJ dysfunction, or aberrant movement or position of the SIJ, may not be painful. Tests of dysfunction are unreliable and should not performed for diagnostic evaluation of SIJ pain. Provocative SIJ examination maneuvers are predictive of response to fluoroscopically guided SIJ diagnostic blocks when multiple tests are positive, because no single test alone is diagnostic of SIJ pain.[10–12]

- Provocative maneuvers: distraction, Gaenslen's Test, thigh thrust, compression, sacral thrust
  - Three or more positive tests = 91% sensitivity and 78% specificity[12]
  - Three or more positive tests in absence of pain centralization during mechanical evaluation = 87% specificity

Diagnostic testing

- Radiographs are often unremarkable in the setting of SIJ pain in the absence of a spondyloarthropathy or other inflammatory arthropathy but can be important for infection, tumor, or fracture evaluation. Early degenerative SIJ changes occur most often on the iliac border. Sclerosis only on the sacral border warrants consideration of an inflammatory arthropathy or metabolic etiology.[13] Radiograph of the pelvis should be performed in the anterior/posterior orientation.
- MRI with short-T1 inversion recovery or T2 fat suppression sequences is the most sensitive modality for detecting early sacroiliitis.[14]
- CT can be helpful to rule out occult fractures, tumors, infectious processes, and inflammatory arthropathies.
- Image-guided SIJ injection remains one of the most helpful diagnostic modalities for SIJ pain as well as an important adjunctive therapeutic modality.

Treatment

- Activity modification: relative rest after a traumatic injury or avoidance of actions that provoke symptoms, especially single-legged activities, can alleviate pain.
- Rehabilitation: core strengthening and obtaining a balance of lower extremity muscular length and strength decrease forces through the SIJ and restore normal lumbopelvic motion. Closed kinetic chain exercises are important components of initial lumbopelvic stabilization. Later, multiplanar exercises facilitate functional activity return. Muscle energy techniques are important for correction of pelvic alignment deficits.
- Medication: anti-inflammatories can be helpful in the acute injury phase.
- SIJ belt: joint compression, decreased pelvic rotation,[15] and gluteal muscle proprioceptive feedback can provide symptomatic relief in the setting of joint hypermobility or significant muscular weakness. The belt is usually worn during activities, such as walking, but in severe presentations can be helpful at rest. As SIJ stabilization improves during rehabilitation, the belt should be weaned. Functional leg length discrepancy (LLD) should be addressed through muscular balance, whereas anatomic LLD may respond to extrinsic correction.
- Injection: adjunctive use of image-guided SIJ injections can be helpful for diagnostic confirmation and to assist with physical therapy when pain limits tolerance or progress.

PUBIC SYMPHYSIS PAIN

Pubic symphysis disorders often occur as a result of traumatic or repetitive forces through the joint. Symptoms commonly present after trauma or infection, in elite athletes, and in the peripartum periods. Minimal shift and rotation are noted through the joint in the nonpregnant population.[16] In pregnancy, hormonal, weight, and center of gravity changes increase joint laxity and mechanical stresses experienced by the joint.[1] In athletes, sports requiring frequent kicking, twisting, pivoting, and sprinting increase shear through the pubic symphysis and may result in injury. Injury to the pubic symphysis may occur alone or in conjunction with surrounding soft tissue injuries.

- Osteitis pubis: a painful overuse injury that leads to pubic symphysis degeneration, demonstrated by radiographic joint abnormalities, including parasymphyseal sclerosis, cortical irregularities, and osteophyte formation.[17] In the acute setting, bone marrow edema and symphyseal fluid are noted on MRI.

Histopathologic evaluation reveals nonspecific inflammatory tissue with areas of fibrosis and cartilaginous mataplasia.[18]

- Pubic symphysis separation (PSS): true separation is a rare obstetric or traumatic diagnosis (**Fig. 2**). During uncomplicated vaginal deliveries, the joint may widen to 9 mm without symptoms,[19] with larger gaps associated with ligamentous injury, instability, and SIJ involvement.[19–21] Separation may be more common in the setting of rapid labor, instrumented delivery, cephalopelvic disproportion, abnormal infant presentation, and forceful hip abduction.[19,22]
- Core muscle injury (CMI)/athletic pubalgia: CMI encompass a spectrum of injuries that are thought to occur secondary to muscular imbalances between adductor and abdominal musculature, which may weaken/tear associated structures. Involved structures vary and may include the rectus abdominus/adductor longus conjoined tendons/insertions, oblique muscles, transversalis fascia, inguinal ligament, and pubic tubercle/symphysis.

Anatomy

- Pubic symphysis: a nonsynovial amphiarthrodial joint composed of a fibrocartilaginous intrapubic disk between hyaline cartilage of the pubic bones. Four ligaments envelope the joint to resist motion in all planes (compression, distraction, superior glide, and inferior glide).
- Muscular attachments: abdominal, pelvic, hip, and thigh musculature/fascia have connections to the pubic symphysis, providing stability and creating forces that are absorbed and transmitted through the joint.
- Innervation: various combined innervations have been proposed, including the pudendal and genitofemoral nerves[23] or pudendal, iliohypogastric, and ilioinguinal nerves.[24]

Clinical Presentation

- Location: anteromedial groin
- Radiation: to the lower abdominal musculature, medial thigh, inguinal region, perineum, and scrotum. May also present with associated SIJ symptoms.
- Provocation: movement may produce crepitus and walking may be limited to a waddling gait when severe. Pelvic motion, transitional movements, single-leg activities/sports, adductor stretching or activation, and abdominal activation may increase pain. Tenderness of the symphysis or pubic rami is common.
- PSS: In pregnancy, symptoms usually occur intrapartum or within 24 hours after delivery, although some patients present later or in the antepartum period.[22]

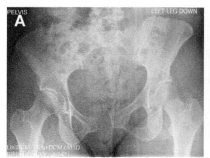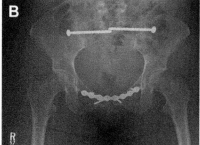

Fig. 2. (A) Plain radiograph demonstrates traumatic separation of the pubic symphysis secondary in the setting of a complicated vaginal delivery. (B) PSS status post–surgical fixation.

Women report sharp pelvic or groin pain and difficulty ambulating. A waddling gait is common in those who can ambulate, and lower extremity weakness has been reported.[19,25,26] A pop or crack may be heard during delivery. Other traumatic etiologies may have similar presentations.

Diagnostic Evaluation

Physical examination

- For suspected PSS, overlying skin should be examined. Palpation of the pubic symphysis and long dorsal ligament may elicit pain. Midline pressure from bilateral greater trochanter (GTs) or hip flexion of extended legs may provoke severe pain and may be deferred.
- For suspected CMI, tenderness of the pubic tubercle or symphysis, inguinal ring, and conjoined tendons/insertions may be present. Pain with resisted sit-ups or hip adduction (in external rotation) should be evaluated. Hip range of motion (ROM) suggestive of femoroacetabular impingement (FAI) may be associated with increased risk for CMI.

Diagnostic testing

- Radiographs: osteitis pubis, fracture, and joint separation can be evaluated with plain films. Flamingo views (alternating single-leg stance views) can demonstrate joint instability.[27] When plain films are diagnostically unrevealing, other imaging modalities are used.
- Ultrasound: in pregnancy, the intrapubic gap may be measured without the use of ionizing radiation. Ultrasound serves as an alternative to MRI in CMI evaluation.
- MRI: special musculoskeletal pelvic magnetic resonance (MR) protocols are used for the evaluation of CMI. MRI is useful for the diagnosis of osteomyelitis and for quantifying soft tissue injury associated with PSS.

Treatment

Evidence for pubic symphysis pain treatment is limited. In general, nonoperative management is the mainstay of treatment with surgical intervention reserved for large separations or recalcitrant CMI.

Pubic symphysis pain

- Activity modification: relative rest or avoidance of actions that provoke pubic symphysis pain symptoms (especially single-legged activities, excessive adductor stretching/activation, or abdominal activation) can alleviate pain.
- Rehabilitation: physical therapy is recommended for nonpregnant and pregnant patients and is associated with strength gains, decreased pain, and more rapid recovery.[28]
- Medication: anti-inflammatories are used commonly with limited research on efficacy.
- Supportive devices: bracing may provide symptomatic relief through joint stabilization, especially during provocative activities. Crutches or walkers may be necessary to offload the joint in severe cases.
- Injection: adjunctive use of image-guided pubic symphysis corticosteroid injections for therapeutic purposes remains controversial but can be considered when pain limits tolerance or progress in rehabilitation.[4,29]

Core muscle injury

Initial treatment of CMI includes a period of rest followed by rehabilitation. Stretching of abdominal, lower limb muscles/tendons is followed by core strengthening (transversus adbominus, multifidus, and pelvic floor) emphasizing neutral spine mechanics. Bilateral lower body exercises should progress to unilateral only after strength and stability improves. Return to play should be supervised and initiated after full lumbar and hip ROM, core stabilization, pain-free activities of daily living, and sport-specific activities are achieved. Surgical consideration is reserved for CMI nonresponsive to conservative management.

PELVIC INSUFFICIENCY FRACTURES/BONE STRESS INJURIES

Pelvic fractures may occur as a result of acute trauma or repetitive overload injury.

- Insufficiency fractures: occur when a normal force is applied to abnormal, weak bones
- Bone stress injuries: occur when a repetitive, submaximal force (ie, distance running) is applied to normal bone with a frequency and intensity that overwhelms the body's bony repair mechanisms. Given the expected resiliency of highly metabolic cancellous pelvic bones to fracture, bone stress injuries in the pelvis should prompt a bone health evaluation, including investigation for the components of the female athlete triad (low energy availability with or without disordered eating, menstrual dysfunction, or low bone mineral density) when appropriate.[30]

Clinical Presentation

Depending on injury location, patients may present with gluteal and/or anterior pelvic pain. With bone stress injuries, pain may be gradual in onset, initially occurring at the end of activity. With progression, pain may be felt throughout activity, at rest, and with activities of daily living. Rarely do radicular symptoms occur with sacral insufficiency and bone stress injuries.[3]

Diagnostic Evaluation

Physical examination

A lumbar and hip examination should be performed to rule out alternative diagnoses. Focal tenderness in addition to pain with provocative SIJ or pubic symphysis maneuvers may occur. Single-leg hop test may be poorly tolerated. SIJ provocative maneuvers, including thigh thrust, pelvic compression/distraction, and the hip flexion, abduction, external rotation (FABER) test may provoke symptoms.[30] Evaluation of contributing biomechanical factors is important for guiding treatment.

Diagnostic testing

- Radiographs: early and mild bone stress injuries may not be evident on plain films, and even complete pelvic fractures are often radiographically occult (**Fig. 3**).
- Nuclear medicine bone scan: although sensitive and able to identify early injury, bone scans are nonspecific, involve radiation, and have largely been replaced by MRI.
- MRI: musculoskeletal MRI has the highest combined sensitivity for pelvic stress injuries, even in early injury, and provides additional information regarding grading and associated soft tissue injuries[31] (see **Fig. 3**).

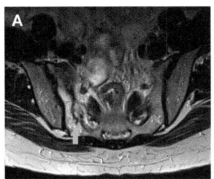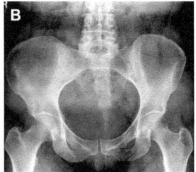

Fig. 3. (*A*) MRI demonstrating sacral bone stress injury (*arrow*). (*B*) Occult sacral bone stress injury on corresponding plain radiograph.

Treatment

Most injuries can be treated conservatively, although fractures involving the SIJ may require operative management.

- Activity modification: relative rest and avoidance of impact activities are critical in the early treatment phase. Swimming and low-impact activities that do not excessively load the pelvis are gradually initiated during rehabilitation.
- Rehabilitation: correction of core stabilization deficits, muscle imbalances, and biomechanical errors are important for recovery and future injury prevention. For athletes, a multidisciplinary return to play protocol should be followed when appropriate.
- Medication: nonsteroidal anti-inflammatory drugs may have a negative affect on early bone healing and should be avoided when possible. Acetaminophen can be helpful in early injury. Calcium and vitamin D supplementation should be instituted when needs cannot be met through dietary sources.
- Assistive devices: often, protected or non–weight-bearing status is maintained with crutches for symptomatic relief. Weight bearing is progressed as pain resolves.
- Risk factor modification: training and biomechanical errors should be addressed. Bone health should be optimized, and multidisciplinary treatment of the female athlete triad instituted when indicated.[30]

HIP DISORDERS

Painful intra-articular hip disorders may result from congenital anatomic variations, overuse injuries, metabolic considerations, and trauma. Recognition of hip disorders may be challenging given the varied presentations of hip pain and symptomatic overlap between lumbar and other pelvic joint/soft tissue diagnoses.

- Hip osteoarthritis (OA): articular cartilage degeneration with associated synovial, subchondral bone, and joint margin changes. Genetically predispositioned primary hip OA is uncommon. Up to 80% of cases result from predisposing pre-arthritic conditions, including trauma, infection, inflammatory arthritis, developmental dysplasia, FAI/labral tears, and avascular necrosis (AVN).[32]
- Developmental dysplasia of the hip (DDH): characterized by acetabular undercoverage of the femoral head; the resultant increased movement and excessive loading of the acetabulum by DDH predispose to early OA and labral tears. Despite routine screening of newborns, many are not diagnosed until adolescence or young adulthood.

- FAI: commonly reported in athletes and occurs as a result of extra bone on the acetabulum (pincer deformity) and/or proximal femur (cam deformity) (**Fig. 4**). Uncertainty persists as to whether this anatomic variation is preexisting or results from demands of certain sports during hip development.
- Hip acetabular labral tear: the acetabular labrum is a densely innervated, hypovascular fibrocartilage ring that deepens the hip socket and provides joint stability and shock absorption from the articular surfaces. Tears occur from acute trauma at hip end ROM or from repetitive microtrauma, especially in conditions such as FAI and DDH.
- Hip AVN: necrosis of the femoral head occurs secondary to blood supply disruption. AVN most commonly results from trauma, childhood hip disorders, corticosteroid use, excessive alcohol use, and blood dyscrasias.
- Femoral neck bone stress injury (FNBSI): although uncommon, FNBSI occurs from repetitive microtrauma accumulation and carries high rates of morbidity due to risk for malunion and AVN. FNBSI is associated with biomechanical factors and training errors as well as the female athlete triad.[30]

Clinical Presentation

Intra-articular hip pain may be insidious or acute and rarely presents without groin pain. Multiple other joint referral patterns exist, including posterior pelvic,

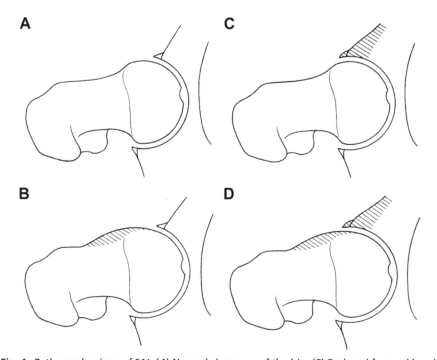

Fig. 4. Pathomechanisms of FAI. (*A*) Normal clearance of the hip. (*B*) Reduced femoral head-neck offset (pincer deformity). (*C*) Excessive overcoverage of the femoral head by the acetabulum (cam deformity). (*D*) Combination of reduced head-neck offset and excessive anterior overcoverage (combined pincer and cam deformity). (*From* Lavigne M, Parvizi J, Beck M, et al. Anterior femoroacetabular impingement. Part 1. Techniques of joint preserving surgery. Clin Orthop 2004;418:62; with permission.)

circumferential thigh, knee, and occasionally calf pain.[33] A history of advanced age and other risk factors for OA should be elucidated. Patients with FAI and/or labral tears may report decreased hip motion or a C sign (where patient cups hand to enclose the anterior groin, lateral hip, and posterior pelvis), whereas DDH is associated with increased hip ROM and instability. Pain severity that prevents weight bearing should elicit concern for fracture, AVN, or high-grade FNBSI.

Diagnostic Evaluation

Physical examination
A thorough lumbosacral and extra-articular evaluation should be completed to rule out alternative symptomatology. Findings suggestive of intra-articular symptomatology include[34]

- Gait: antalgic, Trendelenburg, lateral lurch, decreased/asymmetric stride length, foot internal/external rotation with stance/gait
- ROM: asymmetric or decreased passive ROM
- Provocative tests: internal rotation over pressure (flexion, adduction, and internal rotation [FAIR]) and FABER are the most sensitive hip-specific tests with highest positive predictive value (specificity: 0.91 and 0.82, respectively; PPI: 0.47 and 0.46, respectively) whereas Stinchfield's test is the most specific but with low sensitivity. Other tests include log roll, anterior/posterior hip impingement tests, and hip scour.

Diagnostic testing

- Radiographs: plain films are the initial imaging modality to evaluate fracture, OA, loose bodies, inflammatory arthropathy, and the stigmata of FAI or DDH. In young adult hips, the acetabular shape is best evaluated on antero-posterior pelvis/hip and false-profile views, whereas the femoral shape is best demonstrated with the 45° Dunn, cross-table lateral, and frog-leg lateral views.[35]
- MRI: noncontrast MRI is more useful for the evaluation of radiographically occult FNBSI, hip AVN, and extra-articular soft tissue disease but is limited in evaluation of intra-articular labral and chondral injuries (**Fig. 5**). MR arthrogram improves sensitivity, specificity, and positive predictive value of labral/chrondral injury detection (**Fig. 6**); however, a negative MR arthrogram does not fully exclude intra-articular symptomatology.[32]
- Ultrasound: utility declines for deeper structures and larger body habitus, and labral evaluation is limited. Ultrasound, however, is the only dynamic imaging modality to fully assess for extrinsic causes of snapping hip (iliopsoas, iliotibial band, or gluteus maximus).
- Injection: diagnostic (anesthetic only) image-guided intra-articular injections should be used in conjunction with MR arthrogram for the confirmation of symptomatic intra-articular pathology, because FAI and labral tears are not uniformly symptomatic.

Treatment

Treatment protocols vary depending on the intra-articular etiology:

- Hip OA: initially, a nonoperative trial of activity modification, rehabilitation to address strength and flexibility deficits within a pain-free ROM, low-impact aerobic activity, and specified courses of nonsteroidal anti-inflammatory drugs or acetaminophen can be helpful. Intra-articular steroid injections are considered

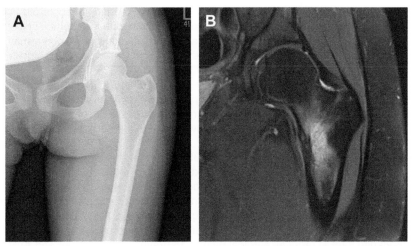

Fig. 5. (*A*) Radiographically occult FNBSI. (*B*) Corresponding MRI with findings consistent with FNBSI.

on a limited basis for symptomatic relief, to delay surgery, or to improve rehabilitation tolerance, although frequent use may contribute to cartilage destruction. Viscosupplementation is not Food and Drug Administration approved for hip OA and benefit remains controversial.[32,36] When conservative measures fail, hip arthroplasty is considered.

- Prearthritic hip disorders: nonoperative management trials should precede operative considerations. Neuromuscular retraining and provocative activity avoidance have been recommended, although no universal protocols exist for

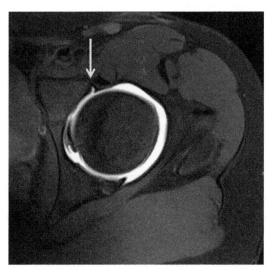

Fig. 6. MR arthrogram demonstrating hip acetabular labral tear (*arrow*). (*From* Jawahara A, Vadea A, Lomasney L, et al. Clinical and surgical correlation of hip MR arthrographic findings in adolescents. Eur J Radiol 2016;85 (6):1193; with permission.)

nonoperative rehabilitation of DDH, FAI, and labral tears. Corticosteroid injections should be avoided if possible in young patients due to potential chondrocyte injury. When pain persists, surgical hip preservation procedures may be considered. Surgical outcomes are more favorable in patients without significant joint degeneration.

- Hip AVN: unfortunately, nonoperative treatment, including modified weight bearing and rehabilitation, has not been proved to alter disease progression. Surgical intervention for early, small lesions may include core decompression and/or osteotomies; however, most patients eventually require arthroplasty for symptomatic AVN.
- FNBSI: compression/medial-sided FNBSI can often be treated with a trial of nonoperative management, including extended non–weight bearing on crutches with gradual progression to full weight bearing. Supervised rehabilitation is critical for recovery and safe return to sport. Signs/symptoms of fracture progression warrant close evaluation. Intrinsic and extrinsic risk factors should be addressed. Tension/lateral-sided FNBSI is considered an orthopedic urgency, because it often requires surgical pinning to prevent displacement and AVN.

PIRIFORMIS SYNDROME

Piriformis syndrome was first described in 1947[37] as a phenomenon wherein the sciatic nerve is compressed by the piriformis muscle. To date, it remains a controversial diagnosis with unsettled diagnostic criteria, and symptoms overlap with lumbosacral radiculopathies and SIJ pain.

Anatomy

Although the piriformis muscle and the sciatic nerve are in close anatomic proximity, true compression/impingement of the nerve in the gluteal region is rare. Piriformis trauma, overuse, and hip musculature imbalances are more commonly involved in this syndrome. Other hip external rotators implicated in similar clinical presentations include the obturator internus and the gemelli muscles.[38]

- Piriformis: originates from the sacrum and inserts on the GT
  ○ Function: external rotation and abduction of the femur
  ○ Innervation: nerve to the piriformis
- Sciatic nerve: arises from the lumbosacral plexus (L4-S3)
  ○ The nerve traverses under the piriformis muscle through the greater sciatic foramen.
  ○ In cadaveric studies, some individuals demonstrated variable anatomy of the piriformis and sciatic nerve (eg, all or part of the sciatic nerve pierces the piriformis).[39–42]

Clinical Presentation

Patients present with gluteal and radicular pain, which may be exacerbated by direct pressure to the affected region, piriformis muscle activation/stretching, hip internal rotation, stair climbing, or prolonged sitting. It is often relieved by resting in hip external rotation.

Diagnostic Evaluation

Physical examination
Given the imperfect criteria for the diagnosis of piriformis syndrome, other etiologies of gluteal pain, including lumbar and SIJ, should be evaluated and excluded.

- ROM, functional movement screen, and biomechanical evaluations should identify compensatory movement patterns that place asymmetric strain on the piriformis.
- Tenderness to palpation may be noted over the sciatic notch, and a taut muscle or gluteal atrophy may be appreciated.[37]
  ○ Maneuvers: FAIR, Lasègue, Freiberg, Beatty, and Pace tests activate or stretch the piriformis to reproduce a patient's typical gluteal pain with or without radiation.

Diagnostic testing

- Piriformis syndrome remains largely a clinical diagnosis.
- MRI, CT, ultrasound, and electromyography may be used to rule out other causes of gluteal pain, such as radiculopathy, intrinsic hip pathology, bursopathies, and tendinopathies as well as soft tissue lesions leading to sciatic nerve compression.
- MR neurography is gaining acceptance in the identification of piriformis syndrome, including responsiveness to surgery.[43]
- Image-guided piriformis muscle injection has been described, suggesting diagnostic and therapeutic utility.[44]

Treatment

- Activity modification: relative rest or avoidance of actions that provoke symptoms can alleviate pain.
- Rehabilitation: initial stretching and ROM exercises should be followed by progressive strengthening of the hip external rotators (including the piriformis), abductors, and extensors.[45] Kinetic chain abnormalities and weakness of the core musculature (lumbopelvic-hip complex) should be addressed. Ultrasound, foam rolling, and myofascial release may also have therapeutic benefit.
- Medication: anti-inflammatories may provide some pain relief, although there is no specific evidence for piriformis syndrome.
- Injection: there is limited evidence supporting mild–moderate symptom improvement after image-guided piriformis injections with local anesthetic, steroid, or botulinum toxin.[44,46,47]
- Surgery: limited evidence for open or endoscopic piriformis release.[48,49] Postsurgical hip external rotation and abduction are largely preserved due to redundant musculature.

HIP FLEXOR TENDINOPATHY

Hip flexor tendinopathy typically results from hip flexor overuse, particularly with running, jumping, or kicking.

Anatomy

Various muscles contribute to flexion at the hip. Of these muscles, the iliopsoas is the most commonly affected, followed by the rectus femoris. The iliopsoas is the primary hip flexor muscle; it also externally rotates the hip and contributes to lumbar and hip stabilization. The rectus femoris flexes the hip and extends the knee.

Clinical Presentation

The anterior hip/inguinal discomfort of hip flexor tendinopathy is exacerbated with active hip flexion, may radiate to the anterior thigh, and may be associated with a snapping sensation. Associated bursal and tendon inflammation is commonly seen in athletes, in the setting of FAI, and after hip surgery/arthroplasty.

Diagnostic Evaluation

Physical examination
Diagnosis of hip flexor tendinopathy is usually made clinically and requires evaluation and exclusion of other etiologies, such as lumbar disk herniation or acetabular labral tears.

- Active hip flexion elicits pain, and decreased hip extension during ambulation may be noted.
- Thomas test may reveal decreased flexibility.
- Provocative maneuvers, including Ludloff's Test and circumduction, may reproduce symptoms

Diagnostic testing

- Imaging is not usually required to make the diagnosis of hip flexor tendinopathy.
- MRI may show muscle/tendon edema of the affected hip flexor muscle(s) and may show associated bursal effusion.[50–52]
- Musculoskeletal ultrasound may demonstrate bursitis and/or tendinopathy and allow for dynamic confirmation of iliopsoas-mediated snapping hip.
- Image-guided iliopsoas injection (anesthetic) under the musculotendinous junction has been suggested to have diagnostic value.[53–56]

Treatment

- Activity modification: relative rest and avoidance of actions that provoke symptoms, such as kicking or stair climbing.
- Rehabilitation: stretching and progressive strengthening of the hip flexors, rotators, and core musculature.[45] In particular, initial psoas inhibition followed by retraining has been described to have therapeutic benefit.[57]
- Medication: anti-inflammatory can be helpful in the acute injury phase.
- Injection: adjunctive use of ultrasound-guided bursal steroid injections may assist with physical therapy when pain limits tolerance or progress.[58]
- Surgery: reserved only for patients who fail conservative management. Arthroscopic release of the iliopsoas tendon may provide relief while preserving function[59] but should be avoided in the setting of increased femoral anteversion due to reliance on the iliopsoas as a secondary hip stabilizer.

GREATER TROCHANTERIC PAIN SYNDROME

GT pain syndrome (GTPS) includes a spectrum of lateral peritrochanteric hip disorders, including gluteus medius and gluteus minimus syndrome, trochanteric bursitis, and/or external snapping hip (iliotibial band or gluteus maximus). It often mimics or coexists with hip and lumbar symptomatology. True bursal inflammation is uncommonly identified on imaging in the absence of direct trauma or repetitive overuse.

Anatomy

- GT insertions:
  - Gluteus medius/minimus underlie the gluteus maximus Iliotibial band and tensor fasciae latae and insert laterally on the GT to function in hip abduction and internal/external rotation.
  - Piriformis and obturator internus/externus muscles insert medially on the GT.

- GT bursae:
  - Several bursae have been described. The largest, most commonly affected is the subgluteus maximus bursa, located on the posterior facet and overlying the gluteus medius tendon.

Clinical Presentation

The discomfort felt in GTPS may occur with functional activities, such as prolonged standing, sitting, walking, crossing legs, sleeping on the affected side, or running.

- Location: pain in the lateral hip/gluteal region, which may radiate to the lateral thigh

Diagnostic Evaluation

Physical examination

Diagnosis of GTPS is made clinically and requires evaluation and exclusion of other etiologies, such as hip pathology, lumbar disk herniation, or other hip abductor symptomatology (ie, gluteus maximus or tensor fascia latae). Tenderness of the GT or gluteal tendon insertions may be elicited. Hip abduction in the extended position preferentially engages the fibers of the gluteus medius/minimus and may demonstrate weakness or elicit pain.

- Provocative maneuvers: single-leg stance and squat may be painful.[45,60]
  - Trendelenburg sign may be seen with significant gluteus medius/minimus weakness.
  - Dropping of the contralateral hip during single-leg squat is more sensitive for mild/moderate weakness.

Diagnostic testing

- Imaging is not usually required to make the diagnosis of GTPS but may be used to rule out other causes of pain.
  - Radiographs may demonstrate enthesopathy, calcific tendinopathy, or underlying joint disease.
  - MRI may show bursitis, calcific tendinitis, and muscle/tendon edema or atrophy of the gluteus medius/minimus.[61] The most sensitive (73%) and specific (95%) finding for tendon tears is T2 hyperintensity superior to the GT.[62]
  - Ultrasound may also demonstrate tendinous and bursal changes similar to MRI and provides a dynamic modality for evaluation for external snapping hip.[63,64]

Treatment

- Activity modification: relative rest and mileage reduction for runners
- Rehabilitation: hip ROM should be maximized and other biomechanical deficits corrected. Lower extremity flexibility (including iliotibial band and tensor fasciae latae), muscular coordination, and progressive strengthening of the gluteal muscles and other hip abductors (including single-leg balance/proprioceptive exercises) should be achieved.[65–67] Other muscle groups of interest include the core, hip external rotators, and hip and knee extensors.
- Medication: anti-inflammatories can be helpful in the acute injury phase.
- Injection: limited adjunctive use of image-guided GT bursal injections may be warranted if there is associated bursitis that limits rehabilitation progress.

ISCHIOFEMORAL IMPINGEMENT SYNDROME

Ischiofemoral impingement (IFI) syndrome describes a phenomenon wherein the quadratus femoris muscle is impinged due to ischiofemoral space narrowing. It is a rare cause of pelvic pain that predominantly affects women.

Anatomy

The quadratus femoris runs through the ischiofemoral space, which is narrowest between the ischial tuberosity and the lesser trochanter.

- Quadratus femoris: originates at the ischial tuberosity and inserts on the posterior aspect of the femoral head. It is often accompanied by a bursa between this muscle and the lesser trochanter.
  ○ Function: external rotation and adduction of the femur
  ○ Innervation: nerve to the quadratus femoris, arising from the lumbosacral plexus (L4-L5)

Clinical Presentation

IFI typically occurs in a posttrauma or postsurgical setting (eg, post–total hip arthroplasty), although some congenital cases have been reported.[68]

- Location: pain in the posterior hip, groin, or gluteal region. May be associated with mechanical symptoms (eg, hip snapping).
- Radiation: to the posterior thigh if the nearby sciatic nerve is irritated.

Diagnostic Evaluation

Physical examination
The diagnosis of IFI through physical examination is not well studied. Alternative diagnoses, including hip and lumbar symptomatology, should be excluded.

- Physical examination maneuvers: reproduction of symptoms with hip ROM
- Provocative maneuvers[69]:
  ○ IFI test (sensitivity 82% and specificity 85%)
  ○ Long-stride walking test (sensitivity 94% and specificity 85%)

Diagnostic testing

- Radiographs may be used as a screening tool for IFI. Proposed cutoff values for ischiofemoral distances include 2.0 cm to 2.1 cm for supine radiographs and 1.7 cm to 1.9 cm for standing radiographs.[70]
- MRI is the current gold standard for detecting IFI.[71–73] Findings include quadratus femoris edema (acute disease) and/or fatty atrophy (chronic disease). A recent meta-analysis[71] proposed cutoff values for the ischiofemoral space (<15 mm, sensitivity 77%, specificity 81%, and overall accuracy 78%) and quadratus femoris space (<10 mm, sensitivity 79%, specificity 74%, and overall accuracy 77%).
- Ultrasound-based measurement of the ischiofemoral space has been shown comparable to MRI-based measurements.[74,75]
- Image-guided quadratus femoris injection has been suggested to have diagnostic value.[76,77]

Treatment

- Activity modification: relative rest or avoidance of actions that provoke symptoms can alleviate pain.

- Rehabilitation: focused on stretching relevant muscle groups (eg, quadratus femoris and piriformis) and increasing hip ROM.[78] Strengthening is generally not a mainstay of treatment given the potential for undesirable muscle hypertrophy.
- Medication: anti-inflammatories may provide some pain relief, although evidence is limited.
- Injection: limited evidence for the adjunctive use of image-guided quadratus femoris injections for diagnostic confirmation and to assist with physical therapy when pain limits tolerance or progress.
- Surgery: limited evidence for relief after open or endoscopic resection of the lesser trochanter, with or without distal advancement.[77]

PELVIC FLOOR DYSFUNCTION

The pelvic floor musculature contributes to core stability as well as bowel, bladder, and sexual function. For more information on painful disorders of the pelvic floor, see the article by Jaclyn H. Bonder and colleagues article, "Myofascial Pelvic Pain and Related Disorders," in this issue.

SUMMARY

Visceral and somatic causes of pelvic pain are vast and often inter-related. Successful diagnosis and treatment of pelvic pain require an appreciation of visceral and somatic anatomy, clinical presentations, and unique diagnostic considerations. A musculoskeletal examination should always be considered in the setting of pelvic pain, because musculoskeletal causes may be the primary or secondary pain generator for pelvic pain.

REFERENCES

1. Prather H, Dugan S, Fitzgerald C, et al. Review of anatomy, evaluation, and treatment of musculoskeletal pelvic floor pain in women. PM R 2009;1(4):346–58.
2. Floyd JR, Keeler ER, Euscher ED, et al. Cyclic sciatica from extrapelvic endometriosis affecting the sciatic nerve. J Neurosurg Spine 2011;14(2):281–9.
3. Hameed F, McInnis KC. Sacral stress fracture causing radiculopathy in a female runner: a case report. PM R 2011;3(5):489–91.
4. Vleeming A, Albert HB, Ostgaard HC, et al. European guidelines for the diagnosis and treatment of pelvic girdle pain. Eur Spine J 2008;17(6):794–819.
5. Vleeming A, Pool-Goudzwaard AL, Hammudoghlu D, et al. The function of the long dorsal sacroiliac ligament: its implication for understanding low back pain. Spine (Phila Pa 1976) 1996;21(5):556–62.
6. Vleeming A, Stoeckart R, Volkers AC, et al. Relation between form and function in the sacroiliac joint. Part I: clinical anatomical aspects. Spine (Phila Pa 1976) 1990;15(2):130–2.
7. Vleeming A, Volkers AC, Snijders CJ, et al. Relation between form and function in the sacroiliac joint. Part II: Biomechanical aspects. Spine (Phila Pa 1976) 1990; 15(2):133–6.
8. Fortin JD, Aprill CN, Ponthieux B, et al. Sacroiliac joint: pain referral maps upon applying a new injection/arthrography technique. Part II: Clinical evaluation. Spine (Phila Pa 1976) 1994;19(13):1483–9.
9. Fortin JD, Dwyer AP, West S, et al. Sacroiliac joint: pain referral maps upon applying a new injection/arthrography technique. Part I: Asymptomatic volunteers. Spine (Phila Pa 1976) 1994;19(13):1475–82.

10. Laslett M. Pain provocation tests for diagnosis of sacroiliac joint pain. Aust J Physiother 2006;52(3):229.
11. Laslett M, Aprill CN, McDonald B. Provocation sacroiliac joint tests have validity in the diagnosis of sacroiliac joint pain. Arch Phys Med Rehabil 2006;87(6):874 [author reply: 874–5].
12. Laslett M, Aprill CN, McDonald B, et al. Diagnosis of sacroiliac joint pain: validity of individual provocation tests and composites of tests. Man Ther 2005;10(3): 207–18.
13. Prather H, Hunt D. Conservative management of low back pain, part I. Sacroiliac joint pain. Dis Mon 2004;50(12):670–83.
14. Madsen KB, Schiøttz-Christensen B, Jurik AG. Prognostic significance of magnetic resonance imaging changes of the sacroiliac joints in spondyloarthritis–a followup study. J Rheumatol 2010;37(8):1718–27.
15. Vleeming A, Buyruk HM, Stoeckart R, et al. An integrated therapy for peripartum pelvic instability: a study of the biomechanical effects of pelvic belts. Am J Obstet Gynecol 1992;166(4):1243–7.
16. Becker I, Woodley SJ, Stringer MD. The adult human pubic symphysis: a systematic review. J Anat 2010;217(5):475–87.
17. Barnes WC, Malament M. Osteitis pubis. Surg Gynecol Obstet 1963;117:277–84.
18. Grace JN, Sim FH, Shives TC, et al. Wedge resection of the symphysis pubis for the treatment of osteitis pubis. J Bone Joint Surg Am 1989;71(3):358–64.
19. Callahan JT. Separation of the symphysis pubis. Am J Obstet Gynecol 1953; 66(2):281.
20. Kharrazi F, Rodgers WB, Kennedy JG, et al. Parturition-induced pelvic dislocation: a report of four cases. J Orthop Trauma 1997;11(4):277–81.
21. Topuz S, Citil I, Iyibozkurt AC, et al. Pubic symphysis diastasis: imaging and clinical features. Eur J Radiol Extra 2006;59(3):127–9.
22. Lindsey R, Leggon RE, Wright DG, et al. Separation of the symphysis pubis in association with childbearing. A case report. J Bone Joint Surg Am 1988;70: 289–92.
23. Gamble JG, Simmons SC, Freedman M. The symphysis pubis. Anatomic and pathologic considerations. Clin Orthop Relat Res 1986;(203):261–72.
24. Gray H, Standring S. Gray's anatomy: the anatomical basis of clinical practice. 40th edition. Churchill-Livingstone, Elsevier; 2008.
25. Kane R, Erez S, O'Leary J. Symptomatic symphyseal separation in pregnancy. Surg Gynecol Obstet 1967;124(5):1032.
26. Snow RE, Neubert AG. Peripartum pubic symphysis separation: a case series and review of the literature. Obstet Gynecol Surv 1997;52(7):438–43.
27. Amorosa LF, Amorosa JH, Wellman DS, et al. Management of pelvic injuries in pregnancy. Orthop Clin North Am 2013;44(3):301–15, viii.
28. Nitsche JF, Howell T. Peripartum pubic symphysis separation: a case report and review of the literature. Obstet Gynecol Surv 2011;66(3):153–8.
29. Fitzgerald CM, Plastaras C, Mallinson T. A retrospective study on the efficacy of pubic symphysis corticosteroid injections in the treatment of pubic symphysis pain. Pain Med 2011;12(12):1831–5.
30. Tenforde AS, Kraus E, Fredericson M. Bone stress injuries in runners. Phys Med Rehabil Clin N Am 2016;27(1):139–49.
31. Nattiv A, Kennedy G, Barrack MT, et al. Correlation of MRI grading of bone stress injuries with clinical risk factors and return to play: a 5-year prospective study in collegiate track and field athletes. Am J Sports Med 2013;41(8):1930–41.

32. Prather H, Cheng A. Diagnosis and treatment of hip girdle pain in the athlete. PM R 2016;8(3):S45–60.
33. Lesher JM, Dreyfuss P, Hager N, et al. Hip joint pain referral patterns: a descriptive study. Pain Med 2008;9(1):22–5.
34. Prather H, Colorado B, Hunt D. Managing hip pain in the athlete. Phys Med Rehabil Clin N Am 2014;25(4):789–812.
35. Clohisy JC, Carlisle JC, Beaulé PE, et al. A systematic approach to the plain radiographic evaluation of the young adult hip. J Bone Joint Surg Am 2008; 90(Suppl 4):47–66.
36. Legre-Boyer V. Viscosupplementation: techniques, indications, results. Orthop Traumatol Surg Res 2015;101(1):S101–8.
37. Robinson DR. Pyriformis syndrome in relation to sciatic pain. Am J Surg 1947; 73(3):355–8.
38. Boyajian-O'Neill LA, McClain RL, Coleman MK, et al. Diagnosis and management of piriformis syndrome: an osteopathic approach. J Am Osteopath Assoc 2008; 108(11):657–64.
39. Beaton LE, Anson JB. The relation of the sciatic nerve and of its subdivisions to the piriformis muscle. Anat Rec 1937;70:1–5.
40. Lee CS, Tsai TL. The relation of the sciatic nerve to the piriformis muscle. Taiwan Yi Xue Hui Za Zhi 1974;73(2):75–80 [in Chinese].
41. Parsons FG, Keith A. Sixth Annual Report of the Committee of Collective Investigation of the Anatomical Society of Great Britain and Ireland, 1895-96. J Anat Physiol 1896;31(Pt 1):31–44.
42. Pokorny D, Jahoda D, Veigl D, et al. Topographic variations of the relationship of the sciatic nerve and the piriformis muscle and its relevance to palsy after total hip arthroplasty. Surg Radiol Anat 2006;28(1):88–91.
43. Filler AG, Haynes J, Jordan SE, et al. Sciatica of nondisc origin and piriformis syndrome: diagnosis by magnetic resonance neurography and interventional magnetic resonance imaging with outcome study of resulting treatment. J Neurosurg Spine 2005;2(2):99–115.
44. Finnoff JT, Hurdle MF, Smith J. Accuracy of ultrasound-guided versus fluoroscopically guided contrast-controlled piriformis injections: a cadaveric study. J Ultrasound Med 2008;27(8):1157–63.
45. Wyss J, Patel A. Therapeutic programs for musculoskeletal disorders. New York: Demos Medical Publishing; 2012.
46. Fowler IM, Tucker AA, Weimerskirch BP, et al. A randomized comparison of the efficacy of 2 techniques for piriformis muscle injection: ultrasound-guided versus nerve stimulator with fluoroscopic guidance. Reg Anesth Pain Med 2014;39(2):7.
47. Jankovic D, Peng P. Brief review: Piriformis syndrome: etiology, diagnosis, and management. Can J Anesth 2013;60(10):10.
48. Martin HD, Reddy M, Gomez-Hoyos J. Deep gluteal syndrome. J Hip Preserv Surg 2015;2(2):99–107.
49. Park MS, Yoon SJ, Jung SY, et al. Clinical results of endoscopic sciatic nerve decompression for deep gluteal syndrome: mean 2-year follow-up. BMC Musculoskelet Disord 2016;17:218.
50. Bui KL, Ilaslan H, Recht M, et al. Iliopsoas injury: an MRI study of patterns and prevalence correlated with clinical findings. Skeletal Radiol 2008;37(3):245–9.
51. Ouellette H, Thomas BJ, Nelson E, et al. MR imaging of rectus femoris origin injuries. Skeletal Radiol 2006;35(9):665–72.
52. Polster JM, Elgabaly M, Lee H, et al. MRI and gross anatomy of the iliopsoas tendon complex. Skeletal Radiol 2008;37(1):55–8.

53. Blankenbaker DG, De Smet AA, Keene JS. Sonography of the iliopsoas tendon and injection of the iliopsoas bursa for diagnosis and management of the painful snapping hip. Skeletal Radiol 2006;35(8):565–71.

54. Koski JM, Anttila PJ, Isomaki HA. Ultrasonography of the adult hip joint. Scand J Rheumatol 1989;18(2):113–7.

55. Rezig R, Copercini M, Montet X, et al. Ultrasound diagnosis of anterior iliopsoas impingement in total hip replacement. Skeletal Radiol 2004;33(2):112–6.

56. Smith J, Finnoff JT. Diagnostic and interventional musculoskeletal ultrasound: part 2. Clinical applications. PM R 2009;1(2):162–77.

57. Edelstein J. Rehabilitating psoas tendonitis: a case report. HSS J 2009;5(1): 78–82.

58. Flanum ME, Keene JS, Blankenbaker DG, et al. Arthroscopic treatment of the painful "internal" snapping hip: results of a new endoscopic technique and imaging protocol. Am J Sports Med 2007;35(5):770–9.

59. Anderson SA, Keene JS. Results of arthroscopic iliopsoas tendon release in competitive and recreational athletes. Am J Sports Med 2008;36(12):2363–71.

60. Chmielewski TL, Hodges MJ, Horodyski M, et al. Investigation of clinician agreement in evaluating movement quality during unilateral lower extremity functional tasks: a comparison of 2 rating methods. J Orthop Sports Phys Ther 2007; 37(3):122–9.

61. Kingzett-Taylor A, Tirman PF, Feller J, et al. Tendinosis and tears of gluteus medius and minimus muscles as a cause of hip pain: MR imaging findings. AJR Am J Roentgenol 1999;173(4):1123–6.

62. Cvitanic O, Henzie G, Skezas N, et al. MRI diagnosis of tears of the hip abductor tendons (gluteus medius and gluteus minimus). AJR Am J Roentgenol 2004; 182(1):137–43.

63. Adler RS, Buly R, Ambrose R, et al. Diagnostic and therapeutic use of sonography-guided iliopsoas peritendinous injections. AJR Am J Roentgenol 2005;185(4):940–3.

64. Connell DA, Bass C, Sykes CA, et al. Sonographic evaluation of gluteus medius and minimus tendinopathy. Eur Radiol 2003;13(6):1339–47.

65. Bewyer DC, Bewyer KJ. Rationale for treatment of hip abductor pain syndrome. Iowa Orthop J 2003;23:57–60.

66. Lachiewicz PF. Abductor tendon tears of the hip: evaluation and management. J Am Acad Orthop Surg 2011;19(7):385–91.

67. Presswood L, Cronin J, Keogh JWL, et al. Gluteus medius: applied anatomy, dysfunction, assessment, and progressive strengthening. Strength Conditioning J 2008;30(5):41–53.

68. Patti JW, Ouellette H, Bredella MA, et al. Impingement of lesser trochanter on ischium as a potential cause for hip pain. Skeletal Radiol 2008;37(10):939–41.

69. Gomez-Hoyos J, Martin RL, Schröder R, et al. Accuracy of 2 clinical tests for ischiofemoral impingement in patients with posterior hip pain and endoscopically confirmed diagnosis. Arthroscopy 2016;32(7):1279–84.

70. Park S, Lee HY, Cuong PM, et al. Supine versus standing radiographs for detecting ischiofemoral impingement: a propensity score-matched analysis. AJR Am J Roentgenol 2016;206(6):1253–63.

71. Singer AD, Subhawong TK, Jose J, et al. Ischiofemoral impingement syndrome: a meta-analysis. Skeletal Radiol 2015;44(6):831–7.

72. Torriani M, Souto SC, Thomas BJ, et al. Ischiofemoral impingement syndrome: an entity with hip pain and abnormalities of the quadratus femoris muscle. AJR Am J Roentgenol 2009;193(1):186–90.

73. Tosun O, Algin O, Yalcin N, et al. Ischiofemoral impingement: evaluation with new MRI parameters and assessment of their reliability. Skeletal Radiol 2012;41(5): 575–87.
74. Finnoff JT, Bond JR, Collins MS, et al. Variability of the ischiofemoral space relative to femur position: an ultrasound study. PM R 2015;7(9):930–7 [quiz: 987].
75. Finnoff JT, Johnson AC, Hollman JH. Can ultrasound accurately assess ischiofemoral space dimensions? A validation study. PM R 2016;7(9):930–7.
76. Backer MW, Lee KS, Blankenbaker DG, et al. Correlation of ultrasound-guided corticosteroid injection of the quadratus femoris with MRI findings of ischiofemoral impingement. AJR Am J Roentgenol 2014;203(3):589–93.
77. Wilson MD, Keene JS. Treatment of ischiofemoral impingement: results of diagnostic injections and arthroscopic resection of the lesser trochanter. J Hip Preserv Surg 2016;3(2):146–53.
78. Lee S, Kim I, Lee SM, et al. Ischiofemoral impingement syndrome. Ann Rehabil Med 2013;37(1):143–6.

Coccydynia: Tailbone Pain

Patrick M. Foye, MD

KEYWORDS

- Coccydynia • Coccygodynia • Coccyx • Pain • Coccyx pain • Tailbone
- Tailbone pain

KEY POINTS

- Coccyx pain (tailbone pain) substantially decreases the quality of life for patients who suffer with this condition.
- Classic symptoms include midline pain located below the sacrum and above the anus. Symptoms are usually worst while sitting or during transitions from sitting to standing.
- Physical examination typically reveals focal tenderness during palpation of the coccyx.
- Diagnostic tests typically should include radiographs (especially sitting-versus-standing radiographs to assess for dynamic instability). Advanced studies may include MRI, computerized tomography scans, or nuclear medicine bone scans.
- Treatments may include the use of cushions, medications by mouth, topical medications, local pain management injections, and (in rare cases) surgical removal of the coccyx (coccygectomy).

INTRODUCTION

The medical term "coccydynia" has multiple synonyms[1,2]:

- Coccygodynia
- Coccyx pain
- Tailbone pain

Coccyx pain has been called "the 'lowest' form of low back pain" because the coccyx is located at the most inferior tip of the spine.[3]

EPIDEMIOLOGY

Coccyx pain is far less common than pain in the lumbar spine, but there is a lack of exact data on its incidence. Although both women and men can suffer from coccyx pain, it occurs more commonly in women. The higher incidence in women may be

The author has nothing to disclose.
Physical Medicine and Rehabilitation, Coccyx Pain Center, Rutgers New Jersey Medical School, 90 Bergen Street, DOC Suite 3100, Newark, NJ 07103-2425, USA
E-mail addresses: Doctor.Foye@gmail.com; Patrick.Foye@rutgers.edu

due to differences in the shape and angles of the female pelvis and, of course, the increased risks while giving birth.

ANATOMY

The coccyx is composed of a series of 3, 4, or 5 coccygeal vertebral bones.[4,5] Thus, it is a misnomer to refer to the coccyx as a single bone.[4] For this article, these bony segments are referred to as C1, C2, C3, C4, and C5. The coccyx is located in the midline, inferior to the sacrum and superior-posterior to the anus.[5]

In addition to the variability in the number of coccygeal bones, there is great variability in whether some or all of these bony segments are fused together.[6,7]

There are many similarities between coccygeal vertebral bones and vertebral bones throughout the cervical-thoracic-lumbar spine, such as the following[4]:

- A vertebral body for each bony segment
- Transverse processes bilaterally (typically only present on the first coccygeal bone, C1)
- Superior articular processes (SAPs) bilaterally (typically only present on C1, where they are referred to as the coccygeal cornua, or horns).

But there are also unique differences at the coccyx region.[4] Unlike the cervical-thoracic-lumbar spine, the coccygeal vertebral bones are unique in the following ways:

- They have no vertebral canal. (The spinal canal ends more superiorly, at the sacral canal. Thus, there is no cerebrospinal fluid at the level of the coccyx.)
- They have no neuroforamina.
- They have no significant superior articular processes, inferior articular processes, or transverse processes (except for the first coccygeal bone).
- Each coccygeal bone is typically smaller (in height and width) than the coccygeal bone above it.

Joints of the coccyx are as follows[4]:

- Sacrococcygeal joint (SCJ): this is actually a collection of joints in which the lower end of the sacrum articulates with the upper end of the coccyx. Similar to intervertebral articulations throughout the cervical-thoracic-lumbar spine, the SCJ includes the following: (1) the articulation between the fifth sacral (S5) vertebral body and the C1 vertebral body, and (2) the bilateral zygapophyseal joints (facet joints). These sacrococcygeal facet joints are composed of the bilateral inferior articular processes (IAPs) from S5 (better known as the sacral cornua, forming the lateral borders of the sacral hiatus) and the bilateral SAPs from C1 (better known as the coccygeal cornua, or horns).
- Intracoccygeal joints (including the intervertebral discs between the coccygeal vertebral bodies).

Ligaments that attach to the coccyx include the following[4]:

- Anterior longitudinal ligament (ALL, also known as the anterior sacrococcygeal ligament) spanning the front of the coccygeal bones
- Posterior longitudinal ligament (PLL, spanning the back of the coccygeal bones)
- Lateral sacrococcygeal ligaments, bilaterally (where the lower sacrum attaches to the ipsilateral transverse process of C1)
- Spinosacral ligaments, bilaterally (attaching the right and left ischial spines to the ipsilateral sacrum and coccyx)

- Sacrotuberous ligament (spanning from the sacrum and coccyx to the ischial tuberosity)

Muscles attaching to the coccyx include the following[4]:

- Bilateral gluteus maximus muscles
- The coccygeus muscle
- The levator ani muscle group. This includes the ileococcygeus muscle, the pubo-coccygeal muscle, and the puborectalis muscle.

Nerves of the coccyx include the following[4]:

- Somatic nerves of the coccyx carry pain and other sensations from the coccygeal bones and ligaments.
- The sympathetic nervous system at the coccyx includes the ganglion impar, which appears to be involved in various forms of "sympathetically maintained pain" in the pelvic region.

CAUSES OF TAILBONE PAIN

There are many known causes of tailbone pain, in addition to idiopathic cases.[8] Some instances are caused by an identifiable episode of blunt trauma, others may be caused gradually by repetitive microtrauma, and some may be nontraumatic.

Coccyx Fractures

Fracture involves disruption of the bony anatomy. Although this seems obvious, clinicians' lack of familiarity with normal coccygeal anatomy (and its variability) can result in the multiple individual nonfractured coccygeal bones being mislabeled as fractures.[9] Coccyx fractures are typically due to blunt trauma (eg, falling onto the coccyx[5,9,10] or giving birth[2,5]).

Coccyx Dislocations

Dislocations involve ligamentous disruption causing 1 or more bones to become displaced from their normal anatomic locations.[5,10,11]

Coccygeal Dynamic Instability

Instability is defined as excessive movement of 1 or more bones relative to other bones. The instability is "dynamic" when it occurs, or becomes visible, only during conditions in which the bones and joints are placed under specific mechanical stresses.[12] At the tailbone, such stress is typically present when a person's coccyx is maximally weight bearing, which occurs when a person is sitting reclining partly backward.[13–15] Coccygeal dynamic instability (an unstable joint at the coccyx) is one of the most common causes of coccydynia.[13–15]

Distal Coccyx Bone Spurs

Bony thickening and elongation at the lowest tip of the coccyx is the classic appearance of a distal coccyx bone spur (also called a bone spicule).[16] The bone spur typically elongates in the inferior-posterior direction, which is opposite to the normal angulation of the distal coccyx (which would angle somewhat anteriorly).[16,17] When a person with a distal coccyx bone spur sits, especially sitting leaning partly backward, the bone spur can pinch the skin and subcutaneous tissue between the spur and the chair, causing pain.[17]

Abnormal Backward Position of Coccygeal Bones

If the coccygeal bones fail to have their normal, slightly forward-flexed position, and instead extend somewhat backward (posteriorly), this can result in abnormal increased weight-bearing forces onto the coccyx while sitting.[18] Also, the skin and subcutaneous tissues can be impinged between the posteriorly tilted distal coccyx and the chair (similar to what occurs with distal coccyx bone spurs).

Abnormally Excessive Forward Flexion of the Coccygeal Bones

If the coccygeal bones are flexed too far forward, they may cause internal obstruction within the pelvis during bowel movements or during childbirth.[18]

Coccygeal Arthritis

As with bones and joints elsewhere throughout the body, degenerative arthritis can occur at the coccyx.[7,19]

Sympathetic Nervous System Pain

Sympathetically maintained pain of the coccyx may occur due to hyperactivity or irritability of the ganglion impar, which is the most anatomically inferior sympathetic nervous system ganglion (located just anterior to the upper coccyx).[7,20]

Pelvic Floor Dysfunction

Hyperactive pelvic floor muscles may contribute to, or exacerbate, coccyx pain in some patients.

Cancer

Cancer at the coccyx can be either primary or metastatic. Chordoma is a primary bone malignancy that has a high tendency to occur at the sacrococcygeal region.[21,22] It is typically fatal even with aggressive surgical treatment.[21,22] Metastatic cancers of the coccyx may originate from distant sites in the body, or from nearby pelvic organs (eg, prostate, ovaries, cervix, colon). It is important to keep malignancy in the differential diagnosis for patients with coccydynia, especially in cases that fail to improve with standard treatments.[7,23]

Osteomyelitis

Bone infection should be considered as a possible underlying cause of coccydynia in patients with the following risk factors: prior history of a deep sacrococcygeal decubitus ulcer, previous coccygeal surgery (eg, coccygectomy), immunodeficiency, prior sepsis, or factors suggesting an underlying infection (local warmth and redness, unexplained fevers, elevated white blood cell count).[24]

SYMPTOMS OF COCCYDYNIA
Pain with Sitting

The classic and most common symptom in patients with coccydynia is pain while sitting.[25] The pain is typically worse while sitting leaning partly backward (partly reclining), because this position puts additional weight-bearing pressure onto the coccyx. Patients usually respond by avoiding sitting, or by sitting leaning forward (flexed at the hips) or by sitting leaning onto one buttock or the other. These adaptations decrease the amount of weight bearing occurring at the tailbone. Individual patients vary regarding whether the pain is worse with sitting on hard surfaces versus soft surfaces.

Pain During Sit-to-Stand

Many patients with coccydynia report exacerbation of the pain while transitioning from sitting to standing.[16,25] Many such cases are thought to be due to coccygeal dynamic instability. Specifically, coccygeal weight bearing during sitting may result in excessive movement (hypermobility) of the coccygeal vertebral bones.[13-16] Then suddenly standing up results in abruptly relieved weight bearing, causing the tailbone to painfully "snap back" into its normal, non–weight-bearing position.

Other Lumbosacral Pain Syndromes, Occurring Concomitantly with Coccydynia

Patients with coccyx pain frequently sit abnormally to avoid causing pain and pressure at the tailbone. Prolonged and recurrent episodes of sitting flexed forward at the hips (or leaning sideways onto one buttock or the other) results in abnormal mechanical forces throughout the lumbosacral and pelvic regions. This can result in a variety of secondary musculoskeletal conditions, including ischial bursitis, piriformis myofascial pain, piriformis syndrome, sciatic nerve irritation, sacroiliac joint pain, lumbosacral zygapophysial (facet) joint pain, and lumbosacral paraspinal myofascial pain.[26] Locally increased muscle tension and guarding due to coccyx pain may result in muscular pain and dysfunction throughout the pelvic floor.

PHYSICAL EXAMINATION FOR COCCYDYNIA
Patient Pointing

One important component of the physical examination is to explicitly ask the patient to point with 1 finger to the site where they experience most of their pain. Patients with coccydynia will, not surprisingly, point to the coccyx. This step can substantially help the clinician to quickly understand that this patient is not reporting generic "low back pain" in the lumbosacral region.

Visual Inspection

The clinician should carefully inspect the skin over the sacral, coccygeal, and perianal regions. Look for any rash, fistula, or discharge that might suggest an underlying pilonidal cyst. Look for any skin redness that might suggest an underlying infection (cellulitis or osteomyelitis). A skin dimple sometimes is seen over a distal coccyx bone spur.

Coccyx Palpation

Careful palpation is a crucial component of the musculoskeletal physical examination, especially for patients with coccydynia.[27] Palpating the sacral hiatus, bordered by the sacral cornua, provides excellent bony landmarks for the lower sacrum. From there, clinicians can "walk" their palpating fingers inferiorly, along the posterior wall of the coccyx. Most patients with coccydynia will have focal reproduction of pain during external, posterior coccyx palpation. The clinician also can appreciate whether the pain seems to be more at the upper, middle, or lower coccyx. A distal coccyx bone spur may be appreciated on direct palpation. Palpation of the anterior coccyx can be accomplished via digital rectal examination, particularly in patients in whom external palpation fails to reproduce their symptoms, or in patients with substantial anal or rectal symptoms. During intrarectal physical examination, pelvic floor muscles can be evaluated for hyperactivity and trigger points.

Adjacent Palpation

Careful palpation includes the para-coccygeal muscles and ligaments, bilateral ischial bursae regions, piriformis muscles, and anococcygeal ligament. Thorough palpation of the pelvic floor muscles and ligaments may be warranted in patients with pelvic floor symptoms.

PHYSICAL EXAMINATION FOR CONCOMITANT LUMBOSACRAL CONDITIONS

Additional physical examination maneuvers may include assessment for concomitant sacroiliac joint pain (eg, FABER [Flexion, Abduction, and External Rotation] test), lumbosacral facet joint pain (worse with facet palpation and with ipsilateral oblique extension), trochanteric bursitis (worse with focal palpation), and lumbosacral radiculopathy (straight leg raise and lower limb neurologic assessment of strength, reflexes, and sensation).[26]

MEDICAL TESTS FOR COCCYDYNIA
Radiographs

Radiographs are typically the first-line imaging study for coccydynia. Note that typical "lumbosacral" radiographs will fail to include the coccyx. Coccyx radiographs should ideally be done using a "coned-down" technique (using a collimator) to decrease the patient's radiation exposure and to improve the quality of the images obtained.[28]

Sitting-Versus-Standing Radiographs

Objective imaging studies to diagnose coccygeal dynamic instability requires comparing images obtained while standing versus images obtained while sitting. These images are done in the lateral view. Normally, in people without coccydynia, sitting results in the coccyx flexing forward by up to an additional 20°,[14] or listhesis at any coccygeal joint by less than 25% (of the coccygeal vertebral body width).[29] Because coccygeal dynamic instability is one of the most common causes of coccydynia, it has been published that "If you suffer from tailbone pain but have not yet undergone coccyx x-rays *while you're sitting*, then your diagnostic workup is *not* complete."[28] Unfortunately, despite more than a quarter century of publications on the value of sitting-versus-standing coccygeal radiographs, many radiology centers are still unfamiliar with performing these studies.[27]

MRI

MRI is superior to radiographs at detecting coccygeal osteomyelitis, primary sacrococcygeal malignancies (eg, chordoma), metastatic cancers of the coccyx, adjacent soft tissue tumors (eg, retrorectal hamartoma or tailgut cyst), and other soft tissue abnormalities (eg, pilonidal cyst).[28,30] Given the relative inability of radiographs to detect these diagnoses, and the high fatality rate of sacrococcygeal chordomas, MRI should be considered in patients with coccydynia with "red flags" suggesting malignancy or patients who fail to get adequate relief despite standard treatment measures.

Computerized Tomography Scans

Computerized tomography (CT) scans can detect some of the same abnormalities as MRI, but are generally less sensitive than MRI at detecting soft tissue abnormalities. Also, unlike MRI, CT scans deliver ionizing radiation to the patient.[28] Such radiation is particularly concerning at the pelvic region, where it may increase the risk of cancers of the reproductive organs and other intrapelvic tissues.

Nuclear Medicine Bone Scans

In select patients in whom there are concerns of osteomyelitis or malignancy despite radiographs and despite MRI or CT scans, a 3-phase nuclear medicine bone scan may be beneficial.[28] This would include looking for increased signal uptake on the third (late) phase of the study. Note that a lateral view of the coccyx is necessary, because otherwise the radioactive material pooling in the urinary bladder will obstruct the view of the coccyx on a standard anterior-posterior view.

See **Fig. 1** for an algorithm of diagnostic tests for patients with coccydynia.

TREATMENT OF COCCYDYNIA
Coccyx Cushions

Using certain types of cushions may help to relieve the pressure placed on the coccyx during sitting. U-shaped or wedge-shaped cushions are often helpful, with the cushion's open area placed at the back of the seat, so that the coccyx essentially "hovers" over the opening (and therefore avoids pressure from the seat).[31] Doughnut-shaped cushions (shaped like an "O") are commonly recommended but are typically far less effective for patients with coccydynia, probably because the back wall of the doughnut causes pressure onto the coccyx.

Modalities and Topical Medications

Local modalities (such as icing) and topical medications (such as topical nonsteroidal anti-inflammatory drugs [NSAIDs]) may provide some relief of coccydynia. However, the tailbone's location between the buttocks and near the anus makes it an inconvenient and somewhat unhygienic area for topical applications, especially when the patient is in public.[32]

Oral Medications

Medications by mouth may provide some relief for coccydynia. However, these medications act systemically, throughout the entire body, providing very little focal activity at the coccyx itself.[32] Meanwhile, the oral administration and systemic distribution of

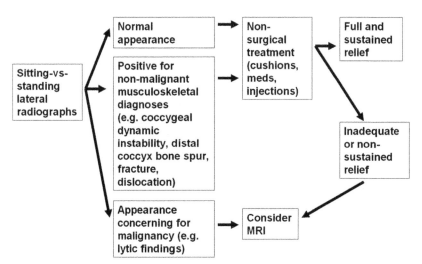

Diagnostic Tests for Tailbone Pain

Fig. 1. Diagnostic imaging studies for coccydynia often include radiographs (especially sitting-versus-standing radiographs) and MRI. (*Courtesy of* Patrick Foye, MD, Newark (NJ).)

the medications may cause gastrointestinal and systemic side effects. Such medications include NSAIDs (such as ibuprofen), acetaminophen, and opioid analgesics (eg, oxycodone and hydrocodone).

Interventional Pain Management Injections

To avoid the systemic side effects of systemically administered medications, and to maximize the local therapeutic benefit at the coccyx, interventional pain management injection techniques can be used to place medications focally at the site of the coccygeal pain generators.[33] These injections are typically done under fluoroscopic guidance, so the clinician can visualize the coccyx and the needle during the procedure and thereby place the medications at the site that matches the abnormalities seen on previous diagnostic tests. Fluoroscopic guidance also helps ensure patient safety, by helping the interventionalist to avoid inadvertently injecting into the rectum, caudal epidural space, or intravascularly.

Typical injections performed for coccydynia include local corticosteroid injections, ganglion impar sympathetic nerve block, and nerve ablation procedures.

- Coccyx steroid injections: injectable corticosteroids can be placed locally[34] at or around the site of a previously diagnosed unstable coccygeal joint or distal coccyx bone spur.[33]
- Ganglion impar sympathetic nerve blocks: these can be helpful for patients with sympathetically maintained pain in the coccyx region.[33,35]
- Nerve ablation: carefully select coccygeal nerves can be intentionally destroyed via radiofrequency ablation[36] or chemical ablation (using ethyl alcohol or phenol).[33] Nerve ablation is typically done only in patients in whom coccyx steroid injections and ganglion impar injections have failed to give adequate relief. Before ablation a "test injection" is performed using local anesthetic to assess whether ablation at that site is likely to provide relief.
- Repeat injections: any of the coccyx injections can be repeated if a given injection fails to give adequate relief (with the additional injection providing a beneficial "second dose" or "additive dose" effect). In cases in which a coccyx injection provides very good relief but the pain eventually returns, the injection can be repeated in hopes of again giving the patient another beneficial response.[33]

Coccygeal Manipulation

Manual medicine techniques at the coccyx can be performed by the clinician inserting 1 or 2 fingers into the patient's rectum and exerting physical manipulation forces onto the coccygeal bones and ligaments. Contraindications against manipulation may include unstable joints (coccygeal dynamic instability), distal coccyx bone spurs, and recent coccygeal fracture.[37] A 2001 French study of coccygeal manipulation for coccydynia found that only 25% of patients had a satisfactory outcome after 6 months, and results were even less favorable after 2 years.[38]

Physical Therapy

In a recent study of pelvic floor physical therapy (PT) for 124 patients with chronic coccydynia or status-post coccygectomy, physical examination revealed pelvic floor myofascial trigger points in 98%, but coccygeal hypermobility in only 10%. Treatment included "downtraining" overactive pelvic floor muscles via a combination of postural retraining exercises, diaphragmatic breathing, stretching, reverse Kegel (perineal bulge), lidocaine 2% jelly for use during internal (vaginal or rectal) PT for myofascial release, use of vaginal or anal dilators, and secondary treatments including oral baclofen for muscle relaxation, ganglion impar sympathetic nerve blocks with local anesthetic, and coccygeus trigger point injections with a combination of local anesthetic and steroid.[39] Patients' pain scores decreased by a mean of 62%.

Coccygectomy

Surgical amputation of the coccyx (coccygectomy) is typically considered only in the relatively uncommon patients who have failed to get adequate relief despite undergoing a valid trial of nonsurgical treatment (including the various injections discussed previously).[40] Postoperative side effects include wound infection (often requiring additional surgery for debridement of the infected postoperative site), bone infection (osteomyelitis), persistent chronic pain, and pelvic floor prolapse.[40]

SUMMARY

Patients suffering with coccydynia deserve a thorough medical evaluation, which includes a careful medical history, a physical examination that includes coccyx palpation, and appropriate diagnostic tests (such as sitting-versus-standing radiographs and in some cases MRI studies). Treatment options for coccydynia include avoiding exacerbating factors, using coccyx cushions while sitting, taking oral analgesics, focal pain management injections at the coccyx, and pelvic floor PT. Uncommonly, recalcitrant cases may require coccygectomy.

REFERENCES

1. Foye PM. Introduction. Tailbone pain relief now! Newark (NJ): Top Quality Publishing; 2015. p. 9–14.
2. Simpson JY. Clinical lectures on the diseases of women. Lecture XVII: coccydynia and diseases and deformities of the coccyx. Med Times Gaz 1859;40:1–7.
3. Foye PM. Overcoming stigma: psychology of tailbone pain. Tailbone pain relief now! Newark (NJ): Top Quality Publishing; 2015. p. 23–8.
4. Foye PM. Anatomy of tailbone pain. Tailbone pain relief now! Newark (NJ): Top Quality Publishing; 2015. p. 29–36.
5. Ryder I, Alexander J. Coccydynia: a woman's tail. Midwifery 2000;16(2):155–60.
6. Postacchini F, Massobrio M. Idiopathic coccygodynia. Analysis of fifty-one operative cases and a radiographic study of the normal coccyx. J Bone Joint Surg Am 1983;65(8):1116–24.
7. De Andres J, Chaves S. Coccygodynia: a proposal for an algorithm for treatment. J Pain 2003;4(5):257–66.
8. Foye PM. Causes of tailbone pain. Tailbone pain relief now! Newark (NJ): Top Quality Publishing; 2015. p. 37–8.
9. Foye PM. Tailbone fractures: the broken coccyx. Tailbone pain relief now! Newark (NJ): Top Quality Publishing; 2015. p. 51–8.
10. Cotton FJ. The sacrum and the coccyx. Dislocations and joint-fractures. Philadelphia: WB Saunders company; 1924. p. 115–7. Chapter VII.
11. Foye PM. Dislocations of the tailbone. Tailbone pain relief now! Newark (NJ): Top Quality Publishing; 2015. p. 59–64.
12. Foye PM. Unstable tailbone joints: dynamic instability. Tailbone pain relief now! Newark (NJ): Top Quality Publishing; 2015. p. 39–50.
13. Maigne JY, Guedj S, Fautrel B. Coccygodynia: value of dynamic lateral x-ray films in sitting position. Rev Rhum Mal Osteoartic 1992;59(11):728–31.
14. Maigne JY, Guedj S, Straus C. Idiopathic coccygodynia. Lateral roentgenograms in the sitting position and coccygeal discography. Spine 1994;19(8):930–4.

15. Maigne JY, Lagauche D, Doursounian L. Instability of the coccyx in coccydynia. J Bone Joint Surg Br 2000;82(7):1038–41.
16. Maigne JY, Doursounian L, Chatellier G. Causes and mechanisms of common coccydynia: role of body mass index and coccygeal trauma. Spine 2000; 25(23):3072–9.
17. Foye PM. Bone spurs of the tailbone. Tailbone pain relief now! Newark (NJ): Top Quality Publishing; 2015. p. 65–70.
18. Foye PM. Abnormal position of the tailbone. Tailbone pain relief now! Newark (NJ): Top Quality Publishing; 2015. p. 75–8.
19. Foye PM. Arthritis of the tailbone. Tailbone pain relief now! Newark (NJ): Top Quality Publishing; 2015. p. 71–4.
20. Foye PM. Sympathetic nervous system pain at the coccyx. Tailbone pain relief now! Newark (NJ): Top Quality Publishing; 2015. p. 79–84.
21. Chandawarkar RY. Sacrococcygeal chordoma: review of 50 consecutive patients. World J Surg 1996;20(6):717–9.
22. Foye PM. Coccydynia (coccyx pain) caused by chordoma. Int Orthop 2007; 31(3):427.
23. Foye PM. Cancer causing tailbone pain. Tailbone pain relief now! Newark (NJ): Top Quality Publishing; 2015. p. 85–92.
24. Foye PM. Bone infection causing tailbone pain. Tailbone pain relief now! Newark (NJ): Top Quality Publishing; 2015. p. 93–102.
25. Foye PM. Symptoms of tailbone pain (coccyx pain). Tailbone pain relief now! Newark (NJ): Top Quality Publishing; 2015. p. 15–22.
26. Foye PM. Back and buttock pain. Tailbone pain relief now! Newark (NJ): Top Quality Publishing; 2015. p. 103–14.
27. Foye PM. Working with your doctors. Tailbone pain relief now! Newark (NJ): Top Quality Publishing; 2015. p. 203–14.
28. Foye PM. Medical tests for tailbone pain. Tailbone pain relief now! Newark (NJ): Top Quality Publishing; 2015. p. 115–30.
29. Maigne JY, Tamalet B. Standardized radiologic protocol for the study of common coccygodynia and characteristics of the lesions observed in the sitting position. Clinical elements differentiating luxation, hypermobility, and normal mobility. Spine 1996;21(22):2588–93.
30. Foye PM. Coccyx pain diagnostic workup: necessity of MRI in detecting malignancy presenting with tailbone pain. AJPMR 2010;89(4):S33.
31. Foye PM. Cushions for tailbone pain. Tailbone pain relief now! Newark (NJ): Top Quality Publishing; 2015. p. 151–8.
32. Foye PM. Medications for tailbone pain. Tailbone pain relief now! Newark (NJ): Top Quality Publishing; 2015. p. 159–68.
33. Foye PM. Injections for tailbone pain. Tailbone pain relief now! Newark (NJ): Top Quality Publishing; 2015. p. 181–94.
34. Finsen V. Corticosteroid injection for coccygodynia. Tidsskr Nor Laegeforen 2001;121(24):2832–3 [in Norwegian].
35. Plancarte R, Amescua C, Patt RB, et al. Presacral blockade of the ganglion of Walther (ganglion impar). Anesthesiology 1990;73(3a):A751.
36. Demircay E, Kabatas S, Cansever T, et al. Radiofrequency thermocoagulation of ganglion impar in the management of coccydynia: preliminary results. Turk Neurosurg 2010;20(3):328–33.
37. Foye PM. Manipulation of the coccyx. Tailbone pain relief now! Newark (NJ): Top Quality Publishing; 2015. p. 169–74.

38. Maigne JY, Chatellier G. Comparison of three manual coccydynia treatments: a pilot study. Spine 2001;26(20):E479–83 [discussion: E484].

39. Scott KM, Fisher LW, Bernstein IH, et al. The treatment of chronic coccydynia and postcoccygectomy pain with pelvic floor physical therapy. PM R 2017;9(4): 367–76.

40. Foye PM. Coccygectomy: surgical removal of the tailbone. Tailbone pain relief now! Newark (NJ): Top Quality Publishing; 2015. p. 195–200.

Neurogenic Pelvic Pain

Nicholas Elkins, DO, Jason Hunt, MD, Kelly M. Scott, MD*

KEYWORDS

- Pelvic pain • Iliohypogastric • Ilioinguinal • Genitofemoral • Pudendal • Tarlov cyst

KEY POINTS

- Neuralgia of the iliohypogastric, ilioinguinal, and genitofemoral nerves typically presents as pain and paresthesia in the groin or upper pubic region.
- Pudendal neuralgia is the most common cause of chronic perineal pain. Its effects often include debilitating and unrelenting pain of the perineal region aggravated by sitting and relieved by standing.
- Tarlov cysts are also known perineural cysts, extradural spinal meningeal cysts, or meningeal diverticula of sacral nerve roots. Tarlov cysts most commonly affect the S1-S3 nerve roots and are one of the most overlooked causes of lumbosacral radiculopathy and pelvic pain.
- Treatment of neurogenic pelvic pain generally consists of starting with conservative measures, such as physical therapy, lifestyle modification, and medications with escalation to more invasive and novel treatments, such as nerve blocks, radiofrequency ablation, cryoablation, neuromodulation, and neurectomy/neurolysis if conservative treatments are ineffective.

INTRODUCTION

Chronic pelvic pain is estimated to affect 7% to 24% of the general population.[1] Neurogenic causes of pelvic pain are among the least well-described in the medical literature, and can be very difficult to diagnose and treat. Many of the conditions described in this article have been recognized only within the past 10 to 15 years, and there are very few published randomized controlled trials for this patient population. Most of what we know is in the form of sparse case reports and retrospective reviews. Neurologic pathology in the pelvic region can produce extreme pain, which greatly affects quality of life by limiting the ability to sit, void/defecate, and engage in sexual intercourse. This review provides an overview of the main causes of neurogenic pelvic pain, along with information on diagnosis and treatment options.

The authors have nothing to disclose.
Department of Physical Medicine and Rehabilitation, UT Southwestern Medical Center, 5323 Harry Hines Boulevard, Dallas, TX 75390-9055, USA
* Corresponding author.
E-mail address: kelly.scott@utsouthwestern.edu

Phys Med Rehabil Clin N Am 28 (2017) 551–569
http://dx.doi.org/10.1016/j.pmr.2017.03.007
1047-9651/17/Published by Elsevier Inc.

ANATOMY OF PELVIC NERVES

The ilioinguinal and the iliohypogastric nerves arise from the anterior rami of L1 with contributions from T12. Both nerves emerge from the lateral border of the psoas major and remain subperitoneal as they cross the quadratus lumborum. These nerves run inferiorly and anteriorly, piercing the internal oblique above the anterior superior iliac spine (ASIS) and giving motor innervation to that muscle. The iliohypogastric nerve then divides into its anterior and lateral cutaneous branches. The anterior branch of the iliohypogastric nerve provides sensory innervation to the skin at the lower abdominal area and the superior portion of the mons pubis. The lateral branch provides sensory innervation to a portion of the lateral gluteal region. The ilioinguinal nerve supplies cutaneous innervation superomedial area of the thigh, the root of the penis, and the anterior scrotum in men or the inferior mons pubis and labia majora in women.

The genitofemoral nerve arises from the L1 and L2 nerve roots and travels through the psoas major muscle at the level of L3-L4 and travels anterior to the psoas muscle in a caudal direction before branching into the genital and femoral branches. The genital branch passes through the internal inguinal ring and then takes differing paths in men and women. In men, it provides sensation to a portion of the scrotum and supplies motor fibers to the cremaster muscle. In women, it provides partial sensation to the labia. The femoral branch descends along with the external iliac artery and pierces the fascia lata entering the femoral sheath lateral to the femoral artery. It supplies sensation to the anterior portion of the upper thigh.

The pudendal nerve originates from the nerve roots of S2-S4. It passes into the gluteal region through the greater sciatic foramen alongside the sciatic nerve, courses over the sacrospinous ligament near its attachment to the ischial spine, and traverses back into the pelvic cavity via the lesser sciatic foramen. The sacrospinous ligament and sacrotuberous ligament, ventrally and dorsally, respectively, border the nerve. The pudendal nerve then passes through the Alcock canal along the medial ischial tuberosity, within the fascia of the obturator internus muscle. From inside and distal to the canal, the terminal branches of the pudendal nerve arise: the inferior rectal nerve, the perineal nerve, and the dorsal nerve of the penis/clitoris. The inferior rectal nerve provides sensory innervation to the distal aspect of the anal canal and the perianal skin and motor innervation to the external anal sphincter. The perineal nerve gives motor innervation to the superficial pelvic floor muscles and urethral sphincter and sensation to the perineum and labia. There is some evidence to suggest that the perineal nerve provides some contribution to the levator ani muscle as well.[2] The dorsal nerve provides sensory innervation to the clitoris or penis. It must be noted that after the pudendal nerve has exited the Alcock canal, many possible variations may occur.[3]

The posterior femoral cutaneous nerve arises from the S2-3 nerve roots in the sacral plexus and exits the pelvic cavity through the greater sciatic foramen just below the piriformis muscle. The inferior cluneal branches turn upward after coursing beneath the gluteus maximus and provide cutaneous innervation to the skin that covers the inferolateral portion of the muscle, as well as sending perineal branches to the ischial region and perineum.

The groin/pubic region has significant overlap of cutaneous innervation shared by the iliohypogastric, ilioinguinal, and genitofemoral nerves, while the perineal region is innervated by the pudendal, inferior cluneal, ilioinguinal, and genitofemoral nerves. This significant cutaneous sensory overlap typically renders the sensory neurologic examination of little use in the diagnosis of these neuropathies. The innervations of the pelvic lumbosacral plexus nerves are summarized in **Table 1**.

Table 1
Innervations of the pelvic lumbosacral plexus nerves

Nerve	Nerve Roots	Cutaneous Innervation	Motor Innervation
Iliohypogastric	T12-L1	• Lower abdomen • Superior mons pubis • Lateral gluteal	• Internal oblique
Ilioinguinal	T12-L1	• Superomedial thigh • Base of penis • Anterior scrotum • Labium majora • Mons pubis	• Internal oblique
Genitofemoral	L1-L2	• Superior anterior thigh • Scrotum • Labia	• Cremaster
Pudendal	S2-S4	• Distal aspect of the anal canal • Perianal • Labia majora • Clitoris • Penis	• External anal sphincter • Transverse perineal muscles • Bulbospongiosus • Ischiocavernosus • Urethral sphincter
Inferior cluneal	S2-S3	• Inferolateral gluteal • Ischial • Perineal	• None

ILIOHYPOGASTRIC, ILIOINGUINAL, AND GENITOFEMORAL NEURALGIA
Introduction

Neuralgia of the iliohypogastric, ilioinguinal, and genitofemoral nerves typically presents as pain and paresthesia in the groin or upper pubic region. Because of overlapping cutaneous sensory distributions, it can be hard to distinguish which of these nerves is the primary pain generator. Furthermore, as these nerves are located in close proximity to each other in the groin region, it is often possible to have damage to more than one nerve concurrently. The term "border nerve syndrome" is sometimes used to refer to neuralgia caused by any of these 3 nerves, either alone or in combination.

Epidemiology and Etiology

The vast majority of both iliohypogastric, ilioinguinal, and genitofemoral neuralgia cases are the result of mechanical insult to the nerve during lower abdominal surgeries. These include appendectomy, hysterectomy, inguinal hernia repair,[4] lumbar sympathetic blocks,[5] lumbar fusion using the minimally invasive lateral retroperitoneal trans-psoas approach,[6] cesarean delivery, and appendectomy.[7] Blunt abdominal trauma and visceral adhesions have also been shown to cause genitofemoral neuralgia[8] Entrapment of the nerves is commonly associated with mesh placement, particularly during inguinal hernia repair. It is hypothesized that the scar tissue formed by the mesh may cause entrapment of the nerves,[8,9] other potential causes include psoas abscess, Pott disease, and prolonged wearing of abdominally constrictive clothing.[10] Data regarding the incidence of isolated neuralgia are lacking, but several studies have examined the incidence of border nerve syndrome (including the iliohypogastric, ilioinguinal, and genitofemoral nerves). One such study demonstrated that the risk of such neuropathy attributable to gynecologic surgery was 1.8%.[11] Another estimated the risk of postoperative neuropathy after major pelvic surgery to be 1.9%, with 73.0%

of those with complete recovery.[12] Shin and Howard[13] found the incidence of ilioingui-nal and iliohypogastric neuropathic pain following closure of laparoscopic incision of the lower abdomen to be 5%. Inguinal hernioplasty with mesh has a higher rate of postoperative inguinodynia, with one study estimating incidence at 10%.[14] Genitofe-moral neuralgia has been shown to have a similar incidence in men and women, and is equally likely to occur on either the right or the left side.[8]

Patient Evaluation

Iliohypogastric, ilioinguinal, and genitofemoral neuralgia present as pain or pares-thesia in their respective cutaneous innervations: the iliohypogastric in the lower abdomen and mons pubis, ilioinguinal in the superomedial thigh, the root of the penis and the anterior scrotum in men or the inferior mons pubis and upper labia majora in women, and the genitofemoral in the inguinal region, upper anterior thigh, and scrotal/labial area.[8] Pain may be described as sharp or burning, and worse with lifting or bending. Neuralgia may refer or mimic pain to the pelvic viscera.[15,16] Weakness is not generally reported as these nerves are largely sensory.

The physical examination may reveal sensory deficits in the cutaneous distribution of the injured nerve, or hyperesthesia to pinprick testing. Patients may exhibit a flexed posture during gait to avoid stretching or tightening the abdominal muscles.[17] They may sit with one leg extended diagonally in front of their chair while leaning away from that leg to minimize compression of the injured nerve in the painful groin. Point tenderness 2 cm medial and 2 to 3 cm inferior to the ASIS may be indicative of ilioin-guinal neuralgia, but this is not diagnostic, as genitofemoral may have similar find-ings.[18] Genitofemoral neuralgia may present with point tenderness where the genital branch passes into the internal ilioinguinal ring.[7,8] Symptoms are exacerbated by walking, running, lifting, stooping, climbing stairs, and hyperextending the hip. Lying down and flexing of the hip can ameliorate the symptoms of border nerve syndrome, although most patients will have significant pain with end-range hip flexion. The anatomic location of these nerves vary enough that patients will not generally have an elicitable Tinel sign.[8]

Magnetic resonance neurography (MRN) of the lumbosacral plexus is emerging as a powerful diagnostic tool to help in the identification of iliohypogastric, ilioinguinal, and genitofemoral neuropathy.[19] Generally performed on a high-resolution, 3 T magnet, this imaging can often show nerve damage or entrapment, particularly in the situation in which these nerves are encased in scar tissue related to prior surgeries. Differential diagnostic nerve blocks are essential to tease out exactly which nerve or nerves are affected in border nerve syndrome.[20,21] These have been described using anatomic landmarks to guide injection placement, but as there is variability in the anatomic course of the nerve, ultrasound or computed tomography (CT) guidance has been found to increase the reliability and accuracy of blocking the nerve in question.[22,23] It is best to perform diagnostic blocks with a small volume of local anesthetic and without any form of sedation, so that the patient can accurately describe whether the nerve block has reduced typical symptoms immediately after the injection. If MRN has previously been performed, the optimal technique is to block the suspected nerve proximal to the location of nerve damage seen on imaging.

Electrophysiologic testing is neither specific nor sensitive enough to accurately di-agnose these neuralgias, although they may be clinically correlated to support the diagnosis.[24,25] Somatosensory evoked potential may be useful in diagnosing the lateral cutaneous branch of the iliohypogastric nerve.[26] Electromyography (EMG), however, has shown value in the evaluation of ilioinguinal neuralgia by providing pre-dictive value in assessing which patients may benefit from neurectomy or neurolysis.[27]

Treatment Options

As with any etiology of neuropathic pain, pharmacologic treatments may be beneficial, including topical anesthetics, tricyclic antidepressants, Pregabalin, Gabapentin, serotonin-norepinephrine reuptake inhibitors, selective serotonin reuptake inhibitors, nonsteroidal anti-inflammatory medications, and N-methyl-D-aspartate receptor antagonists.[20,28]

Serial therapeutic nerve blocks with local anesthetic and corticosteroid have shown to be successful in many patients.[29,30] Again, ultrasound and CT guidance techniques have been proven to be more accurate at targeting the specific nerve as opposed to using only anatomic landmarks.[20,22,31] Radiofrequency ablation has provided long-term pain relief without causing risk of neuroma formation.[20,32] One study found radiofrequency ablation to be superior to local nerve infiltrations when comparing mean visual analog scores 1 year after the procedure.[21] Another study showed that 80% of patients reported pain relief for up to 9 months after undergoing pulsed radiofrequency ablation.[33] Peripheral nerve stimulation has also been shown to provide pain reduction in 70% of patients with genitofemoral neuralgia.[34] Cryoablation (also known as cryoanalgesic ablation or cryoneurolysis) is another intervention reported to have success for painful neuropathies.[4] Cryoablation involves freezing the nerve to create axonotmesis and resultant Wallerian degeneration, preserving the epineurium and perineurium to avoid neuroma formation, with the hope that subsequent nerve regeneration will create a healthier axon.[20,29]

Surgical treatment should be reserved for symptoms not controlled by more conservative methods.[20,29] Surgical treatment should not be performed until 6 to 12 months after a surgery that resulted in ilioinguinal, iliohypogastric, or genitofemoral neuralgia, as the decrease in the inflammatory response may result in symptom cessation without intervention.[20] Extraperitoneal excision of the nerve is successful in treating cases caused by entrapment,[7] and some experts consider it the treatment of choice.[8] Minimally invasive endoscopic retroperitoneal neurectomy of the genitofemoral nerve has been described.[35] A more definitive treatment of generalized refractory inguinodynia would be a triple neurectomy, which removes the proximal branches of the ilioinguinal, genitofemoral, and iliohypogastric nerves.[36] For any treatment involving a neurectomy, research shows that it is more effective when longer segments of the nerve are removed.[14,37] Neurectomy has been shown to be effective in multiple studies, which report long-term pain relief between 62.5% and 77.0%.[38–40] However, one study showed that neurectomy was less effective in treating genitofemoral neuralgia than it was in treating ilioinguinal and iliohypogastric neuralgia.[41] Endoscopic retroperitoneal neurectomy has been shown to allow patients to be pain-free 12 months after the procedure 69.2% of the time.[35] It is likely important to implant the proximal cut end of the nerve into the muscle of the abdominal wall to avoid painful neuroma formation after neurectomy.[42] It is important to consider neuroma formation in any patient who has continued pain after neurectomy of the iliohypogastric, ilioinguinal, or genitofemoral nerves.

PUDENDAL NEURALGIA
Introduction

Pudendal neuralgia is the most common cause of chronic perineal pain.[43] Its effects often include debilitating and unrelenting pain of the perineal region aggravated by sitting and relieved by standing. Other symptoms can include urinary hesitancy, frequency, urgency, constipation, sexual dysfunction, loss of libido, altered sensation of ejaculation, and impotence.[1]

Epidemiology and Etiology

It is estimated that approximately 4% of all cases of chronic pelvic pain are caused by pudendal neuralgia.[44] Although the condition is most commonly seen in women, it is likely that it is underdiagnosed in men, as it is estimated that approximately 11% of men in the United States have experienced chronic prostatitislike pain, with 95% of those men having no evidence of bacterial infection or inflammatory cells in the prostatic fluid.[1] Pudendal neuralgia has an average age at onset of 50 to 70 years.[43]

The etiology of pudendal neuralgia can be broken down into extrinsic and intrinsic causes. Mechanical insult causes most pudendal neuralgia cases. This includes iatrogenic injury during pelvic surgery, stretching of the nerve during vaginal childbirth, compression from prolonged sitting (most commonly in cycling), and prolonged positions of stretching, which have been documented in orthopedic surgical cases involving traction.[11,45–48] Chemoradiation, tumors, and endometriosis have also been documented as causes of nerve compression.[49] The proximity of the pudendal nerve to the sacrospinous ligament can leave the pudendal nerve vulnerable to iatrogenic damage during the sacrospinous ligament fixation (SSLF) colpopexy for pelvic organ prolapse,[46,50] where a slightly misplaced suture may entrap or damage the nerve. Surgeries done for pelvic organ prolapse repair using mesh and midurethral slings (particularly with transobturator tape) also have been implicated as potential causes of pudendal neuropathy.[51,52] Anatomic variation of the falciform process of the sacrotuberous ligament may also predispose the nerve to stretching in some individuals.[53] Intrinsic causes are much less common than entrapment, but there have been documented cases caused by autoimmune or inflammatory illness.

There are thought to be 4 primary sites for entrapment of the pudendal nerve.[54] The first site is the exit of the greater sciatic notch in concert with piriformis muscle spasm. The second is at the level of the ischial spine, sacrotuberous ligament, and the lesser sciatic notch entrance. The third location is at the entrance of the Alcock canal in association with obturator internus muscle spasm. The fourth site is entrapment of the terminal branches distal to the Alcock canal. In many cases, the nerve is not truly entrapped at these sites along its winding course, but rather under traction due to biomechanical factors, such as pelvic floor muscle spasm or the presence of a pelvic obliquity. It has been hypothesized that repetitive flexion of the hip, such as in sports or strength training, may cause hypertrophy of the muscles of the pelvic floor as well as elongation and posterior remodeling of the ischial spine causing stretch of the nerve over the sacrospinous ligament.[45]

Patient Evaluation

Patients with pudendal neuralgia present with pain in the perineum, penis, scrotum, labia, or anorectal region and may be described as burning, tearing, sharp, shooting, or a foreign body sensation.[24,25,55] In most cases, symptoms are unilateral.[56] It is common for patients to develop associated pelvic floor and other myofascial dysfunctions, and so with time the pain can spread to the opposite side or begin to encompass the deep pelvis, gluteal region, groin, lower abdomen, and leg.[57] Pain may be accompanied by urinary hesitancy, frequency, urgency, constipation, sexual dysfunction, loss of libido, altered sensation of ejaculation, impotence, dyspareunia or hyperarousal.[1] Sitting is an almost universal aggravating factor. Most patients will find relief when standing or sitting on a toilet seat.[45] In most cases, patients will not complain of numbness in the perineal region (in part, due to overlapping sensory cutaneous nerve distributions, as described previously). It is uncommon for pudendal neuralgia to present with urethral incontinence unless the nerve is affected bilaterally. Anal spasm, defecatory pain, or proctalgia fugax also can be associated with pudendal neuralgia.[58]

The Nantes criteria for the diagnosis of pudendal neuralgia were developed in 2006 (**Box 1**).[59] To make the diagnosis, all 5 of the inclusion criteria must be met without exhibiting any of the exclusion criteria. The Nantes criteria have not been shown to be specific for pudendal neuralgia; however, as patients with significant pelvic floor dysfunction and pelvic floor myofascial pain will typically meet all the Nantes criteria while having no pain originating from the pudendal nerves.

Although pudendal neuralgia is a clinical diagnosis and has no specific, reliable confirmatory examination, a thorough pelvic examination focusing on pelvic floor muscles is necessary in any suspected case.[49] This includes external, transvaginal, and/or transrectal palpitation of the pelvic floor muscles to assess for overactivity and myofascial pain, as well as pelvic muscle function testing. Sensory testing of the sacral dermatomes and perineum should be done with light touch and pinprick. Patients with pudendal neuralgia typically do not have numbness, but may have hyperesthesia to pinprick sensation, particularly in the labial or posterior scrotal/perineal regions. The vaginal introitus can be gently touched with a cotton swab to determine if there is unilateral vulvodynia, which can be another sign of pudendal neuralgia. Palpation at the ischial spine internally or over the Alcock canal internally or externally may reproduce pain or cause paresthesia, known as a Tinel sign. Examination also may reveal anal deviation to the unaffected side due to ipsilateral perineal muscle atrophy.[1] Favoring of one side while sitting may also be observed.

MRN is a useful tool in the diagnosis of pudendal neuropathy, and can help with localization of the lesion along the nerve course, helping to guide decision-making for the placement of diagnostic or therapeutic injections.[60] Findings may include asymmetry of piriformis or obturator internus muscles or swelling of the neurovascular bundle in the Alcock canal or at the ischial spine. MRN is thought to be sensitive enough to rule out pudendal entrapment of the mainstem nerve and proximal terminal branches, but should be followed with confirmatory nerve block.[54]

Pudendal nerve blocks serve as an essential step in objective testing for pudendal neuralgia and are essential for diagnosis according to the Nantes criteria. Relief of the

---

Box 1
Nantes criteria for the diagnosis of pudendal neuralgia

- Pain in the area innervated by the pudendal nerve extending from the anus to clitoris
- Pain is more severe when sitting
- Pain does not awaken patients from sleep
- Pain with no objective sensory impairment
- Pain relieved by diagnostic pudendal block

Exclusion criteria

- Pain located exclusively in the coccygeal, gluteal, pubic, or hypogastric area (without pain in the area of distribution of pudendal nerve)
- Pruritus
- Exclusively paroxysmal pain
- Abnormalities on any imaging test (eg, MRI, computed tomography) that might explain the pain

pain after an accurately placed injection of local anesthetic signifies possible pudendal involvement, but does not absolutely implicate the nerve as the pain generator, because the nerve innervates the superficial pelvic floor muscles and sphincters. Therefore, a pudendal nerve block will also block pain that is generated in those structures and not within the nerve itself. A negative guided block, however, is thought to rule out pudendal neuralgia. As with the border nerves discussed previously, it is best to do the nerve blocks with a small amount of local anesthetic and with no sedation. Steroids also may be used in combination with local anesthetic for therapeutic benefit. Several approaches are available, including transperineal, transgluteal, transrectal, and transvaginal. Ultrasound guidance has been proven to increase accuracy compared with injections using palpated landmarks as guides,[22] although the efficacy depends largely on the skill level of the machine operator. CT, fluoroscopic, and MRN guidance have also been described.[60,61] Advantages of ultrasound when compared with other imaging guides is its cost-effectiveness, availability, and lack of radiation exposure, but the nerve can be very difficult to see clearly on ultrasound, as it runs on the inside of the pelvic bones for much of its course. CT-guided pudendal blocks are now recommended as the standard of care for improved accuracy and the ability to target the nerve not only at the ischial spine but through the Alcock canal.[60]

Neurophysiology tests, such as electromyography and terminal motor latency tests, have a complementary role in diagnosing pudendal neuralgia but are not specific enough to be considered confirmatory, because asymptomatic stretching of the nerve is common in multiparous women or in patients with chronic constipation, which will give a false-positive result.[62] Because these tests assess only the motor function of the nerve, they are not sensitive enough to rule out pudendal neuralgia. EMG may be useful for assessing motor function of the nerve, but is not capable of localizing the site of entrapment.[63]

Treatment Options

There are several treatment options for pudendal neuralgia. Early treatment is associated with better prognosis. Behavior modifications should be tried first, especially with etiologies like cycling or repetitive hip flexion. As with most conditions, it is recommended to begin with conservative treatment.

Physical therapy may be beneficial, as excessive spasm of the pelvic floor muscles, especially the levators and obturator internus, is common. A therapist with specialized training in pelvic rehabilitation and pudendal neuralgia is recommended. The focus of physical therapy is generally aimed at what is termed "downtraining" of the overactive pelvic floor muscles, with the goal of easing traction/compression on the irritated or damaged pudendal nerve. Stretches that may be beneficial include bringing the affected side knee to the chest in the supine position and sitting in the lotus position and bringing the head toward the ground.[1,64]

Pharmacologic agents commonly used in chronic and neuropathic pain may be beneficial. Gabapentin, Pregabalin, tricyclic antidepressants, and muscle relaxers may provide relief.[44] These medications (often compounded into suppository form or creams) also may be delivered vaginally, which for some patients provides better relief with fewer systemic side effects. Vaginal valium or baclofen suppositories are commonly used and well tolerated.

CT-guided or ultrasound-guided nerve blocks are the mainstay of pudendal neuralgia treatment. Corticosteroid (triamcinolone or methylprednisolone) mixed with bupivacaine is a common combination used for injections, although evidence for the efficacy of the addition of corticosteroid is lacking.[64] There are several described injection protocols, but most involve a series of 3 injections spread over 3 to 6 weeks.[62]

One study of CT-guided perineural injections for pudendal neuralgia reported 78% of patients had significant pain relief 24 hours after the injection.[65] The same study revealed pain relief in 89% of subjects at 12-month follow-up and a 20% improvement in quality of life index. Another study showed that pudendal block under MR neurography guidance resulted in 87% good to excellent outcomes.[54] Studies of nerve blocks with botulinum toxin and/or hyaluronidase have shown to be effective[22,54]; however, bilateral treatment may cause urinary and fecal incontinence.

Neuromodulation is based on gate control theory, which hypothesizes that if large nerve fibers are being stimulated, small fibers carrying pain signals will be unable to transmit their signal. Case studies have shown neuromodulation of the sacral nerve roots and conus medullaris to be effective in controlling pain associated with pudendal neuralgia.[66,67] In one prospective study of 27 cases, 74% had significant improvement of pain.[68] The pudendal nerve itself also can be directly stimulated.[69] Although promising, more research is needed to confirm sacral or pudendal neuromodulation efficacy.

Cryoablation and pulsed radiofrequency ablation are other options to consider. One study of CT-guided cryoablation of 11 patients showed decrease of pain on a 10-point scale from an average of 7.6 pre-procedure to 3.1 at 6 months posttreatment.[70] A recent study of 26 patients undergoing pulsed radiofrequency ablation of the pudendal nerve under CT guidance demonstrated a decrease of pain on a 10-point scale from an average of 9 pre-procedure to 1.9 at 1 year posttreatment.[71] Again, more research is needed to confirm the efficacy of both cryoablation and pulsed radiofrequency ablation.

If the conservative measures fail to improve symptoms, surgery is an option for some patients. Surgical approaches include transperineal, transgluteal, transischiorectal and laparoscopic.[54] Decompressive surgery has been reported successful in one-third to two-thirds of patients.[56,72,73] Patients post-SSLF colpopexy with confirmed entrapment have shown improvement or resolution of symptoms with removal of the suture, even up to 2 years after the initial surgery.[42,46]

CLUNEALGIA
Introduction

Clunealgia refers to pain and paresthesia along the nerve distribution of the inferior cluneal nerves.[74] This is the result of pathology to these terminal branches of the posterior femoral cutaneous nerve (PFCN). The 2 most common anatomic regions in which pathology occurs are at the level of the sacrotuberous ligament and the passage under the ischium.

Epidemiology and Etiology

Isolated clunealgia is thought to be rare; pudendal neuralgia is likely much more common. Most of the published literature is limited to case studies and a true epidemiology is not available. Known etiologies include venous malformation surrounding the nerve, iatrogenic from hematoma evacuation from a coronary angiography in the femoral artery, and gluteal intramuscular injections or idiopathic.[75–77]

Patient Evaluation

Clunealgia usually presents with pain and paresthesia along the nerve distribution, including lower gluteal area, inferior perineum, and ischium. Pain also may radiate to the ipsilateral hip. Because of the pure cutaneous sensory function of the nerve, patients typically do not present with weakness or bladder, bowel, or sexual dysfunction.

The pain and paresthesia location is often very similar to that of pudendal neuralgia and may be difficult to distinguish. Physical examination findings rarely include pain and rarely sensory abnormalities in the distribution of the nerve.

Clunealgia is largely diagnosed based on high clinical index of suspicion. As it is difficult to distinguish clinically from pudendal pathology, misdiagnosis is common.[78] As with the nerves discussed previously, the best diagnostic approach is to do a CT-guided PFCN block using local anesthetic and no sedation.[79] MRN can be used to visualize abnormalities within the PFCN proper, but the inferior cluneal branches are typically too small to be seen reliably.[80] Nerve conduction studies have shown benefit in confirming the diagnosis of PFCN neuropathy proper, but the inferior cluneal branches are not isolatable.[76,77,81] Therefore, if there is isolated damage to the inferior cluneal branches in the lower gluteal, ischial, or perineal regions, the PFCN nerve conduction studies will still be normal. High-resolution ultrasound has also emerged as a tool for diagnosing PFCN neuropathy.[78] Both nerve conduction studies and ultrasound reliability are highly operator dependent.

Treatment

Neuropathic medications and therapeutic nerve blocks are the most common treatment of clunealgia. MRI guidance has been shown to be effective in targeting the PFCN[82]; however, high cost may limit the feasibility of this guidance technique. CT guidance has been shown to be a cheaper and more convenient method with similar efficacy to MRI guidance.[79] Surgical neurectomy of the inferior cluneal branches or PFCN proper may also be considered as a last resort.[74]

TARLOV CYSTS
Introduction

Tarlov cysts are also known as perineural cysts, extradural spinal meningeal cysts, or meningeal diverticula of sacral nerve roots. They are cysts filled with cerebrospinal fluid (CSF) and are often located near the dorsal root ganglion of the sacral nerves, between the perineurium and the endoneurium.[83] Although most common in the sacral area, they are also rarely found throughout the spine. Tarlov cysts most commonly affect the S1-S3 nerve roots and are one of the most overlooked causes of lumbosacral radiculopathy and pelvic pain.[84–87]

Epidemiology and Etiology

The prevalence of Tarlov cysts has been estimated to be between 1% and 5% of the population.[84,85,88,89] Twenty percent to 26% of Tarlov cysts are thought to be symptomatic, accounting for about 1% of the population, so it is important to not discount them as purely incidental when patients have corresponding symptoms.[84,86,88] Tarlov cysts are significantly more common in women, and women are also more likely to be symptomatic.[83,89]

The origin of Tarlov cysts is unclear and controversial, but there is causal evidence supporting traumatic hemorrhage, pseudomeningoceles, hydrostatic CSF pressures, congenital diverticula from persistent embryonic fissures, inflammation in the subarachnoid space, inflammation within the nerve root cysts leading to inoculation of fluid, arachnoidal proliferation along and around the exiting sacral nerve root, and from hemosiderin deposits breaking down venous drainage in the epineurium and perineurium after trauma.[86,87,90]

Tarlov cysts can increase in size but the pathogenesis is unclear. One theory is the ball-valve mechanism wherein CSF enters the cyst during systole, but is unable to leave in the same amount during diastole.[91] Another potential etiology is that the increased hydrostatic pressure of CSF forces CSF into the normally obliterated perineural space. As the cysts grow, they stretch the nerves and ganglia within them, resulting in symptoms.[92] Tarlov cysts can erode the sacrum and lead to formation of a meningocele.[93,94] Due to the growth of Tarlov cysts, there can be sacral bone remodeling and dilatation of the intervertebral foramina.[95]

Patient Evaluation

The clinical presentation of a patient with Tarlov cysts varies depending on cyst size and location. They are often found incidentally on radiological imaging and are frequently small and asymptomatic, but have been reported to be as large as 8 × 9 × 11 cm.[96,97] Tarlov cysts are generally considered large if they are greater than or equal to 1.5 cm in diameter.[98] As with any cause of spinal nerve root pathology or compression, only those patients with symptoms from their Tarlov cysts require treatment. As they are located near the dorsal root, sensory symptoms are more likely to occur than motor symptoms.[99] Symptoms may include low back or sacral pain, buttock pain, coccydynia, radicular leg pain and paresthesia, and pain throughout the pelvis, genitals, and perineum.[83,100] Dyspareunia and bladder and bowel dysfunction also can occur.[101] Tarlov cysts also can cause cauda equina syndrome and can present as such.[86] Tarlov cysts have been shown to cause persistent genital arousal disorder.[102] Tarlov cysts can mimic disc herniation symptomatology.[103] Patients may specifically complain of pain while sitting, standing, walking, or bending, and relief is often only achieved by lying on their side.[104] There may be a history of infertility and retrograde ejaculation if the Tarlov cysts affect the sacral and cauda equina areas.[105]

The physical examination for a patient with suspected sacral radiculopathy related to Tarlov cysts should include a thorough spine examination including detailed neurologic testing of the lower extremities and pelvis. Particular attention should be paid to sensory testing with light touch and pinprick in the sacral dermatomes and genital/perineal regions. Anal sphincter tone should be assessed, as should pelvic floor muscle function and tonicity. Sacral dermatome numbness and decreased anal sphincter tone are signs of significant sacral nerve root compromise.

Imaging is the primary form of diagnosis, as there is no symptomatology unique to Tarlov cysts alone. Tarlov cysts can be found on MRI and it is recommended to perform with and without contrast.[106] MRN of the lumbosacral plexus can help to differentiate whether the sacral roots are neuropathic in relation to the cysts or whether they remain largely unaffected.[107] Tarlov cysts can be confused with adnexal cysts on ultrasound imaging.[108] Data are equivocal on being able to detect nerves affected by Tarlov cysts with electromyography, which makes sense given that Tarlov cysts typically affect the sensory more than motor fibers of the sacral nerve roots, which are not easily tested via electrodiagnostics.[83] Tarlov cysts do not usually communicate freely with the subarachnoid space, so they can fill with a delay on myelography.[87]

Treatment

It is important to remember that asymptomatic Tarlov cysts do not need treatment.[92] Oral steroids have been shown to be helpful in treatment of Tarlov cysts.[101,109] Nonsteroidal anti-inflammatory drugs and neuropathic pain medications were shown to give mild improvement in pain symptoms.[83] Pelvic physical therapy may play a role in helping to calm down any associated pelvic floor myofascial pain or dysfunction.

Epidural steroid injections have been shown to be helpful in the treatment of sacral radiculopathy associated with Tarlov cysts,[101,109] and have been shown specifically to help treat pelvic pain caused by Tarlov cysts.[110] Some experts believe that high volumes of triamcinolone, such as 8 mL instead of the usual 3 mL is more effective in treatment to reduce inflammation.[111] One case report found that electroacupuncture relieved symptoms by decreasing inflammation within the cyst.[112] Spinal cord stimulation has been shown to be effective in treating neuropathic pain originating in the spinal cord, and could be considered in cases of sacral radiculopathy associated with Tarlov cysts, just as it is used for patients with lumbar radicular pain.[113] Minimally invasive fluoroscopy-guided percutaneous gel injection therapy has been shown to be effective in treating symptomatic Tarlov cysts that cause pain.[114] Tarlov cysts can also be successfully treated with aneurysm clips or percutaneous drainage.[115,116] Percutaneous drainage of the cyst has been shown at times to offer only temporary relief.[109] CT-fluoroscopic–guided needle aspiration and fibrin injection has shown excellent results in reducing symptoms, although this carries a potential risk of aseptic meningitis.[92,117]

Surgical treatment has been reported effective if performed on symptomatic Tarlov cysts larger than 1.5 cm in diameter.[118,119] It may be wise not to consider surgery unless the patient has at least a temporary response to epidural steroid injections, implicating the Tarlov cyst as the likely pain generator.

Complications of interventional or surgical treatment for Tarlov cysts may be quite significant. Ruptured Tarlov cysts have been shown to cause cerebral fat embolisms.[120] Positional headaches, CSF leaks, and aseptic meningitis have been reported with various interventions, including percutaneous aspiration.[117,121,122] Surgical decompression of Tarlov cysts can be complicated by the development of a postoperative pseudomeningocele.[109] Surgical treatment also may carry the risk of further damage to the sacral nerve roots, with resultant lower motor neuron bladder or bowel dysfunction.

CAUDA EQUINA SYNDROME
Introduction

The adult spinal cord terminates at the conus medullaris at the level of the L1-L2 vertebrae.[123] Nerves continue to travel individually through the lumbar spinal canal as the cauda equina. Compression on the nerve roots of the cauda equina causes cauda equina syndrome, characterized by a triad of saddle anesthesia, bowel or bladder dysfunction, and lower extremity weakness.[124] Additional symptoms are sciatica and low back or pelvic pain.[107,123,125] Presentation can be acute or chronic. If the presentation is acute, action needs to be taken quickly to avoid permanent loss of neural function.

Epidemiology and Etiology

Midline disc herniation is the most common cause of cauda equina syndrome,[124] and L4-L5 is the most common site.[123] Other causes include spinal metastases, spinal hematoma or seroma, epidural abscess, traumatic compression, or acute transverse myelitis.[124] Scar tissue can accumulate around the cauda equina nerve roots after lumbar surgery complicated by a dural tear, with subsequent arachnoiditis formation.[107] Bilateral[116] or unilateral[109] Tarlov cysts also can cause cauda equina syndrome.

The incidence rate of cauda equina syndrome in the general population is 3.4 per million. The prevalence is 8.9 per 100,000.[126] Among patients with low back pain, the prevalence is much higher at 4 in 10,000.[124]

Patient Evaluation

Similar to patients with sacral radiculopathy related to Tarlov cysts, patients with cauda equina syndrome can present with lower extremity radicular symptoms (including weakness, numbness, and pain), as well as pelvic pain, saddle or perineal anesthesia, and bladder, bowel, and sexual dysfunction. The physical examination for suspected cauda equina syndrome should be the same as is detailed previously in the Tarlov cyst section of this review, with particular attention paid to lower extremity strength testing, sensory deficits in the sacral dermatomes, and anal sphincter tone.

MRI of the lumbar spine is the mainstay for diagnosis, and should be ordered emergently for patients with an acute presentation. MRN of the lumbosacral plexus (preferably done with and without contrast) has been shown to improve likelihood of diagnosis of cauda equina nerve root pathology over conventional MRI, particularly in cases in which the nerve roots are entrapped in scar tissue without large mass lesion, like an epidural hematoma or large herniated disk.[107]

Treatment

For an acute presentation, high dose intravenous steroids are recommended, followed quickly by surgical consultation.[124] Surgical decompression is the definitive treatment, and should be sought without delay. Laminectomy with gentle traction of the cauda equina and discectomy is the treatment of choice.[123]

Outcome is determined by the patient's state of functionality at presentation, with earlier detection and treatment being important. Patients who can ambulate with assistance at presentation have a 50% chance of walking again, and patients with urinary retention have a 79% chance of needing a urinary catheter afterward.[123]

Unfortunately, those patients with chronic cauda equina syndrome generally have only symptomatic treatment options, as the nerve damage is typically past the point of reversibility. Neuropathic and opioid pain medications are useful for the severe pelvic and lower extremity pain that many of these patients can develop. Some patients will require a lower motor neuron bladder and bowel program, including bladder catheterization and manual removal of stool. General or pelvic floor physical therapy may play a limited role in improving functionality and ability to compensate for neurologic deficits, as can assistive devices to aid with ambulation. Spinal cord stimulators can be considered for pain relief.[113]

SUMMARY

Pelvic neuralgias frequently cause severe pain and may be accompanied by bladder, bowel, or sexual dysfunctions that can significantly impact quality of life. In general, these neuropathies are difficult to treat and most patients deal with symptoms chronically. As with all painful conditions that affect quality of life, it is important to remember the psychological well-being of patients with pelvic neuropathies, and referrals to counseling and support groups (which are most easily found online) are usually of utmost importance. Treatment strategies are evolving: many novel procedures and approaches are being developed, but study into this field is truly just beginning and more research is sorely needed.

REFERENCES

1. Possover M, Forman A. Voiding dysfunction associated with pudendal nerve entrapment. Curr Bladder Dysfunct Rep 2012;7(4):281–5.
2. Stein TA, DeLancey JO. Structure of the perineal membrane in females: gross and microscopic anatomy. Obstet Gynecol 2008;111(3):686–93.
3. Schraffordt SE, Tjandra JJ, Eizenberg N, et al. Anatomy of the pudendal nerve and its terminal branches: a cadaver study. ANZ J Surg 2004;74(1–2):23–6.

4. Fanelli RD, DiSiena MR, Lui FY, et al. Cryoanalgesic ablation for the treatment of chronic postherniorrhaphy neuropathic pain. Surg Endosc 2003;17(2):196–200.

5. Dirim A, Kumsar S. Iatrogenic ureteral injury due to lumbar sympathetic block. Scand J Urol Nephrol 2008;42(4):395–6.

6. Tender GC, Serban D. Genitofemoral nerve protection during the lateral retroperitoneal transpsoas approach. Neurosurgery 2013;73(2 Suppl Operative): ons192–6 [discussion: ons196–7].

7. Harms BA, DeHaas DR Jr, Starling JR. Diagnosis and management of genitofemoral neuralgia. Arch Surg 1984;119(3):339–41.

8. Murovic JA, Kim DH, Tiel RL, et al. Surgical management of 10 genitofemoral neuralgias at the Louisiana State University Health Sciences Center. Neurosurgery 2005;56(2):298–303 [discussion: 298–303].

9. Demirer S, Kepenekci I, Evirgen O, et al. The effect of polypropylene mesh on ilioinguinal nerve in open mesh repair of groin hernia. J Surg Res 2006; 131(2):175–81.

10. Rauchwerger J, Giordano J, Rozen D, et al. On the therapeutic viability of peripheral nerve stimulation for ilioinguinal neuralgia: putative mechanisms and possible utility. Pain Pract 2008;8(2):138–43.

11. Bohrer JC, Walters MD, Park A, et al. Pelvic nerve injury following gynecologic surgery: a prospective cohort study. Am J Obstet Gynecol 2009;201(5): 531.e1-7.

12. Cardosi RJ, Cox CS, Hoffman MS. Postoperative neuropathies after major pelvic surgery. Obstet Gynecol 2002;100(2):240–4.

13. Shin JH, Howard FM. Abdominal wall nerve injury during laparoscopic gynecologic surgery: incidence, risk factors, and treatment outcomes. J Minim Invasive Gynecol 2012;19(4):448–53.

14. Zannoni M, Luzietti E, Viani L, et al. Wide resection of inguinal nerves versus simple section to prevent postoperative pain after prosthetic inguinal hernioplasty: our experience. World J Surg 2014;38(5):1037–43.

15. Choi PD, Nath R, Mackinnon SE. Iatrogenic injury to the ilioinguinal and iliohypogastric nerves in the groin: a case report, diagnosis, and management. Ann Plast Surg 1996;37(1):60–5.

16. Balasubramanian S, Morley-Forster P. Chronic pelvic pain due to peripheral neuropathy: a case report. J Obstet Gynaecol Can 2006;28(7):603–7 [Erratum appears in J Obstet Gynaecol Can. 2006;28(10):862].

17. Kopell HP, Thompson WA, Postel AH. Entrapment neuropathy of the ilioinguinal nerve. N Engl J Med 1962;266:16–9.

18. ter Meulen BC, Peters EW, Wijsmuller A, et al. Acute scrotal pain from idiopathic ilioinguinal neuropathy: diagnosis and treatment with EMG-guided nerve block. Clin Neurol Neurosurg 2007;109(6):535–7.

19. Chhabra A, Rozen S, Scott K. Three-dimensional MR neurography of the lumbosacral plexus. Semin Musculoskelet Radiol 2015;19(2):149–59.

20. Cesmebasi A, Yadav A, Gielecki J, et al. Genitofemoral neuralgia: a review. Clin Anat 2015;28(1):128–35.

21. Kastler A, Aubry S, Piccand V, et al. Radiofrequency neurolysis versus local nerve infiltration in 42 patients with refractory chronic inguinal neuralgia. Pain Physician 2012;15(3):237–44.

22. Peng PW, Tumber PS. Ultrasound-guided interventional procedures for patients with chronic pelvic pain—a description of techniques and review of literature. Pain Physician 2008;11(2):215–24.

23. Wadhwa V, Scott KM, Rozen S, et al. CT-guided perineural injections for chronic pelvic pain. Radiographics 2016;36(5):1408–25.

24. Labat JJ, Delavierre D, Sibert L, et al. Electrophysiological studies of chronic pelvic and perineal pain. Prog Urol 2010;20(12):905–10 [in French].

25. Rabie M, Drory VE. A test for the evaluation of the lateral cutaneous branch of the iliohypogastric nerve using somatosensory evoked potentials. J Neurol Sci 2005;238(1–2):59–63.

26. Dias RJ, Souza L, Morais WF, et al. SEP-diagnosed neuropathy of the lateral cutaneous branch of the iliohypogastric nerve: case report. Arq Neuropsiquiatr 2004;62(3B):895–8.

27. Viswanathan A, Kim DH, Reid N, et al. Surgical management of the pelvic plexus and lower abdominal nerves. Neurosurgery 2009;65(4 Suppl):A44–51.

28. Benito-Leon J, Picardo A, Garrido A, et al. Gabapentin therapy for genitofemoral and ilioinguinal neuralgia. J Neurol 2001;248(10):907–8.

29. Acar F, Ozdemir M, Bayrakli F, et al. Management of medically intractable genitofemoral and ilioingunal neuralgia. Turk Neurosurg 2013;23(6):753–7.

30. Suresh S, Patel A, Porfyris S, et al. Ultrasound-guided serial ilioinguinal nerve blocks for management of chronic groin pain secondary to ilioinguinal neuralgia in adolescents. Paediatr Anaesth 2008;18(8):775–8.

31. Campos NA, Chiles JH, Plunkett AR. Ultrasound-guided cryoablation of genitofemoral nerve for chronic inguinal pain. Pain Physician 2009;12(6):997–1000.

32. Mitra R, Zeighami A, Mackey S. Pulsed radiofrequency for the treatment of chronic ilioinguinal neuropathy. Hernia 2007;11(4):369–71.

33. Rozen D, Ahn J. Pulsed radiofrequency for the treatment of ilioinguinal neuralgia after inguinal herniorrhaphy. Mt Sinai J Med 2006;73(4):716–8.

34. Walter J, Reichart R, Vonderlind C, et al. Neuralgia of the genitofemoral nerve after hernioplasty. Therapy by peripheral nerve stimulation. Chirurg 2009; 80(8):741–4 [in German].

35. Giger U, Wente MN, Buchler MW, et al. Endoscopic retroperitoneal neurectomy for chronic pain after groin surgery. Br J Surg 2009;96(9):1076–81.

36. Chen DC, Hiatt JR, Amid PK. Operative management of refractory neuropathic inguinodynia by a laparoscopic retroperitoneal approach. JAMA Surg 2013; 148(10):962–7.

37. Zannoni M, Nisi P, Iaria M, et al. Wide nervous section to prevent post-operative inguinodynia after prosthetic hernia repair: a single center experience. Hernia 2015;19(4):565–70.

38. Kennedy EM, Harms BA, Starling JR. Absence of maladaptive neuronal plasticity after genitofemoral-ilioinguinal neurectomy. Surgery 1994;116(4):665–70 [discussion: 670–1].

39. Starling J, Harms B. Diagnosis and treatment of genitofemoral and ilioinguinal neuralgia. World J Surg 1989;13(5):586–91.

40. Starling JR, Harms BA, Schroeder ME, et al. Diagnosis and treatment of genitofemoral and ilioinguinal entrapment neuralgia. Surgery 1987;102(4):581–6.

41. Lee CH, Dellon AL. Surgical management of groin pain of neural origin. J Am Coll Surg 2000;191(2):137–42.

42. Dellon AL, Mackinnon SE. Treatment of the painful neuroma by neuroma resection and muscle implantation. Plast Reconstr Surg 1986;77(3):427–38.

43. Labat JJ, Robert R, Delavierre D, et al. Symptomatic approach to chronic neuropathic somatic pelvic and perineal pain. Prog Urol 2010;20(12):973–81 [in French].

44. Pereira A, Perez-Medina T, Rodriguez-Tapia A, et al. Chronic perineal pain: analyses of prognostic factors in pudendal neuralgia. Clin J Pain 2014;30(7): 577–82.

45. Antolak SJ Jr, Hough DM, Pawlina W, et al. Anatomical basis of chronic pelvic pain syndrome: the ischial spine and pudendal nerve entrapment. Med Hypotheses 2002;59(3):349–53.

46. Alevizon SJ, Finan MA. Sacrospinous colpopexy: management of postoperative pudendal nerve entrapment. Obstet Gynecol 1996;88(4 Pt 2):713–5.

47. Pailhe R, Chiron P, Reina N, et al. Pudendal nerve neuralgia after hip arthroscopy: retrospective study and literature review. Orthop Traumatol Surg Res 2013;99(7):785–90.

48. Leibovitch I, Mor Y. The vicious cycling: bicycling related urogenital disorders. Eur Urol 2005;47(3):277–86 [discussion: 286–7].

49. Elahi F, Callahan D, Greenlee J, et al. Pudendal entrapment neuropathy: a rare complication of pelvic radiation therapy. Pain Physician 2013;16(6):E793–7.

50. Bohrer JC, Chen CC, Walters MD. Pudendal neuropathy involving the perforating cutaneous nerve after cystocele repair with graft. Obstet Gynecol 2008; 112(2 Pt 2):496–8.

51. Marcus-Braun N, Bourret A, von Theobald P. Persistent pelvic pain following transvaginal mesh surgery: a cause for mesh removal. Eur J Obstet Gynecol Reprod Biol 2012;162(2):224–8.

52. Paulson JD, Baker J. De novo pudendal neuropathy after TOT-O surgery for stress urinary incontinence. JSLS 2011;15(3):326–30.

53. Loukas M, Louis RG Jr, Hallner B, et al. Anatomical and surgical considerations of the sacrotuberous ligament and its relevance in pudendal nerve entrapment syndrome. Surg Radiol Anat 2006;28(2):163–9.

54. Filler AG. Diagnosis and treatment of pudendal nerve entrapment syndrome subtypes: imaging, injections, and minimal access surgery. Neurosurg 2009; 26(2):E9.

55. Calabro RS, Gervasi G, Marino S, et al. Misdiagnosed chronic pelvic pain: pudendal neuralgia responding to a novel use of palmitoylethanolamide. Pain Med 2010;11(5):781–4.

56. Benson JT, Griffis K. Pudendal neuralgia, a severe pain syndrome. Am J Obstet Gynecol 2005;192(5):1663–8.

57. Stav K, Dwyer PL, Roberts L. Pudendal neuralgia. Fact or fiction? Obstet Gynecol Surv 2009;64(3):190–9.

58. Damphousse M, Jousse M, Verollet D, et al. Evidence of pudendal neuropathy in proctalgia fugax: perineal neurophysiological assessment in 55 patients. Prog Urol 2012;22(4):220–4 [in French].

59. Labat J, Riant T, Robert R, et al. Diagnostic criteria for pudendal neuralgia by pudendal nerve entrapment (Nantes criteria). Neurourol Urodyn 2008;27(4): 306–10.

60. Wadhwa V, Hamid AS, Kumar Y, et al. Pudendal nerve and branch neuropathy: magnetic resonance neurography evaluation. Acta Radiologica 2016. [Epub ahead of print].

61. Schelhorn J, Habenicht U, Malessa R, et al. Magnetic resonance imaging-guided perineural therapy as a treatment option in young adults with pudendal nerve entrapment syndrome. Clin Neuroradiol 2013;23(2):161–3.

62. Khoder W, Hale D. Pudendal neuralgia. Obstet Gynecol Clin North Am 2014; 41(3):443–52.

63. Lefaucheur JP, Labat JJ, Amarenco G, et al. What is the place of electroneuro-myographic studies in the diagnosis and management of pudendal neuralgia related to entrapment syndrome? Neurophysiol Clin 2007;37(4):223–8.
64. Labat JJ, Riant T, Lassaux A, et al. Adding corticosteroids to the pudendal nerve block for pudendal neuralgia: a randomised, double-blind, controlled trial. BJOG 2017;124(2):251–60.
65. Fanucci E, Manenti G, Ursone A, et al. Role of interventional radiology in pudendal neuralgia: a description of techniques and review of the literature. Radiol Med 2009;114(3):425–36.
66. Valovska A, Peccora CD, Philip CN, et al. Sacral neuromodulation as a treatment for pudendal neuralgia. Pain Physician 2014;17(5):E645–50.
67. Rigoard P, Delmotte A, Moles A, et al. Successful treatment of pudendal neuralgia with tricolumn spinal cord stimulation: case report. Neurosurgery 2012; 71(3):E757–63.
68. Buffenoir K, Rioult B, Hamel O, et al. Spinal cord stimulation of the conus medullaris for refractory pudendal neuralgia: a prospective study of 27 consecutive cases. Neurourol Urodyn 2015;34(2):177–82.
69. Peters KM, Killinger KA, Boguslawski BM, et al. Chronic pudendal neuromodulation: expanding available treatment options for refractory urologic symptoms. Neurourol Urodyn 2010;29(7):1267–71.
70. Prologo JD, Lin RC, Williams R, et al. Percutaneous CT-guided cryoablation for the treatment of refractory pudendal neuralgia. Skeletal Radiol 2015;44(5): 709–14.
71. Masala S, Calabria E, Cuzzolino A, et al. CT-guided percutaneous pulse-dose radiofrequency for pudendal neuralgia. Cardiovasc Intervent Radiol 2014; 37(2):476–81.
72. Mauillon J, Thoumas D, Leroi A, et al. Results of pudendal nerve neurolysis-transposition in twelve patients suffering from pudendal neuralgia. Dis Colon Rectum 1999;42(2):186–92.
73. Robert R, Labat JJ, Riant T, et al. Neurosurgical treatment of perineal neuralgias. Adv Tech Stand Neurosurg 2007;32:41–59.
74. Darnis B, Robert R, Labat JJ, et al. Perineal pain and inferior cluneal nerves: anatomy and surgery. Surg Radiol Anat 2008;30(3):177–83.
75. Chutkow JG. Posterior femoral cutaneous neuralgia. Muscle Nerve 1988;11(11): 1146–8.
76. Gomceli YB, Kapukiran A, Kutlu G, et al. A case report of an uncommon neuropathy: posterior femoral cutaneous neuropathy. Acta Neurol Belg 2005;105(1): 43–5.
77. Kim JE, Kang JH, Choi JC, et al. Isolated posterior femoral cutaneous neuropathy following intragluteal injection. Muscle Nerve 2009;40(5):864–6.
78. Meng S, Lieba-Samal D, Reissig LF, et al. High-resolution ultrasound of the posterior femoral cutaneous nerve: visualization and initial experience with patients. Skeletal Radiol 2015;44(10):1421–6.
79. Kasper JM, Wadhwa V, Scott KM, et al. Clunealgia: CT-guided therapeutic posterior femoral cutaneous nerve block. Clin Imaging 2015;38(4):540–2.
80. Weissman E, Boothe E, Wadhwa V, et al. Magnetic resonance neurography of the pelvic nerves. Seminars in Ultrasound, CT, and MRI, in press.
81. Tong HC, Haig A. Posterior femoral cutaneous nerve mononeuropathy: a case report. Arch Phys Med Rehabil 2000;81(8):1117–8.
82. Fritz J, Bizzell C, Kathuria S, et al. High-resolution magnetic resonance-guided posterior femoral cutaneous nerve blocks. Skeletal Radiol 2013;42(4):579–86.

83. Marino D, Carluccio MA, Di Donato I, et al. Tarlov cysts: clinical evaluation of an Italian cohort of patients. Neurol Sci 2013;34(9):1679–82.

84. McEvoy SD, DiLuna ML, Baird AH, et al. Symptomatic thoracic Tarlov perineural cyst. Pediatr Neurosurg 2009;45(4):321–3.

85. Kim K, Chun SW, Chung SG. A case of symptomatic cervical perineural (Tarlov) cyst: clinical manifestation and management. Skeletal Radiol 2012;41(1): 97–101.

86. Cattaneo L, Pavesi G, Mancia D. Sural nerve abnormalities in sacral perineural (Tarlov) cysts. J Neurol 2001;248(7):623–4.

87. Baek WS, Rezania K. Tarlov cysts masquerading as peripheral neuropathy. Arch Neurol 2006;63(12):1804–5.

88. Badshah A, Hussain N, Janjua M. Bilateral Tarlov cysts: a rare cause of peripheral neuropathy. South Med J 2009;102(9):986–7.

89. Burdan F, Mocarska A, Janczarek M, et al. Incidence of spinal perineurial (Tarlov) cysts among East-European patients. PLoS One 2013;8(8):e71514.

90. Guo D, Shu K, Chen R, et al. Microsurgical treatment of symptomatic sacral perineurial cysts. Neurosurgery 2007;60(6):1059–65 [discussion: 1065–6].

91. Zubizarreta IK, Menoyo JL, Ojeda JR, et al. Cerebral fat embolisms secondary to rupture of a Tarlov cyst. J Neuroimaging 2014;24(4):432–3.

92. Acosta FL Jr, Quinones-Hinojosa A, Schmidt MH, et al. Diagnosis and management of sacral Tarlov cysts. Case report and review of the literature. Neurosurg Focus 2003;15(2):E15.

93. Ostojic P. Sacral perineural cyst mimicking inflammatory low back pain. Z Rheumatol 2015;74(1):75–7.

94. Hefti M, Landolt H. Presacral mass consisting of a meningocele and a Tarlov cyst: successful surgical treatment based on pathogenic hypothesis. Acta Neurochir (Wien) 2006;148(4):479–83.

95. Manara R, Severino M, Mandari R, et al. Chronic cystic lesion of the sacrum: characterisation with diffusion-weighted MR imaging. Radiol Med 2008;113(5): 739–46.

96. Ishii K, Yuzurihara M, Asamoto S, et al. A huge presacral Tarlov cyst. Case report. J Neurosurg Spine 2007;7(2):259–63.

97. Langdown AJ, Grundy JR, Birch NC. The clinical relevance of Tarlov cysts. J Spinal Disord Tech 2005;18(1):29–33.

98. Sajko T, Kovac D, Kudelic N, et al. Symptomatic sacral perineurial (Tarlov) cysts. Coll Antropol 2009;33(4):1401–3.

99. Hwang DS, Kang C, Lee JB, et al. Arthroscopic treatment of piriformis syndrome by perineural cyst on the sciatic nerve: a case report. Knee Surg Sports Traumatol Arthrosc 2010;18(5):681–4.

100. Fernandes C, Pinho R, Veloso R, et al. Tarlov cysts: an unusual case of perianal pain. Tech Coloproctol 2012;16(4):319–20.

101. Cantore G, Bistazzoni S, Esposito V, et al. Sacral Tarlov cyst: surgical treatment by clipping. World Neurosurg 2013;79(2):381–9.

102. Komisaruk BR, Lee HJ. Prevalence of sacral spinal (Tarlov) cysts in persistent genital arousal disorder. J Sex Med 2012;9(8):2047–56.

103. Gunduz OH, Sencan S, Kokar S. A rare cause of lumbar radiculopathy: perineural cyst. Pain Med 2015;16(1):199–200.

104. Peart O. A real pain in the back. Radiol Technol 2008;80(2):183.

105. Singh PK, Singh VK, Azam A, et al. Tarlov cyst and infertility. J Spinal Cord Med 2009;32(2):191–7.

106. Chaiyabud P, Suwanpratheep K. Symptomatic Tarlov cyst: report and review. J Med Assoc Thai 2006;89(7):1047–50.

107. Petrasic JR, Chhabra A, Scott K. Impact of magnetic resonance in patients with chronic cauda equina syndrome presenting as chronic pelvic pain and dysfunction. AJNR Am J Neuroradiol 2017;38(2):418–22.

108. Hirst JE, Torode H, Sears W, et al. Beware the Tarlov cyst. J Minim Invasive Gynecol 2009;16(1):78–80.

109. Mitra R, Kirpalani D, Wedemeyer M. Conservative management of perineural cysts. Spine (Phila Pa 1976) 2008;33(16):E565–8.

110. Freidenstein J, Aldrete JA, Ness T. Minimally invasive interventional therapy for Tarlov cysts causing symptoms of interstitial cystitis. Pain Physician 2012;15(2): 141–6.

111. Hur W, Choi SS, Lee JJ. Caudal epidural injections for the treatment of Tarlov cysts: suggestions for the better results. Pain Physician 2012;15(3):E351–3 [author reply: E353].

112. Chia KL. Symptomatic Tarlov cyst and electroacupuncture: more studies required. J Integr Med 2015;13(1):58–60.

113. Hiers RH, Long D, North RB, et al. Hiding in plain sight: a case of Tarlov perineural cysts. J Pain 2010;11(9):833–7.

114. Jiang W, Qiu Q, Hao J, et al. Percutaneous fibrin gel injection under C-arm fluoroscopy guidance: a new minimally invasive choice for symptomatic sacral perineural cysts. PLoS One 2015;10(2):e0118254.

115. Wang B, Moon SJ, Olivero WC, et al. Pelvic pain from a giant presacral Tarlov cyst successfully obliterated using aneurysm clips in a patient with Marfan syndrome. J Neurosurg Spine 2014;21(5):833–6.

116. Baker JF, Fitzgerald CW, O'Neill SC, et al. Cauda equina syndrome secondary to bilateral sacral Tarlov cysts. Spine J 2014;14(6):1065–6.

117. Murphy KJ, Nussbaum DA, Schnupp S, et al. Tarlov cysts: an overlooked clinical problem. Semin Musculoskelet Radiol 2011;15(2):163–7.

118. Tanaka M, Nakahara S, Ito Y, et al. Surgical results of sacral perineural (Tarlov) cysts. Acta Med Okayama 2006;60(1):65–70.

119. Voyadzis JM, Bhargava P, Henderson FC. Tarlov cysts: a study of 10 cases with review of the literature. J Neurosurg 2001;95(1 Suppl):25–32.

120. Duja CM, Berna C, Kremer S, et al. Confusion after spine injury: cerebral fat embolism after traumatic rupture of a Tarlov cyst: case report. BMC Emerg Med 2010;10:18.

121. Guest JD, Silbert L, Casas CE. Use of percutaneous endoscopy to place syringopleural or cystoperitoneal cerebrospinal fluid shunts: technical note. J Neurosurg Spine 2005;2(4):498–504.

122. Smith ZA, Fessler RG, Batjer HH. Perspective–sacral Tarlov cyst: surgical treatment by clipping. World Neurosurg 2013;79(2):285.

123. Ahad A, Elsayed M, Tohid H. The accuracy of clinical symptoms in detecting cauda equina syndrome in patients undergoing acute MRI of the spine. Neuroradiol J 2015;28(4):438–42.

124. Small SA, Perron AD, Brady WJ. Orthopedic pitfalls: cauda equina syndrome. Am J Emerg Med 2005;23(2):159–63.

125. Fraser S, Roberts L, Murphy E. Cauda equina syndrome: a literature review of its definition and clinical presentation. Arch Phys Med Rehabil 2009;90(11):1964–8.

126. Podnar S. Epidemiology of cauda equina and conus medullaris lesions. Muscle Nerve 2007;35(4):529–31.

Urologic and Gynecologic Sources of Pelvic Pain

Dominique R. Malacarne, MD[a,b], Kimberly L. Ferrante, MD[c,d],
Benjamin M. Brucker, MD[e,f,g],*

KEYWORDS

- Genitourinary syndromes • Urogynecologic pain sources • Pelvic pain

KEY POINTS

- Infectious or inflammatory sources make up a large portion of genitourinary etiologies of pelvic pain and should be ruled out.
- Chronic pain syndromes involving the gynecologic or genitourinary syndromes can be complex and often requires multimodal treatments.
- Malignancy of gynecologic or genitourinary origin often does not cause pain until it is in advanced stages.
- A multidisciplinary approach is favored when deciphering between gynecologic and urologic sources of pelvic pain, as this allows experts of both fields to contribute to a more timely and accurate diagnosis.

In recent years, a great deal of knowledge has been acquired regarding various genitourinary etiologies for pelvic pain in both male and female patients. Despite this, there is still vast ground to gain regarding diagnosis and treatment for these medical disorders. Chronic pelvic pain affects more than 15% of the population and accounts for

The authors have nothing to disclose.
[a] Department of Urology, NYU Langone Medical Center, 150 East 32nd Street, 2nd Floor, New York, NY 10016, USA; [b] Female Pelvic Medicine and Reconstructive Surgery, Department of Obstetrics and Gynecology, NYU Langone Medical Center, 150 East 32nd Street, 2nd Floor, New York, NY 10016, USA; [c] Female Pelvic Medicine and Reconstructive Surgery, Department of Obstetrics and Gynecology, New York University School of Medicine, 462 1st Avenue, Room 9 E2, New York, NY 10016, USA; [d] Department of Urology, New York University School of Medicine, 462 1st Avenue, Room 9 E2, New York, NY 10016, USA; [e] Female Pelvic Medicine and Reconstructive Surgery, Neurourology and Voiding Dysfunction, Tisch Hospital, NYU Langone Medical Center, 12 East, New York, NY 10016, USA; [f] Department of Urology, NYU Langone Medical Center, 150 East 32nd Street, 2nd Floor, New York, NY 10016, USA; [g] Department of Obstetrics and Gynecology, NYU Langone Medical Center, 150 East 32nd Street, 2nd Floor, New York, NY 10016, USA
* Corresponding author. Department of Urology, Department of Obstetrics and Gynecology, NYU Langone Medical Center, 150 East 32nd Street, 2nd Floor, New York, NY 10016.
E-mail address: Benjamin.Brucker@nyumc.org

Phys Med Rehabil Clin N Am 28 (2017) 571–588
http://dx.doi.org/10.1016/j.pmr.2017.03.008
1047-9651/17/© 2017 Elsevier Inc. All rights reserved.

more than $800 million in annual US medical costs, which reveals the overall impact of pelvic pain as a disease process.[1,2] Gynecologic and urologic etiologies are discovered in most patients with pelvic pain and oftentimes recognition and treatment require a multidisciplinary approach. The growing practice in the field of female pelvic medicine and reconstructive surgery is to promote integration of both gynecologic and urologic knowledge to care for patients with pelvic pain through a more comprehensive method. We use this multidisciplinary practice and recommend collaboration to provide the highest quality care to patients affected by genitourinary sources of pelvic pain.

This article aims to provide a comprehensive review of the various genitourinary sources of pelvic pain, categorized by anatomic arrangement. Although often these patients are referred to specialists for treatment, practitioners from various backgrounds will ultimately encounter patients with pelvic pain, and it is crucial to understand the range of genitourinary causes of pain to provide patients with optimal avenues of referral when necessary. It is important to recognize that although these disorders predominantly affect women, there are various conditions discussed that span across genotypic sex and should be considered in the differential diagnosis in both male and female patients presenting with pelvic pain.

VULVAR AND VAGINAL PAIN

Various disorders affecting the vulvar and vaginal epithelium can contribute to symptoms of pelvic pain. These conditions can range from topical skin disorders to infectious processes, neurologic disorders, and even malignancy. Performing a thorough medical history and physical examination are paramount to arriving at the correct diagnosis for vulvovaginal syndromes causing pelvic pain. Vulvar skin disorders are not uncommon and can oftentimes be chronic entities with a relapsing and remitting course. Many patients afflicted with these disorders will primarily complain of vulvar pain and itching before noting any physical skin changes.[3] Time course can be very helpful when deciphering causes of vulvar pain, as infections and contact dermatoses tend to be acute in onset, whereas chronic dermatoses (eg, lichen sclerosis, psoriasis) and neoplastic lesions may cause progressively worsening discomfort for weeks to months. Patients may first notice pain with intercourse and many times dyspareunia is a presenting symptom in these cases. Vulvar and vaginal examinations are of distinct importance regardless of sexual activity level, as inspection may prompt diagnosis of a vulvar disorder that would be otherwise missed in its earlier stages.

Up to 60% of patients with vulvar symptoms may be experiencing atopic dermatitis, which usually appears as an erythematous demarcated area that has come in contact with an inciting allergen.[4] Typical culprits are laundry detergents, new soaps or shampoos, latex products, lubricants, and new topical medications, such as corticosteroids or antimycotic agents.[5] If a temporal relationship is noted with the introduction of a new product, contact dermatitis should be strongly considered. Sanitary products may also be a source of contact dermatitis causing urogenital or vulvar discomfort. Patients with genitourinary pain should routinely be screened for symptoms of incontinence, as incontinence dermatitis can ensue in these instances. Practitioners also should inquire about routine sanitary product use and reasons for this practice. Patients may experience discomfort due to an allergy to an anti-incontinence product used, or simply due to irritation caused by a moist environment that can accompany urinary or bowel leakage. In these cases, vulvovaginal hygiene practices should be reviewed and patients can be referred to incontinence specialists for further evaluation and treatment.

In contrast to acute dermatoses, chronic dermatologic conditions of the vulva can oftentimes require more in-depth evaluation and may necessitate lifelong treatment. The 3 most commonly seen vulvar dermatoses are described as follows and are best characterized by visual appearance.

- Lichen simplex chronicus: chronic eczematous disease often in response to long-term contact with environmental factors (can be caused by untreated contact dermatitis).
  - Scaling and lichenified plaques are present and itching usually precede pain; leathery or thickened appearance can be seen with long-standing disease.
  - Occurs in mid-adulthood and childhood.
- Lichen sclerosis: chronic skin disorder most commonly seen on the vulva, thought to be autoimmune or genetic in origin.
  - Skin appears whitened and thinned (often described as "cigarette paper") with papules and plaques common (**Fig. 1**); labial fusion can occur as well as reabsorption of the labia minor. This process generally spares vaginal epithelium, but may lead to a stenotic and narrowed introitus.
  - Occurs in fifth to sixth decade of life most often but can occur at any age.
- Lichen planus: inflammatory disorder of oral or genital mucosa, thought to be immune mediated. Erosive form is the most common morphology.
  - Purple, pruritic, shiny papules are hallmark sign; erosive disease can present with deep, painful erosion and denuded vulvar and vaginal epithelium that appears red and inflamed.
  - Occurs in third and fourth decades of life most commonly; 1% long-term malignancy transformation.

The variations in these dermatologic conditions can be subtle and further evaluation by a specialist, most often in conjunction with a vulvar biopsy, is required to make the diagnosis.

Psoriasis of the vulva can occur, appearing as a smooth, nonscaly erythema. Patients are more prone to genital psoriasis if it also occurs in other areas and can be treated similarly, although psoriasis can occur solely in the genital region in 1% to

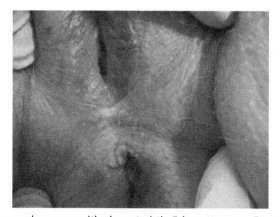

Fig. 1. Postmenopausal woman with characteristic "cigarette paper" appearance of perineal and perianal tissue, consistent with lichen sclerosis. (*From* Goldstein I. Female urology. 3rd edition. Philadelphia: SAUNDERS ELSEVIER; 2008. p. 513. http://dx.doi.org/10.1016/B978-1-4160-2339-5.50099-9; with permission.)

2% of individuals. Psoriasis of the genitourinary area will spare mucus membranes and so will not be found in vaginal or urethral regions.[6] Another chronic inflammatory skin condition to be aware of is hidradenitis suppurativa. Patients typically present with painful sores or "boils" in the groin region. The condition is more likely to be found in women, although if found in men is more common in gluteal and perianal regions. Women are more likely to have inguinal lesions and the condition is also positively correlated with smoking and family history.[7] The clinical manifestation can vary and venereal disease workup including herpes simplex virus, syphilis, bacterial culture, and Gram stain should be considered in anyone who is high risk, as some sexually transmitted infections, such as granuloma inguinale, can present similarly. Usually patients will have painful recurring nodules and abscesses with sinus tract drainage. With healing of these lesions, severe scars can form. It is important to also distinguish this process from a vulvar manifestation of Crohn disease, which can also present with abscess and ulcer formation. In patients with suspected bowel disease, this differential diagnosis should be strongly considered.

Genitourinary syndrome of menopause or vulvovaginal atrophy is often overlooked as a potential source of vulvar and vaginal pain. It is imperative to be cognizant of a patient's hormonal status when performing an evaluation for pelvic pain. The low levels of circulating estrogen associated with menopause and breastfeeding result in lower elastin levels, alteration of smooth muscle function, and decrease in blood vessels. The urethral meatus becomes more prominent with retraction of surrounding tissues, increasing vulnerability to irritation and trauma (**Fig. 2**) These changes promote friability and weakness of vulvar and vaginal tissues and skin breakdown is common with any type of friction.[8] Intercourse can become extremely painful and bleeding is not uncommon. Petechiae may be noted at the peri-urethral tissues and fissures may also be present. Although many women respond to estrogen replacement alone, a multimodal treatment approach can be helpful for these patients, such as that of topical estrogen and pelvic floor physical therapy, especially in the settings of dyspareunia and lower urinary tract dysfunction.

Vaginitis, although most typically associated with abnormal vaginal discharge, can at times cause vaginal pain, especially during sexual intercourse. Women who complain of dyspareunia accompanied by abnormal vaginal discharge should be

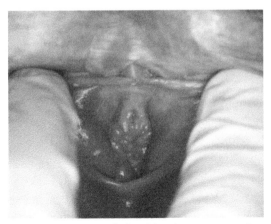

Fig. 2. Severe atrophy of the vulvar vestibule with subsequent prominent urethral meatus. (*From* Goldstein AT, King MA. Ospemifene may not treat vulvar atrophy: a report of two cases. Sex Med 2016;4(3):e218; with permission.)

screened for sexually transmitted infections. The 3 most common causes of vaginitis include the following:

- Vulvovaginal candidiasis: symptoms including itching and burning, exacerbated with urination. A thick white discharge is often noted.
- Bacterial vaginosis: polymicrobial sexually associated infection. Symptoms include malodorous, gray discharge; may have dyspareunia.
- Trichomoniasis: sexually transmitted infection; prototypical symptoms include itching, burning, dyspareunia and postcoital bleeding; cervix appears inflamed and erythematous.

Vaginal and oral formulations are used to treat these underlying causes of vaginitis and treatment course can vary from one to 7 days for uncomplicated infections.[9] Although microscopy may be sufficient for diagnosis, vaginal culture can be helpful if a particular organism is suspected but not identified. Patients should receive timely treatment for these conditions to reduce risk of long-term sequelae, such as various vulvar dermatologic conditions and vulvar pain syndrome.[10]

Two major glands of the vulva that can become blocked and infected are the Bartholin gland, which is known as the major vestibular gland on either side of the vaginal vestibule, and the Skene gland, a periurethral gland located on the left and right sides of the urethra (**Fig. 3**). The Bartholin ducts are the source of drainage for the Bartholin glands and are located at the 4 and 8 o'clock positions with respect to the vaginal introitus. The Skene ducts are located just lateral and inferior to the urethral meatus. Both sets of glands are prone to cyst and even abscess formation if blockage occurs, which can often be accompanied by pain. Bartholin gland abscesses are the more common vulvar abscesses, and treatment can range from drainage of these collections to excision of glands if the condition is persistent. Antibiotics also may be warranted if the clinical picture is consistent with an infected gland.[11] Mindfulness of the exact location of these ducts can assist with appropriate diagnosis and treatment. Awareness and understanding of the clinical presentation of other periurethral masses, such as a urethral diverticulum, which is discussed later, can be crucial to arriving at a correct diagnosis.

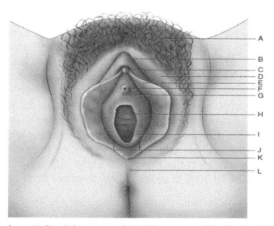

Fig. 3. The external genitalia: (A) mons pubis, (B) prepuce, (C) clitoris, (D) labia majora, (E) labia minora, (F) urethral meatus, (G) Skene ducts, (H) vagina, (I) hymen, (J) Bartholin glands, (K) posterior fourchette, (L) perineal body. (*Reproduced from* Townsend CM, Beauchamp RD, Evers BM, et al: Sabiston Textbook of Surgery, 17th ed. Philadelphia, W.B. Saunders, 2004; with permission.)

Vulvodynia, described as either generalized or localized burning pain and vulvar irritation, contrasts vulvar pain syndrome in that there is no identifiable clinical finding or infectious or neurologic cause for the symptom profile. Vulvodynia can be very distressing, as it is a diagnosis of exclusion and the true etiology is unknown, and likely multifactorial. Patients often complain of vulvar pain that is provoked; however, unprovoked disease also can be present. It is important to distinguish generalized vulvodynia from that which is localized to a specific area, usually at the site of the introitus. This can be done with a cotton swab test so that distinct areas of disease are identified.[12] This diagnostic technique can prove helpful especially when conservative treatments fail and patients may resort to vestibular surgery for relief. These patients should be counseled on vulvar care, which includes use of only cotton underwear, avoidance of douching and vulvar irritants, proper hygiene techniques after urination and defecation, and application of cold compresses to the vulvar area, among other practices.[13] When evaluating these patients, clinicians should inquire about any previous pelvic or spinal surgeries or spinal injury or disease (ie, spinal stenosis). If pain is localized to perineal and vulvar regions in this setting, pudendal neuralgia should be considered. This condition is usually associated with worsening of symptoms in the seated position, intact sensation, and relief of symptoms is typically noted with pudendal nerve block.[14] Patients with spinal stenosis also can present with pain and pruritus in clitoral or vulvar regions as a result of nerve entrapment. If symptoms are noted in close temporal relationship to vaginal prolapse repair surgery, removal of apical suspension sutures may be considered.

Another vulvar pain disorder to be cognizant of when evaluating patients with vulvar and vaginal pain is vaginismus. Traditionally referred to as a disorder of involuntary muscle spasm around the vaginal orifice, this condition causes aversion to any type of penetration and patients are often averse to both sexual and nonsexual (vaginal examination, tampon) encounters due to actual pain or anticipation of pain. There are various subcategories of vaginismus, which describe varying degrees of penetration tolerability and disease progression.[15] Studies have shown that pain patterns of vaginismus are very similar to those of provoked vulvodynia and patients often do well with desensitization techniques, which include muscle retraining and relaxation.[16,17]

Vulvar pain is not a primary symptom associated with vulvar malignancy; however, can be present if premalignant and malignant lesions are exhibited in the form of ulcers or are accompanied by enlarged inguinal lymph nodes. Vulvar intraepithelial neoplasia is used to denote high-grade squamous lesions of the vulva and often is identified as a hyperpigmented vulvar lesion, although lesions can be flat or raised and range from white to brown or black in color. All pigmented vulvar lesions require biopsy for accurate diagnosis. Vulvar malignancy can occur in melanoma, sarcoma, and vulvar Paget disease, as well as squamous cell carcinomas, which account for 90% of vulvar cancers.[18] Vulvar Paget disease exhibits distinct clinical findings of a well-demarcated eczematous lesion with slightly raised edges. Although pruritus is the most common symptom, vulvar and vaginal pain can occur. More often than not, patients exhibit multifocal lesions and present in the seventh or eighth decade of life. Synchronous neoplasms occur in 20% to 30% of patients and so whole body surveillance should be common practice.[19]

UTERINE AND CERVICAL SOURCES OF PAIN

In female patients with pelvic pain accompanied by abnormal uterine bleeding, the diagnosis of leiomyomas or adenomyosis should be contemplated. Patients may commonly note a midline pelvic mass that may have grown overtime, consistent with an enlarged uterus. Leiomyomas (also called fibroids) are classified as benign uterine soft tissue tumors arising from the myometrium and are the most common indication for hysterectomy, with cumulative prevalence in women approaching 80%, with slightly earlier occurrence in black women.[20] Symptoms most often described are pelvic pressure and dyspareunia; however, patients are more likely to describe intense pelvic pain if fibroids are in a degenerating phase or if they are aborting through the cervix. With growth impinging on adjacent structures, patients may experience discomfort or urgency with defecation or urination. Pain also can be a secondary component of degeneration of leiomyomas. This can occur at any point, but usually closer to perimenopausal status. When blood supply is diminished, whether naturally or iatrogenically (with embolization or ablation of myomas), necrosis of the fibroid tissue can cause pain secondarily. Physical examination may reveal an enlarged uterus with irregular shape and contour if fibroids are subserosal in nature. If the uterus is more uniform but globular in character, adenomyosis should be considered. This condition arises when endometrial glands are present in the uterine musculature and promotes hypertrophy of the surrounding myometrium. The uterus may be enlarged but is usually smaller in size than that of a fibroid uterus, although these 2 processes frequently occur in conjunction. Patients with adenomyosis report painful menstruation or dysmenorrhea as a common symptom, and this is noted in approximately 25% of patients afflicted with the disease.[21] A pelvic ultrasound should be considered if an enlarged uterus is palpated on physical examination, or if the examination is limited by habitus of the patient.

Another common disorder of ectopic endometrial tissue causing pain is that of endometriosis and although this can commonly be associated with uterine pain, endometriosis can affect multiple pelvic organs, such as bowel and bladder and should frequently be in the differential diagnosis of pelvic pain in a woman. In contrast with adenomyosis, endometrial tissue is endometriosis is extrauterine, and these ectopic cells elicit an inflammatory response causing pelvic pain. Endometriosis is an estrogen-dependent inflammatory process and usually affects women of reproductive age in their third decade of life. In a recent study of women with a diagnosis of endometriosis, the most common presenting symptoms were dysmenorrhea (79%) and generalized pelvic pain (69%).[22] Oftentimes pain is cyclical in nature and relieved with use of oral contraceptive pills. Endometriosis can be diagnosed clinically; however, definitive diagnosis is through histopathologic examination of a pelvic lesion biopsied during surgery (generally laparoscopy).

Uterine infections such as pelvic inflammatory disease (PID) should be considered in sexually active patients with dyspareunia and lower abdominal pain of acute onset. PID results from ascending vaginal or cervical bacteria and can affect the cervix and uterus as well as adnexa. The most common causes of PID are sexually transmitted infections such as *Chlamydia trachomatis* and *Neisseria gonorrhoeae,* which together with *Gardnerella vaginalis* (bacterial vaginosis) comprise 85% of all infections causing PID.[23] Patients at higher risk for this condition are those with history of an STI, multiple sexual partners, age 25 or younger, and history of PID in the past. If left untreated, PID has been known to cause infertility, ectopic pregnancy, and long-term chronic pelvic pain.

Uterovaginal prolapse symptoms are thought to affect many women, especially those who have had 1 or more vaginal births, women with a body mass index greater than 25, and those with a history of a hysterectomy. In one recent prevalence study, more than 6% of the female population admitted to symptoms of pelvic organ prolapse and 50% of those women reported moderate or great distress due to these symptoms.[24] Most women with symptomatic prolapse will complain of pelvic pressure or "pulling" sensation and many can have difficulty with urinating and bowel movements. Other patients may describe organs falling out of the vagina and many times this can be seen to varying degrees on pelvic examination. Discrete pelvic pain as well as lower back pain, although historically thought to be attributable to pelvic organ prolapse, has not been distinctly linked to the disorder, and so if persistent pelvic pain is of primary concern, other etiologies should be explored, even in the setting of concomitant prolapse.[25,26] In patients who present with pelvic pain with a history of prior surgery for prolapse, it is crucial to understand the type of surgery performed and whether any synthetic material was used. Vaginal mesh can be the source of pain due to perforation, fistula formation, or inflammatory reaction, and mesh extrusion also should be ruled out as a potential cause of pelvic pain (**Fig. 4**). Oftentimes if mesh is the source of pain, surgical intervention is required.[27]

In premenopausal patients with pelvic pain, it is important to be aware of congenital or iatrogenic factors that could cause hematometra, which is the collection or retention of blood in the uterus. This commonly causes cyclical pelvic pain accompanied by amenorrhea. In younger women, this disorder is most commonly caused by an imperforate hymen or transverse vaginal septum, but can also be due to cervicovaginal agenesis or other Mullerian anomalies.[28,29] An abdominal mass also may be present, representing an enlarged uterus filled with blood. Examination and pelvic ultrasound, in addition to clinical history, can assist with arrival at this diagnosis and patients should be referred to a clinician who specializes in management of congenital anomalies. Hematometra may also occur after endometrial ablation, and incidence can reach more than 2% of those who undergo this procedure.[30] In instances in which endometrium is adherent, some endometrial tissue can be inadvertently missed in the ablative procedure. If this occurs behind the occlusion, hematometra will result. This phenomenon can occur remote from the ablative procedure itself and so premenopausal women with cyclical pelvic pain and a history of endometrial ablation should be evaluated for this condition.[31]

Last, uterine and cervical malignancies, although more likely to cause abnormalities in bleeding patterns, also can be the source of pelvic pain in certain instances. Uterine cancers are often diagnosed in early stages and confined to the endometrium, in which case pain is not typically present. In the case of uterine sarcomas, however, abdominal pain can be a common presenting symptom, and this is likely secondary to the rapid growth patterns and overall mass effect of this type of tumor.[32] Similarly, cervical cancer may not incite symptoms of pelvic pain until in its more advanced stages. Dyspareunia and postcoital bleeding can occur with manipulation of a cervical

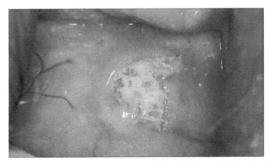

Fig. 4. Mesh erosion noted at the posterior vaginal wall. (*From* Jelovsek JE, Maher C, Barber MD. Pelvic organ prolapse. Lancet 2007;369(9566):1035; with permission.)

mass. Pelvic and lower back pain related to cervical malignancy tend to occur most frequently in the case of bone metastases and hydronephrosis caused by tumor mass effect.

OVARIAN AND ADNEXAL PAIN

Ovarian sources of pelvic pain tend to be more acute in nature. In some instances, pain can be intermittent, but this is less common. Chronic pain tends to be more often related to musculoskeletal disorders that invariably are mistaken for ovarian etiologies. One significant source of adnexal pain, which is managed emergently in many instances, is that of ectopic pregnancy. This occurs when a pregnancy forms outside of the uterus, and approximately 98% of the time these pregnancies will be found in the fallopian tube.[33] Patients commonly present with abdominal pain as their initial symptom, which may be associated with vaginal bleeding. The pain is commonly described as sharp and intense in quality and discomfort can significantly intensify with ectopic rupture. Clinical manifestations usually appear 6 to 8 weeks after the last menstrual period; however, this time course can vary.[34] This diagnosis should be considered in any patient with a positive pregnancy test and unconfirmed intrauterine pregnancy, or in which pregnancy cannot be ruled out. If rupture occurs, exploratory laparoscopy or laparotomy is necessary and hemoperitoneum can be the source of excruciating pain in these life-threatening instances.

Ovarian cysts tend to be found incidentally, and are not typically associated with pelvic pain, unless rupture or ovarian torsion occurs. Ovarian cyst rupture can ensue at any time and is common in women of reproductive age.[35] Cysts can form during regular cycles of menstruation and typically resolve without any symptoms. In some cases, cyst rupture can cause pain, as the fluid released tends to irritate the peritoneal cavity. Pain is usually sudden in onset and unilateral and most patients can be managed conservatively. It is imperative to differentiate cyst rupture from ovarian torsion, or rotation of the ovary on its ligamentous supports, often impeding blood supply. This can occur due to ovarian enlargement caused by an ovarian cyst. This contrasts with ovarian cyst rupture in that it is a surgical emergency. Ovaries are more likely to twist if a cyst is larger than 5 cm, and benign cysts are more likely than malignant neoplasms to be involved in torsion.[36] Ovarian torsion does not always occur secondary to a singular ovarian cyst, however. Torsion is more likely in the settings of ovulation induction whereby the ovary itself is stimulated and can become enlarged, in pregnancy, and even in setting of tubal ligation or hydrosalpinx, which can occur as a result of longstanding PID. Patients usually describe pain as sharp or "stabbing" in nature and pain often radiates to the lower back. Nausea and vomiting are common concomitant symptoms, as well as rebound and guarding.[37]

Tubal or ovarian infections also can cause pain, and these frequently result from further seeding of ascending uterine infections. As mentioned previously, fallopian tubes can become damaged as a result of previous infection and this results in blockage or clubbing of the tube. Fluid can become trapped, and a hydrosalpinx can form. The tube does not have to be twisted to cause pain, and in many instances tubal blockage itself can cause patients discomfort. Commonly, however, tubal factor infertility is the only sequelae. Another infectious etiology for adnexal pain is that of a tubo-ovarian abscess (TOA). A TOA is defined as an inflammatory mass or complex (if agglutination occurs) involving the fallopian tube, ovary, and not infrequently various other pelvic organs, such as bowel or bladder. A TOA is thought to be a progression of PID, so many times will present similarly with acute-onset abdominal pain and signs of systemic illness, such as fever, nausea, and vomiting. Historically, a TOA presentation can have a less abrupt course, and chronic lower abdominal pain has also been documented in the setting of this condition in approximately one-quarter of a large cohort of patients evaluated and treated for the disease.[38] There is always a risk for rupture of a TOA, and in the setting of this occurrence, symptoms are likely to be more acute and life-threatening. Again, in patients at high risk of contracting sexually transmitted infections, this diagnosis always should be considered.

Another condition thought to contribute to chronic pelvic pain is pelvic congestion syndrome. This entity has remained controversial in the literature, as it is thought to occur due to dilation of uterine and ovarian veins, causing pelvic varicosities. These varicosities display reduced blood flow leading to reflux, which it turn causes deep dyspareunia, postcoital pain, and exacerbation of pelvic symptoms with prolonged standing.[39] In many instances, this finding is thought to be the source of pelvic pain in many women in whom no other etiologies have been uncovered. In contrast, there has been documentation of incompetent and dilated pelvic vessels in many women who are completely asymptomatic.[40]

Adnexal malignancy, like many other genitourinary malignancies, tends to cause various nonspecific symptoms, which may or may not include pelvic pain, until disease is in its advanced stages. That being said, it is crucial to be aware of symptoms that tend to occur concurrently in the setting of ovarian malignancy, and at greater frequency than in that of the general population. These include bloating, pelvic or abdominal pain, difficulty with eating or early satiety, and urinary urgency or frequency.[41] In many studies, these symptoms were found to occur in clusters and were present even in early stages of disease. Women tend to explain these symptoms as persistent and a stark contrast from their normal behavior.[42] As a practitioner, one should order abdominal and pelvic imaging if patients present with daily occurrences of these symptoms for a duration of more than a few weeks.

Although many conditions involving fallopian tubes and ovaries have been outlined previously as potential causes of adnexal pain, it is imperative to be mindful of the notion that many times musculoskeletal causes of lower abdominal pain can be mistaken for conditions affecting the reproductive organs themselves. Pelvic floor musculoskeletal dysfunction should not be underestimated as a source of chronic pelvic pain. Referred pain from spasm of the pelvic floor muscles should always be contemplated after more acute pathophysiology has been ruled out and can be diagnosed on physical examination.

BLADDER PAIN

There are many possibilities for the underlying cause of bladder pain, and in explaining bladder pain many patients will be more specific in their description, characterizing their pain as midline and suprapubic in location. With any similar complaint, it is always best to first obtain a urinalysis and urine culture to check for a urinary tract infection (UTI). Some women, especially those who are perimenopausal, may contract recurrent UTIs as part of a more global genitourinary syndrome of menopause. Patients often will have UTI symptoms and suprapubic pain as part of this constellation, which may become chronic in nature. Patients may find relief with topical estrogen therapy or medical prophylaxis via acidification of the urine; however, some patients will require suppressive antibiotic therapy in the immediate postdiagnosis period. Postmenopausal women are more likely to experience recurrent UTIs if they experienced UTIs before menopause, and this condition is more likely to be associated with urinary incontinence and uterovaginal prolapse.[43] For these reasons it is important to be aware that pelvic pain associated with recurrent UTIs can be the result of a multifactorial process.

If infection has been ruled out, another fairly noninvasive, in-office diagnostic procedure would be to check a postvoid residual after a patient has emptied the bladder. This can be done by using a bladder scanner or by catheterizing the patient for residual urine. Urinary retention can frequently cause lower abdominal or suprapubic pain and is commonly associated with the feeling of incomplete bladder emptying.[44] Acute urinary retention is much more common in men, and is most often the result of benign prostatic hyperplasia.[45] Patients can have large amounts of residual urine volume, often exceeding 200 mL, and in cases of chronic urinary retention, a bladder ultrasound can detect enlarged bladder capacities of greater than 1000 mL. Urinary retention is not always secondary to obstructive causes, however, and can be due to neurogenic causes or insufficient detrusor muscle activity. If urinary retention is uncovered as a source of bladder pain, the bladder should be decompressed first and foremost. Patients should be referred to a urologist or urogynecologist for further workup.

Foreign bodies also can be the cause of bladder pain. Pain or discomfort usually results from recurrent bladder spasm that often occurs as the bladder's response to a foreign body present. This can happen in the setting of mesh perforation or extrusion after mid-urethral sling placement. Mesh extrusion is associated with bladder and vaginal pain, as well as dyspareunia. Mesh can often be palpated or visualized on pelvic examination or office cystoscopy. Patients usually have persistence of symptoms in this setting and most symptomatic mesh complications require one or more surgical revision procedures; however, pain secondary to the presence of mesh also can occur without extrusion or erosion.[46] Pain may be reproducible if mesh is palpated; however, may not be visible or malpositioned. In most cases, the presence of mesh and even the palpation of mesh produce no such symptoms; however, in the case of pain related to mesh, removal should be considered or injection at the site of pain with local anesthetic. This can occur with any type of mesh from vaginal mesh kits to sling mesh. Sacrocolpopexy mesh also can be the source of discomfort, either in the bladder, the vagina, or both locations. Obtaining an operative report of the patient's prior surgery is crucial when attempting to identify if previously placed mesh is associated with pelvic pain. Bladder stones can form as a result of exposed foreign material in the bladder. *Proteus mirabilis* is the bacteria most commonly associated with formation of bladder stones, and pain associated with persistent bladder infections can be a primary suggestion of mesh extrusion in the setting of a recent sling procedure. Patients with diabetes and bleeding complications at time of a sling procedure are at higher risk for postoperative mesh exposures.[47] Practitioners should be knowledgeable of the characteristics of any recent surgical procedures, as this can assist with timely diagnosis of mesh complications.

Bladder pain syndrome (BPS), which is also referred to as interstitial cystitis (IC), is defined as "an unpleasant sensation (pain, pressure, discomfort) perceived to be related to the urinary bladder, associated with lower urinary tract symptoms of more than 6 weeks duration, in the absence of infection or other identifiable causes."[48] BPS significantly impairs function of daily activities, is associated with decreasing ability to perform activities of daily living, and is often refractory to treatment.[49] A complete medical history, including urinary and bowel symptoms, history of reproductive tract disease, psychoneurological disorders, and musculoskeletal syndromes, is key in patients who suffer from this disorder.[50] It is important to consider psychological and social factors associated with BPS, in addition to possible physical causes. BPS is a diagnosis of exclusion, and the symptoms cited are variable and have a wide range. How to effectively treat IC/BPS has remained a major challenge and a large cohort of patients is obliged to resort to using a combination of therapies.[51] Sources of infection, malignancy, and inflammation leading to bladder symptoms should be ruled out before arriving at this diagnosis.[52,53] Additionally, one should consider pelvic floor physical therapy as a primary treatment option, as there is evidence that many of the symptoms of BPS may be caused by associated pelvic floor dysfunction, and pelvic floor physical therapy has been shown to be effective for many of these patients.[52]

Bladder cancer, like many other gynecologic and genitourinary malignancies, tends to not be associated with pain until in its later stages. Pain associated with bladder cancer is usually indicative of metastatic disease or a tumor with local invasion into adjacent tissue. The localization of the pain symptoms oftentimes will direct identification of the site of tumor invasion. Flank pain is frequently associated with obstruction in the setting of a bladder malignancy, and this can occur with growth at any level of the renal system from the kidney itself, the ureters, or the bladder. Obstruction is more often related to invasion into the musculature, although similar symptoms can ensue if tumors involve the ureteral orifices. Suprapubic pain may be present with local tumor invasion into the soft tissues or nerves. This can also occur if the bladder tumor is located near the bladder outlet, which can cause obstruction leading to urinary retention. It is important to recognize that women tend to present with more advanced disease than men, so significant symptomatology may occur in the earlier stages of disease in men, allowing workup and diagnosis to occur sooner.[54] Regardless of gender, symptoms are usually intermittent and progress to persistent in nature, like most malignancies previously described. Patients with carcinoma in situ (CIS) may present with irritative bladder symptoms but sometimes can be described as a vague pain. Urine cytology and or cystoscopy can be a good tools if CIS is suspected. The biggest risk factor for bladder cancer is smoking. As with many malignancies, incidence increases with increasing age. Hematuria microscopic or gross in patients will pelvic pain deserves a complete workup in most cases.

URETHRAL PAIN

A common cause of urethral pain in adult women is the presence of a urethral diverticulum, which is an outpouching of urethral mucosa into surrounding tissues, usually causing a symptomatic midline vaginal mass. This condition typically presents in women between the ages of 20 and 60 years, and is often associated with dysuria and dyspareunia.[55] Although the etiology of this condition is not clearly understood, the thought is that the diverticulum forms as a result of recurrent infection and inflammation of the periurethral glands, causing enlargement and eventually obstruction.[56] There is an approximately 6% to 9% risk of malignancy, and this should be suspected if a hard mass is noted within the diverticulum.[57] Imaging is very helpful to best characterize this condition if the diagnosis is unclear.

In men, urethral pain is most commonly associated with acquisition of a sexually transmitted infection. Similar to those discussed previously, the typical pathogens responsible for this illness are C trachomatis and N gonorrhoeae. Men are typically younger and of reproductive age and commonly present with a complaint of urethral pain with urination as well as persistent burning or pruritus, and many may notice a urethral discharge as well. In a symptomatic man, the diagnosis can be made with presence of 1 of the following[58]:

- Mucopurulent discharge noted on urethral examination
- More than 2 white blood cells (WBCs) per field on Gram stain from a urethral swab
- Positive leukocyte esterase on the first-void urine or more than 10 WBCs per field on first-void urine

Men diagnosed with urethritis should refrain from any sexual intercourse for 7 days after initiation of treatment for their condition and should be counseled on safe sex practices for prevention of recurrence.

Last, urethral pain can be caused by urethral prolapse in women, or the presence of a urethral caruncle. This condition is specific to women, and in that subgroup is generally found in women of postmenopausal status.[59] Although the terms are sometimes used interchangeably, urethral prolapse generally refers to mucosa that is circumferentially everted at the meatus (**Fig. 5**), whereas a urethral caruncle is used most often to describe eversion of only a portion of the distal urethra, often at the posterior edge. Patients' symptoms are generally that of dysuria, pain or burning at the site of the urethra, vaginal spotting, or sometimes detection of a "lump" around the urethral opening.[60] Patients also may report "spraying" or delay of urine stream, due to obstruction caused by the caruncle itself. Although topical estrogen may promote resolution of symptoms and is considered first-line treatment for urethral prolapse, patients should be referred to a specialist for a full evaluation to ensure proper diagnosis and rule out the possibility of malignancy. Urethral cancer, although extremely rare, does occur. The presence of malignancy should be considered in the setting of urethral pain, especially after more common sources of pain have been ruled out.

URETER/KIDNEY/PROSTATE PAIN

As reviewed previously, suprapubic pain radiating to the flank may denote the presence of obstruction along the genitourinary tract, and this can be a result of many different disease processes. Although malignancy does cause obstruction, a much more widespread process is that of renal or ureteral stones, which can commonly cause obstruction leading to pain symptoms spanning from a dull ache to intense discomfort requiring parenteral analgesia.[61] It is not uncommon for patients to experience waves of pain with nephrolithiasis with or without significant obstruction, and intense symptoms can usually occur for approximately 20 to 60 minutes, followed by a pain-free or significantly less symptomatic period. Included in the differential diagnosis of flank pain is pyelonephritis. In contrast to nephrolithiasis, pyelonephritis symptoms are more similar to those of a UTI, and fever is oftentimes present. Laboratory evidence of pyuria or bacteriuria supports the diagnosis. Other

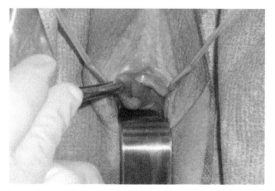

Fig. 5. Urethral prolapse in a postmenopausal woman. (*From* Bradley LD. Chapter 11 – investigation of abnormal uterine bleeding in postmenopausal women. Hysteroscopy. Philadelphia: MOSBY Elseveir; 2009. p. 118; with permission.)

frequent symptoms include costvertebral angle tenderness and nausea and vomiting. In men, these symptoms are much rarer; however, men may be at higher risk of UTIs and pyelonephritis if uncircumcised or engage in insertive anal intercourse.[62] In women, this constellation of symptoms may mimic that of PID, and it is important to differentiate these diagnoses, as treatment may be different and delay in accurate diagnosis and treatment could lead to negative long-term health effects in both instances.

The prostate is subject to inflammatory disorders that can cause pain and these can be acute or chronic in nature. Acute bacterial prostatitis is often followed by some type of prostatic manipulation, although can ensue from an ascending urethritis or other bacterial infection, most frequently gram-negative bacteria. Recent instrumentation, such as intermittent catheterization or chronic indwelling catheterization, may be associated with the diagnosis. Patients are at an increased risk as well in the setting of a recent prostatic biopsy, and providers should be aware of a rising fluoroquinolone resistance of these inciting organisms, which can lead to acute prostatitis.[63] Resistance has been directly linked to prior use of fluoroquinolones in these patients and clinicians should be aware of any antibiotic treatments a patient has been given around the time of a prostate biopsy. Symptoms are often acute and serious and may include fevers, chills, pain at the tip of the penis, and/or swelling in the groin area, which may or may not lead to voiding dysfunction.

Chronic prostatitis can be due to bacterial causes, as mentioned previously, or may be associated with chronic pelvic pain of unclear etiology. Chronic prostatitis/chronic pelvic pain syndrome (CP/CPPS) is a clinical syndrome in men that is diagnosed based on the presence of pelvic pain (penile, testicular, urethral, perineal) in the absence of a clinical infection or malignancy. Patients also may have difficulty or discomfort with ejaculation, blood in the semen, and voiding difficulties. Sexual dysfunction associated with this syndrome is often significant and can substantially impact a patient's quality of life.[64] Similar to BPS, this condition is a diagnosis of exclusion, and is thought by many experts to be closely correlated, and may be of the same pathophysiologic process as BPS. There is still much knowledge to acquire surrounding both of these syndromes; however, patients can often present similar and respond to similar treatment modalities. It is also important to consider pelvic floor physical therapy as a treatment option, as CP/CPPS has been known to be associated with pelvic floor dysfunction and pelvic floor myofascial pain, both which can be alleviated with a pelvic floor physical therapy treatment program.[65] Prevalence of CP/CPPS disorder tends to peak in the fifth decade of life; however, can be present in men of all ages.

Overall, it is important to be aware of the multitude of gynecologic and genitourinary causes of pelvic pain, not limited to those reviewed previously. Providers who encounter patients with pelvic pain should attempt to localize these symptoms and obtain a comprehensive history from the patient to help direct diagnostic evaluation. Providers should be aware of possible infectious causes and these processes should be ruled out, as delay in diagnosis of infectious processes could impede future reproductive function in various instances, in both men and women. Additionally, malignancy causing pelvic pain should be excluded in a timely fashion, as genitourinary and gynecologic malignancies can be locally destructive and metastasis is not uncommon at the time of symptomatic presentation of these cancers. Last, it is imperative to be conscious of the various chronic pain syndromes that can affect patients, and important to recognize appropriate resources for long-standing nonsurgical treatment modalities that may be available for patients.

REFERENCES

1. Jarrell JF, Vilos GA, Allaire C, et al. Consensus guidelines for the management of chronic pelvic pain. J Obstet Gynaecol Can 2005;27(8):781–826.

2. Mathias SD, Kuppermann M, Liberman RF, et al. Chronic pelvic pain: prevalence, health-related quality of life, and economic correlates. Obstet Gynecol 1996; 87(3):321–7.

3. Hansen A, Carr K, Jensen JT. Characteristics and initial diagnoses in women presenting to a referral center for vulvovaginal disorders in 1996-2000. J Reprod Med 2002;47(10):854–60.

4. Crone AM, Stewart EJ, Wojnarowska F, et al. Aetiological factors in vulvar dermatitis. J Eur Acad Dermatol Venereol 2000;14(3):181–6.

5. ACOG Practice Bulletin No. 93: diagnosis and management of vulvar skin disorders. Obstet Gynecol 2008;111(5):1243–53.

6. Meeuwis KA, de Hullu JA, Massuger LF, et al. Genital psoriasis: a systematic literature review on this hidden skin disease. Acta Derm Venereol 2011;91(1):5–11.

7. Schrader AM, Deckers IE, van der Zee HH, et al. Hidradenitis suppurativa: a retrospective study of 846 Dutch patients to identify factors associated with disease severity. J Am Acad Dermatol 2014;71(3):460–7.

8. Yen SSC, Jaffe R. Reproductive endocrinology. 2nd edition. Philadelphia: W.B. Saunders Co; 1986.

9. ACOG Practice Bulletin. Clinical management guidelines for obstetrician-gynecologists, Number 72, May 2006: Vaginitis. Obstet Gynecol 2006;107(5): 1195–206.

10. Nguyen RH, Swanson D, Harlow BL. Urogenital infections in relation to the occurrence of vulvodynia. J Reprod Med 2009;54(6):385–92.

11. Pundir J, Auld BJ. A review of the management of diseases of the Bartholin's gland. J Obstet Gynaecol 2008;28(2):161–5.

12. Haefner HK. Critique of new gynecologic surgical procedures: surgery for vulvar vestibulitis. Clin Obstet Gynecol 2000;43(3):689–700.

13. ACOG Committee Opinion: Number 345, October 2006: vulvodynia. Obstet Gynecol 2006;108(4):1049–52.

14. Labat JJ, Riant T, Robert R, et al. Diagnostic criteria for pudendal neuralgia by pudendal nerve entrapment (Nantes criteria). Neurourol Urodyn 2008;27(4): 306–10.

15. Crowley T, Goldmeier D, Hiller J. Diagnosing and managing vaginismus. BMJ 2009;338:b2284.

16. Reissing ED, Binik YM, Khalifé S, et al. Vaginal spasm, pain, and behavior: an empirical investigation of the diagnosis of vaginismus. Arch Sex Behav 2004; 33(1):5–17.

17. Ter Kuile MM, Van Lankveld JJ, Vlieland CV, et al. Vulvar vestibulitis syndrome: an important factor in the evaluation of lifelong vaginismus? J Psychosom Obstet Gynaecol 2005;26(4):245–9.

18. ACOG Committee Opinion No. 509: Management of vulvar intraepithelial neoplasia. Obstet Gynecol 2011;118(5):1192–4.

19. Feuer GA, Shevchuk M, Calanog A. Vulvar Paget's disease: the need to exclude an invasive lesion. Gynecol Oncol 1990;38(1):81–9.

20. Baird DD, Dunson DB, Hill MC, et al. High cumulative incidence of uterine leiomyoma in black and white women: ultrasound evidence. Am J Obstet Gynecol 2003;188(1):100–7.

21. McElin TW, Bird CC. Adenomyosis of the uterus. Obstet Gynecol Annu 1974;3(0): 425–41.
22. Sinaii N, Plumb K, Cotton L, et al. Differences in characteristics among 1,000 women with endometriosis based on extent of disease. Fertil Steril 2008;89(3): 538–45.
23. Brunham RC, Gottlieb SL, Paavonen J. Pelvic inflammatory disease. N Engl J Med 2015;372(21):2039–48.
24. Rortveit G, Brown JS, Thom DH, et al. Symptomatic pelvic organ prolapse: prevalence and risk factors in a population-based, racially diverse cohort. Obstet Gynecol 2007;109(6):1396–403.
25. Swift SE, Tate SB, Nicholas J. Correlation of symptoms with degree of pelvic organ support in a general population of women: what is pelvic organ prolapse? Am J Obstet Gynecol 2003;189(2):372–7 [discussion: 377–9].
26. Heit M, Rosenquist C, Culligan P, et al. Predicting treatment choice for patients with pelvic organ prolapse. Obstet Gynecol 2003;101(6):1279–84.
27. Crosby EC, Abernethy M, Berger MB, et al. Symptom resolution after operative management of complications from transvaginal mesh. Obstet Gynecol 2014; 123(1):134–9.
28. Grover S. Pelvic pain in the female adolescent patient. Aust Fam Physician 2006; 35(11):850–3.
29. Miller RJ, Breech LL. Surgical correction of vaginal anomalies. Clin Obstet Gynecol 2008;51(2):223–36.
30. Lethaby A, Hickey M, Garry R, et al. Endometrial resection/ablation techniques for heavy menstrual bleeding. Cochrane Database Syst Rev 2009;(4):CD001501.
31. McCausland AM, McCausland VM. Long-term complications of endometrial ablation: cause, diagnosis, treatment, and prevention. J Minim Invasive Gynecol 2007;14(4):399–406.
32. Nordal RR, Thoresen SO. Uterine sarcomas in Norway 1956-1992: incidence, survival and mortality. Eur J Cancer 1997;33(6):907–11.
33. Bouyer J, Coste J, Fernandez H, et al. Sites of ectopic pregnancy: a 10 year population-based study of 1800 cases. Hum Reprod 2002;17(12):3224–30.
34. Casanova BC, Sammel MD, Chittams J, et al. Prediction of outcome in women with symptomatic first-trimester pregnancy: focus on intrauterine rather than ectopic gestation. J Womens Health (larchmt) 2009;18(2):195–200.
35. Bottomley C, Bourne T. Diagnosis and management of ovarian cyst accidents. Best Pract Res Clin Obstet Gynaecol 2009;23(5):711–24.
36. Oltmann SC, Fischer A, Barber R, et al. Cannot exclude torsion–a 15-year review. J Pediatr Surg 2009;44(6):1212–6 [discussion: 1217].
37. Houry D, Abbott JT. Ovarian torsion: a fifteen-year review. Ann Emerg Med 2001; 38(2):156–9.
38. Landers DV, Sweet RL. Tubo-ovarian abscess: contemporary approach to management. Rev Infect Dis 1983;5(5):876–84.
39. Koo S, Fan CM. Pelvic congestion syndrome and pelvic varicosities. Tech Vasc Interv Radiol 2014;17(2):90–5.
40. Rozenblit AM, Ricci ZJ, Tuvia J, et al. Incompetent and dilated ovarian veins: a common CT finding in asymptomatic parous women. AJR Am J Roentgenol 2001;176(1):119–22.
41. Goff BA, Mandel LS, Drescher CW, et al. Development of an ovarian cancer symptom index: possibilities for earlier detection. Cancer 2007;109(2):221–7.
42. Yawn BP, Barrette BA, Wollan PC. Ovarian cancer: the neglected diagnosis. Mayo Clin Proc 2004;79(10):1277–82.

43. Raz R, Gennesin Y, Wasser J, et al. Recurrent urinary tract infections in postmenopausal women. Clin Infect Dis 2000;30(1):152-6.

44. Thomas K, Chow K, Kirby RS. Acute urinary retention: a review of the aetiology and management. Prostate Cancer Prostatic Dis 2004;7(1):32-7.

45. Curtis LA, Dolan TS, Cespedes RD. Acute urinary retention and urinary incontinence. Emerg Med Clin North Am 2001;19(3):591-619.

46. Abbott S, Unger CA, Evans JM, et al. Evaluation and management of complications from synthetic mesh after pelvic reconstructive surgery: a multicenter study. Am J Obstet Gynecol 2014;210(2):163.e1-8.

47. Osborn DJ, Dmochowski RR, Harris CJ, et al. Analysis of patient and technical factors associated with midurethral sling mesh exposure and perforation. Int J Urol 2014;21(11):1167-70.

48. Hanno P, Dmochowski R. Status of international consensus on interstitial cystitis/bladder pain syndrome/painful bladder syndrome: 2008 snapshot. Neurourol Urodyn 2009;28(4):274-86.

49. Hanno PM, Erickson D, Moldwin R, et al. Diagnosis and treatment of interstitial cystitis/bladder pain syndrome: AUA guideline amendment. J Urol 2015;193(5):1545-53.

50. Everaert K, Devulder J, De Muynck M, et al. The pain cycle: implications for the diagnosis and treatment of pelvic pain syndromes. Int Urogynecol J Pelvic Floor Dysfunct 2001;12(1):9-14.

51. Sairanen J, Leppilahti M, Tammela TL, et al. Evaluation of health-related quality of life in patients with painful bladder syndrome/interstitial cystitis and the impact of four treatments on it. Scand J Urol Nephrol 2009;43(3):212-9.

52. FitzGerald MP, Payne CK, Lukacz ES, et al. Randomized multicenter clinical trial of myofascial physical therapy in women with interstitial cystitis/painful bladder syndrome and pelvic floor tenderness. J Urol 2012;187(6):2113-8.

53. FitzGerald MP, Anderson RU, Potts J, et al. Randomized multicenter feasibility trial of myofascial physical therapy for the treatment of urological chronic pelvic pain syndromes. J Urol 2013;189(1 Suppl):S75-85.

54. Mitra AP, Skinner EC, Schuckman AK, et al. Effect of gender on outcomes following radical cystectomy for urothelial carcinoma of the bladder: a critical analysis of 1,994 patients. Urol Oncol 2014;32(1):52.e1-9.

55. Burrows LJ, Howden NL, Meyn L, et al. Surgical procedures for urethral diverticula in women in the United States, 1979-1997. Int Urogynecol J Pelvic Floor Dysfunct 2005;16(2):158-61.

56. Foley CL, Greenwell TJ, Gardiner RA. Urethral diverticula in females. BJU Int 2011;108(Suppl 2):20-3.

57. Thomas AA, Rackley RR, Lee U, et al. Urethral diverticula in 90 female patients: a study with emphasis on neoplastic alterations. J Urol 2008;180(6):2463-7.

58. Workowski KA, Bolan GA. Sexually transmitted diseases treatment guidelines, 2015. MMWR Recomm Rep 2015;64(RR-03):1-137.

59. Conces MR, illiamson SR, Montironi R, et al. Urethral caruncle: clinicopathologic features of 41 cases. Hum Pathol 2012;43(9):1400-4.

60. Marshall FC, Uson AC, Melicow MM. Neoplasma and caruncles of the female urethra. Surg Gynecol Obstet 1960;110:723-33.

61. Fwu CW, Eggers PW, Kimmel PL, et al. Emergency department visits, use of imaging, and drugs for urolithiasis have increased in the United States. Kidney Int 2013;83(3):479-86.

62. Hooton TM, Stamm WE. Diagnosis and treatment of uncomplicated urinary tract infection. Infect Dis Clin North Am 1997;11(3):551-81.

63. Mosharafa AA, Torky MH, El Said WM, et al. Rising incidence of acute prostatitis following prostate biopsy: fluoroquinolone resistance and exposure is a significant risk factor. Urology 2011;78(3):511–4.
64. Sonmez NC, Kiremit MC, Güney S, et al. Sexual dysfunction in type III chronic prostatitis (CP) and chronic pelvic pain syndrome (CPPS) observed in Turkish patients. Int Urol Nephrol 2011;43(2):309–14.
65. Dirk-Henrik Z, Ishigooka M, Doggweiler R, et al. Chronic prostatitis: a myofascial pain syndrome? Infect Urol 1999;12(3):84–8, 92.

Physical Therapy Treatment of Pelvic Pain

Michelle H. Bradley, PT, DPT, WCS, CLT-LANA, Ashley Rawlins, PT, DPT*,
C. Anna Brinker, PT, MHS

KEYWORDS

- Pelvic health physical therapy • Chronic pelvic pain • Functional restoration
- Underactivity • Overactivity • Trigger points • Biopsychosocial model

KEY POINTS

- Chronic pelvic pain can have many musculoskeletal and neuromuscular manifestations.
- The pelvic girdle is functionally connected to both trunk and legs, an important area of force transfer.
- Physical therapists are in a unique position to affect the multisystem component of pelvic pain, particularly concerning functional restoration.
- In chronic pelvic pain, it is imperative to understand a patient's entire pain story and how it affects them physiologically, anatomically, emotionally, mentally, physically, and socially.
- Physical therapists are a key part of the multidisciplinary team helping to treat chronic pelvic pain.

INTRODUCTION

Chronic pelvic pain (CPP) in the absence of malignancy is the perception of a noxious stimulus in the pelvic area of either men or women that persists either intermittently or continuously for 6 months or longer.[1] CPP encompasses a wide range of diagnoses including, but not limited to, dyspareunia, vaginismus, vulvodynia or vestibulodynia, endometriosis, interstitial cystitis or painful bladder syndrome, chronic nonbacterial prostatitis or prostadynia, chronic proctalgia, piriformis syndrome, hip dysfunction, and pudendal neuralgia. CPP can affect as many as 1 in 4 women.[2] CPP in men is believed to affect from 2% to 10% of men, noting that the term CPP and chronic prostatitis are typically interchanged terms.[3,4]

Pelvic pain can affect many systems in the body, including the nervous, endocrine, urinary, reproductive, gastrointestinal, and immune systems (**Table 1**). The influence

The authors have nothing to disclose.
Physical Therapy, Outpatient PM&R, Physical Medicine and Rehabilitation Clinic, UT Southwestern Medical Center of Dallas, 5151 Harry Hines Boulevard, Dallas, TX 75390-9055, USA
* Corresponding author.
E-mail address: ashley.rawlins@utsouthwestern.edu

Phys Med Rehabil Clin N Am 28 (2017) 589–601
http://dx.doi.org/10.1016/j.pmr.2017.03.009
1047-9651/17/© 2017 Elsevier Inc. All rights reserved.

Table 1
Summary of system effects of pelvic pain

Affected System	Effects on Pelvic Pain
Nervous system	• Abnormal impulse generating sites in the peripheral nerves[5,6] • Dorsal horn changes[5,6] • Cortical changes leading to increased sensitivity in a protective response[5,6] • Autonomic response changes that affect the visceral organs[5,6]
Endocrine system	• Increased cortisol secondary to chronic stress response in the body[7] • Decreased estrogen leading to urogenital atrophy, osteoporosis, and increased density of pain-sensing neurons in the female genitalia[8]
Urinary system	• Altered detrusor activity[6] • Muscular irritation to the lower urinary tract system[6]
Reproductive system	• Endometriosis, polycystic ovarian syndrome and uterine fibroids contributing to muscular irritation and inflammation process
Gastrointestinal system	• Altered smooth muscle activity[9]
Immune system	• Overproduction of proinflammatory cytokines[6] • Alterations in the immune responses[6]

of pelvic pain on the musculoskeletal and neuromuscular systems is of paramount importance, and is discussed in depth elsewhere in this review.

CPP can affect persons of all ages, socioeconomic status, and race.[9] Owing to the complex interactions of these systems, it often takes a team of specialists to comprehensively diagnose and treat the patient with CPP. This is why the biopsychosocial model for the treatment of chronic pain is so important for these patients. Pain is emotional, and it is rare that pain affects only the adjacent tissues. In CPP, it is imperative to understand a patient's entire pain story, and how it is affecting them physiologically, anatomically, emotionally, mentally, physically, and socially.[10]

In health care, physical therapists are among the experts in the treatment of musculoskeletal and neuromuscular dysfunction. Musculoskeletal and neuromuscular pelvic pain originates from any of the soft tissues, nerves, joints, or muscles of the lumbopelvic, abdominopelvic, and hip complex in the pelvic girdle. When there is dysfunction in any one of these components, pain can occur. In the absence of infection, malignancy, or visceral sources, pelvic pain is commonly myofascial, musculoskeletal, neuromuscular, or any combination of these in nature.[11,12] One particular study discovered that endometriosis was found in fewer than 25% of women undergoing a hysterectomy for treatment of CPP.[13]

Medications provide pain and visceral management, surgery provides correction of structure, but physical therapy's research-based approach provides functional restoration. This is why physical therapy is an important component of comprehensive treatment. Better known in the orthopedic spectrum, physical therapists specialize in the treatment of musculoskeletal and neuromuscular dysfunction, and therefore offer a specialization of care for those with pelvic pain. Traditionally the role of physical therapy in pelvic floor treatment has been with the pregnant patient with regard to body mechanics, posture, gait mechanics, and balance. In the past 20 years, however, physical therapy has grown to include a more comprehensive treatment of the pelvic girdle for both female and male because internal examination of the pelvic floor muscles is within the scope of practice for physical therapists.[14] Owing to the complexities of CPP, physical therapists play a vital role in helping to treat those suffering from this prevalent health condition.

Physical therapy treatment for pelvic pain differs depending on the dysfunctions present when evaluated. It is the physical therapy evaluation of the total body, including an internal pelvic (vaginal and/or rectal) examination, that determines the activity level of the muscles involved, whether overactive or underactive, and their relationship with the trunk, pelvic girdle, and hip structures.

Pelvic floor physical therapy will often include a variety of treatments including:

- Therapeutic exercises to help normalize muscle length, strength, and function;
- Neuromuscular reeducation to help teach pain-free movement and optimize coordination of associated muscles with correction of posture and body mechanics;
- Manual therapy to help reduce soft tissue restrictions, normalize muscle activity, encourage normal blood flow, and normalize joint alignment and movement; and
- Self-care management training and education to teach patients behavioral and lifestyle changes that can help to minimize and manage their pain.

ROLE OF PHYSICAL THERAPY IN THE ASSESSMENT OF PELVIC GIRDLE FUNCTION IN THE PRESENCE OF PAIN

Functionally, the pelvic girdle is the bottom of the trunk and the top of the legs. The pelvic diaphragm muscles are a group of muscles that run from the pubic bone to coccyx, wrapping around the pelvic openings to support the pelvic organs in maintaining their optimal functional positions. The pelvic diaphragm muscles are surrounded by the soft tissue to support the abdominal contents, blood vessels, and lymphatics for nutrient/waste exchange, and nerves to supply motor and sensation to the pelvic girdle and lower extremities. When there is dysfunction in any one of these components, pain can occur. In some cases, a patient does not respond to core stabilizer muscle strengthening for treatment of lumbar spine pain until coordination of the pelvic floor is addressed.[15] There is evidence of a functional link between pelvic floor muscle underactivity and hip weakness, but this is quite reasonable as the obturator internus is both a member of the pelvic floor muscle group and a hip rotator coupled posteriorly with the piriformis muscle.[16] There may also be a link between hip joint dysfunction and pelvic pain, but this has yet to be studied methodically.

The pelvic girdle is a key transitional area of the body that must:

- Provide support for the viscera;
- Allow for both storage of and elimination of waste;
- Allow for sexual function and childbirth; and
- Provide dynamic stability of the trunk and hips for balance and ambulation.

Diane Lee has stated,

The primary function of the lumbopelvic-hip complex is to transfer loads safely while fulfilling the movement and control requirements of any task in a way that ensures that the objectives of the task are met, musculoskeletal structures are not injured...and that the organs are supported/protected in concert with optimal respiration. Optimal function will, therefore, require both mobility and stability.[17]

To understand the role of the pelvic girdle in the development and persistence of pelvic pain, one must remember the laws of mechanical physics. The body is a series of mechanical levers (bones) turning on fulcrums (joints) by a force that is both active (muscles and tendons) and passive (joint capsules, ligaments, connective tissue). The rules governing these structures include the muscle length–tension relationship, which dictates the amount of force that muscles can exert on the lever arm. Changes in the passive forces brought on by repetitive or acute injury can also weaken the stability of the fulcrums. It is important to remember that pelvic musculoskeletal structures must support and provide the inferior stability to the trunk, but also be able to translate forces to lower limbs for locomotion.

Dysfunction in the muscle can occur when its length–tension relationship is suboptimal. For optimal function, a muscle be able to contract and shorten as well as relax and lengthen. When we look at the length–tension relationship of skeletal muscles, we know that a muscle in its most shortened position and a muscle in its most lengthened position are incapable of its maximal contraction strength.[18] The strength of the contraction is optimal in the middle of the curve (**Fig. 1**).

When a muscle is placed in a state of continuous activation, the connective tissue surrounding the muscle fibers will also eventually shorten to fit. To illustrate this, consider an elbow that has been in a brace or cast at a certain degree of flexion for several weeks. When the brace or cast is removed, the elbow does not automatically straighten without tissue resistance, but will have a passive shortening of the biceps muscle. This passive tissue shortening will then reduce the potential length of the muscle upon relaxation. Should similar overactivity persist in the levator ani, the muscle will reach a point in which the resting length is inadequate to provide the contraction strength required to function optimally, whether that function is to prevent urine or fecal loss or to stabilize the trunk while transferring force to the hip joints. Eventually, this muscle is at risk of going into spasm because this increasing tissue resistance slows the blood flow.

When muscles in the pelvic floor are shortened, reducing the length of the associated connective tissue, there is also a risk of compressing the structures supported by the connective tissue, including the pelvic nerves. Overactive muscles frequently lead to the development of shortened, taut bands within the muscle called trigger points, which have the ability to refer pain to other areas. Within the pelvis, the viscera (bladder, vagina, uterus, prostate, rectum) are innervated at the same spinal levels as the supportive muscle and bone structures, leading to a potential overlap in communication called viscerosomatic convergence.[19] The patient may have a sensation of a visceral pain when there is a musculoskeletal or neuromuscular dysfunction either coactive with a visceral problem or mimicking a visceral problem altogether.

Ultimately, the brain has the responsibility to keep the rest of the body safe. A bladder infection, for instance, if left alone can potentially lead to death. A cramp in

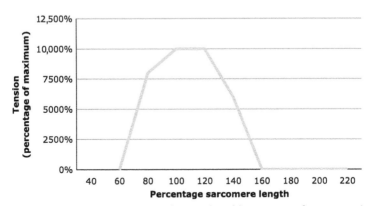

Fig. 1. Length tension curve: percent tension produced by percent of sarcomere length.

the levator ani, however, will not be fatal. The "warning" messages in each scenario, however, are both sent along the same pathways of S2, S3, and S4 to the brain. There are noted instances of an inflammatory response in the bladder of rats when an actual source of infection could not be found.[20] It is also known that those with pain conditions such as interstitial cystitis have tender points and myofascial changes in the abdominal, pelvic floor, and even hip intrinsic muscles.[21] When pelvic floor musculoskeletal abnormalities are treated, the sensation of bladder pain is typically reduced.[19]

The pelvic girdle, then, should not be thought of only in anatomic proximity of the trunk and legs in its position of transition, but rather as a part of the whole, within the body and controlled by the brain that senses, processes, and guides physical responses to noxious stimuli produced by dysfunction. A comprehensive treatment approach includes addressing nervous system sensitization and psychological responses to pain that would perpetuate and intensify pelvic pain.[22] The brain's perception of pain and its ability to become more sensitive to neural inputs in a further attempt to protect the body is integral to the understanding and treatment of pelvic pain. The development of neural hypersensitivity can potentially lead to central sensitization in which a greater amount of change in the abnormal myofascial tissues must occur before a reduction in pain is perceived.[6]

To better understand the relationship between CPP and emotional distress, anxiety, and catastrophization, it is important to look at the brain itself. In mapping of the sensory cortex, termed the homunculus, it has been found that the sensory input from the genital area is directly below the area of foot sensory reception.[23] This area lies directly over the cingulate gyrus, an important part of the limbic system that is involved in the emotional response to pain, particularly in fear avoidance and anxiety. As would be anticipated by the close anatomic proximity of these cerebral structures, a relationship between a stressful stimulus and the immediate motor response of levator ani activation has been demonstrated.[24] This suggests that, in the presence of existing pelvic pain, stress and anxiety can lead to greater muscle overactivity that, in turn, feeds back into the already painful condition.

An example may serve well to illustrate. Take, for example, a patient with sexual pain that begins to hinder sexual function. Relationship distress may then develop. What may start as dyspareunia may quickly develop into vaginismus. It has been shown that the stress of chronic pain can also have a significant effect on gastrointestinal function.[9] If the patient with vaginismus is at risk of losing her marriage, the stress could then lead to gastrointestinal dysfunction such as irritable bowel syndrome, manifesting as diarrhea. In the face of chronic diarrhea, the already shortened pelvic floor muscles may not be able to adequately mount a strong contraction, putting the patient at risk for fecal incontinence. The patient may well experience increasing activity of the pelvic floor muscles to avoid accidents, which further shortens the tissues and intensifies her pain. In the study of chronic pain in a functional area, the biopsychosocial model is needed to encompass all pain generators.

It is the pelvic floor physical therapist's role to identify presence of muscle overactivity involved in the patient's pain, the mechanical inducers of the pain, and the treatment approach that best addresses the patient's pain. The ultimate goal of pelvic floor physical therapy is to equip the patient with a home program of self-management of pelvic pain to allow for return to function in daily activities.

PHYSICAL THERAPY TREATMENT OF PELVIC PAIN

Physical therapy management of pelvic pain is based on the principles of other forms of musculoskeletal pain found elsewhere in the body, in both men and women. First, the physical therapist performs a total body systems review based on the patient's needs, age, and medical diagnosis, including a postural and gait assessment.[25] Evaluation and later treatment are guided by distinct symptoms reported by the patient. As evaluation of the specific pelvic floor muscles is performed, either vaginally or rectally for the female patient and rectally for the male patient, the therapist must accurately evaluate and assess the musculoskeletal condition underlying the pelvic pain. At the basic level, muscles can be overactive, underactive, or a combination of both (**Fig. 2**).

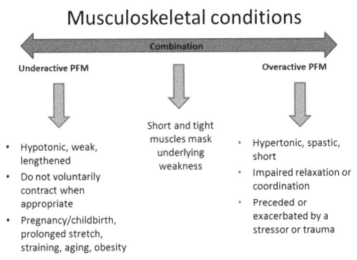

Fig. 2. Characteristics of muscle dysfunction by type. PFM, pelvic floor muscles.

- An overactive skeletal muscle is one that is characterized by poor flexibility (shortened), having a suboptimal length tension relationship (weakness) resulting in a lack of coordination (inability to relax). The overactive muscle can potentially have poor health secondary to the reduced blood flow and neurologic mobility restrictions present in its chronically shortened state. Once this muscle is returned to its optimal resting length, functional strength of the muscle is restored.
- An underactive muscle is functionally weakened with a suboptimal length–tension relationship, but has excessive length, providing poor support to the pelvic girdle structures. Because an underactive muscle is not a shortened muscle, it is not typically painful.
- A muscle can exhibit a combination of overactivity and underactivity. In this scenario, the muscle will have over activity and shortness at baseline, but once a normal length is restored, the muscle is inherently deficient in the ability to produce force (weakened).

Many who are unfamiliar with pelvic floor physical therapy may think only of levator ani contractions, known as "Kegel" exercises. Physical therapy, however, is concerned of restoration of function, and strengthening is not always warranted. If a biceps muscle is tight and overactive, the correct treatment would not be to put a weight in the patient's hand and exercise the muscle with biceps curls. Instead a physical therapist would work to improve the flexibility of the muscle, straighten the elbow, and then determine if strengthening is required. The levator ani and other pelvic floor muscles are similar in structure to any other skeletal muscle in the body and, therefore, should be rehabilitated in the same manner. Similarly, without an accurate diagnosis of muscle activity, the plan of care may potentially increase rather than decrease symptoms.[26] Pelvic floor physical therapy should therefore not be associated with automatic instruction in the "Kegel" exercise for all patients, regardless of their type of muscle dysfunction (**Fig. 3**).

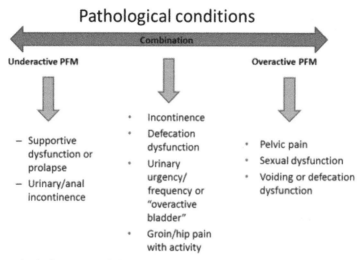

Pathological conditions

Combination

Underactive PFM

Overactive PFM

− Supportive dysfunction or prolapse

− Urinary/anal incontinence

- Incontinence
- Defecation dysfunction
- Urinary urgency/ frequency or "overactive bladder"
- Groin/hip pain with activity

- Pelvic pain
- Sexual dysfunction
- Voiding or defecation dysfunction

Fig. 3. Muscle dysfunction and development of pathology. PFM, pelvic floor muscles.

Physical therapy treatment of acute or CPP is directed toward immediate pain management, correcting musculoskeletal problems and postural malalignment with strategies to correct muscle length and aid in flexibility while improving the ability of the muscle to relax. Although this review more commonly describes pain in women, CPP can occur in men as well, with the same sequelae of dysfunction. Treatment can differ in that the levator ani muscle is treated intrarectally, but the guiding principles are the same.

Postural Correction and Muscle Flexibility Restoration

Postural correction and muscle flexibility restoration are required to reduce the recurring pattern of passive strain across the lower trunk, pelvic girdle, and hip intrinsic musculature. Typical posture in standing as related to pelvic pain includes exaggerated thoracic kyphosis and lumbar lordosis, anterior pelvic tilt, and external rotation of the hips. The patient benefits from learning correct postural alignment and symmetry for sitting and standing with encouragement to make these posture corrections habit. In the case of coccydynia, the patient often sits off to one side, further facilitating muscle maladaptation.

Treatment involves muscle length restoration of muscle groups that are typically shortened, including the abdominals, quadratus lumborum, lumbar extensors, hip internal and external rotators, hip adductors, hip flexors, hip extensors, hamstrings, and even the plantar flexors of the lower leg. When lower extremity and hip muscles are shortened, they exert an unequal force on the pelvic girdle. This increases involvement of the pelvic floor stabilizers, thereby potentially placing strain on the lumbosacral spine, leading to altered activity in the lumbar extensors and abdominals. This strain continues up the kinetic chain to the head and neck. Stretching exercises directed at the involved muscle groups are integral to normalize posture and joint motion in restoring strength and mobility.

Specific stretching of the pelvic floor muscles that are imbedded within the bony pelvis offers a particular challenge. Instruction in deep and sustained squats up to 60 seconds, for instance, can decrease the tension and tightness of the levator ani muscles, but caution must be taken to position the squat to allow for relaxation rather than contraction of the levator ani. As previously mentioned, the levator ani is the inferior border of the trunk stabilizers, so strength and stabilization training involving contracting the pelvic floor muscles may, in fact, exacerbate symptoms.

Some forms of strength training that facilitate a short pelvic floor, particularly those that call for transverse abdominal concentric contractions or "core training," may need to be temporarily suspended until muscle length restoration is complete.[27] Continued strengthening of these stabilizing muscle groups can, therefore, become a pain generator and are to be avoided during rehabilitation of the short pelvic floor. Specific yoga positions are helpful during the transition from muscle lengthening to trunk stabilization in maintaining pelvic floor muscle flexibility when muscle length has been maximally restored.

BIOFEEDBACK TRAINING

Pelvic floor patients are often referred with a prescription for biofeedback training. Biofeedback has been defined as "a group of experimental procedures where an external sensor is used to give an indication on bodily processes, usually in the purpose of changing the measured quality."[28] A variety of biofeedback apparatuses designed for pelvic floor training are available to the therapist, and portable biofeedback devices are also available, which can be used as home units for patient practice. High-tech devices are not always necessary, though, because biofeedback can be as simple as the use of a mirror.

Physician orders calling for biofeedback as the sole mode of treatment can imply instrumentation repeated over time as the complete means to solve muscle dysfunction. This technique is often confused with the works by A.H. Kegel (1948), where the emphasis was on strength training of the pelvic floor muscles. Biofeedback for strength training used in isolation can be detrimental in the treatment of the overactive levator ani muscles. However, biofeedback can instead be used to note when the muscles are relaxing well.[29] Surface electromyography (sEMG) using intravaginal sensors, intrarectal sensors, or surface sensors map the motor recruitment of the muscle and activity level. Decreasing pain and overactivity of pelvic floor muscles centers around reducing electrical activity in the overactive muscle as the patient is receiving an ongoing visual, auditory, or tactile feedback. Biofeedback is best used as an adjunct component of a comprehensive treatment plan, and should not be thought of as the sole or even most important aspect of a pelvic floor physical therapy prescription (**Fig. 4**).

As the patient improves, their understanding of how to relax can be carried over functionally for use in reducing pain with sexual dysfunction, prolonged sitting, and muscle coordination for voiding and other activities. This emphasis on reducing muscle over activity is called "down-training." Down-training encompasses many techniques to improve and retrain relaxation of a muscle contraction, which may include any of the following:

- Reducing muscle activity during a sEMG session,
- Diaphragmatic breathing,
- Visualization to encourage relaxation,
- Perineal bulges for conscious lengthening of the pelvic floor muscles,[30] and
- Thermotherapy to improve circulation, healing, and soft tissue extensibility.

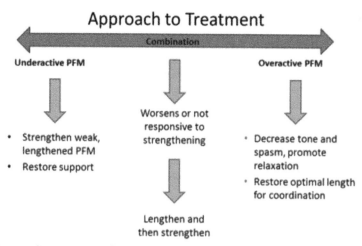

Fig. 4. Approach to treatment by muscle dysfunction present. PFM, pelvic floor muscles.

MANUAL THERAPY, MYOFASCIAL RELEASE, AND TRIGGER POINT MASSAGE

Soft tissue mobilization and myofascial and connective tissue release are used to improve circulation, restore tissue integrity, decrease ischemia, and decrease adverse neural tension of peripheral nerve branches. Skin rolling along the anatomic pathway of the pudendal nerve and other peripheral nerves in the pelvic region can improve neural flexibility and decrease stretch tension. Joint mobilization or muscle energy techniques may be used to restore motion by placing the lumbar spine, pelvic girdle, and hip joints in their ideal positions for optimal mobility or, in the case of the sacroiliac joint, optimal shock absorption.

In many states, physical therapist practice includes intramuscular dry needling when the noninvasive manual approaches are limited. This involves the use of small needles to deactivate trigger points and improve local and referred pain to loosen shortened muscles.

THERAPEUTIC EXERCISE

Therapeutic exercise is also incorporated into treatment, but prescribed for very specific muscles to promote posture and joint muscle balance while avoiding exacerbation of pelvic floor muscle overactivity and the recurrence of pain. Of course, after the muscle tissue length has been restored and the patient is proficient in completely relaxing these once overactive muscles, if true weakness persists, levator ani strengthening is then performed in a very controlled manner. Usually, sEMG biofeedback is added as an adjunct to ensure full relaxation of the involved muscles after recruitment for a certain exercise.

DESENSITIZATION

Physical therapy treatment can also help to reduce the effects of nervous system sensitization with desensitization techniques involving light touch, graded motor imagery[31] techniques, and progressive relaxation meditation in promoting further muscle relaxation by interrupting the reflexive protective muscle contraction brought on by the perception of stress and anxiety. The emotional connection cannot be ignored, as discussed previously concerning the concept of central sensitization. Exercises have been developed to assist with desensitization by restoring the normal pathways of the communication between sensory receptors and the brain. Desensitization is most effective when introduced gradually, including visualization exercises to improve tolerance to touch in a painful region without eliciting an emotional reaction. Partner exercise is also taught and encouraged. Relaxation techniques to overcome the sympathetic response of flight or fight can be taught to normalize limbic responses.[32] Again, sEMG biofeedback is useful during desensitization techniques, particularly with regard to sexual dysfunction. Although simple relaxation techniques may be enough, these more involved techniques can be helpful. A full description of these techniques, however, is beyond the scope of this review.

PHYSICAL THERAPY TECHNIQUES FOR SEXUAL DYSFUNCTION

Physical therapy for sexual dysfunction requires creating a supportive setting with privacy and emotional support to evaluate, treat, and educate the patient. If the practitioner is able to convey an understanding of the pelvic anatomy and the musculoskeletal involvement that plays a role in difficult vaginal penetration and avoidance behaviors, the patient will often feel reassured and be more amenable to participation in treatment.[33] Painful conditions that limit a woman's sexual function include dyspareunia, vulvar pain, and vulvodynia. Dyspareunia can, at least in part, develop after tissue damage from vaginal births, trauma, or surgery. The goals of physical therapy in the treatment of sexual dysfunction typically include the following[34]:

- Desensitization of soft tissues,
- Normalization of muscle activity and compliance,
- Improve muscle discrimination and muscle relaxation,
- Improved elasticity of the introital tissues,
- Reduction of fear associated with vaginal penetration, and
- Referral to sex therapy/counseling as appropriate.

Manual therapy techniques include Thiele's massage, scar and connective tissue mobilization, and the use of dilator therapy to stretch both the superficial and deep muscles of the pelvic floor. Thiele's massage can be used intravaginally or intrarectally to stretch the levator ani muscles and reduce scar tissue or trigger points and reduce pain with intercourse.[35] Vaginal and anal dilator sets have a variety of increasing sizes to stretch and desensitize muscles. Dilators have been especially helpful in the treatment of dyspareunia in women.[36] Dilators are also helpful in patients with CPP, both women and men, used as a form of graded exposure in helping to reduce functional, social, and relationship-associated limitations that are common in chronic pain.[37] Both vaginal and anal dilators are available, allowing for a home self-management program for both male and female patients. Perineal massage and manual desensitization are techniques taught for improving perineal length in preparation for vaginal child birth delivery, but can be used to decrease vulvodynia and dyspareunia.

The patient is taught home methods to use a finger sweep and sustained pressure with or without dilators to stretch vaginal muscles. Recommended lubricants, warm baths, and often a mirror are helpful for self-care instruction. A partner may be taught to assist with this these techniques and this may help to address intimacy issues and provide a treatment plan that feels supportive for the client.

LIFESTYLE AND BEHAVIOR MODIFICATIONS

Additionally, increasing activity (such as walking and other cardiovascular exercise) can play a role in recovery via improvement of blood flow and release of the body's natural endorphins, leading to a reduction of chronic pain. Lifestyle and behavioral modifications are often used to help the patient minimize factors that aggravate their symptoms. This may include exercise modification, dietary changes including caffeine reduction and increased water intake, hygiene recommendations, and skin protection. This may also include education on healthy bowel and bladder habits, body mechanics to optimize posture to facilitate voiding, and bowel and bladder training. When patients understand the benefit of these changes, willingness to modify behavior increases.

EVIDENCE FOR PELVIC FLOOR PHYSICAL THERAPY

The addition of pelvic floor physical therapy to treatment has been shown to be beneficial for many conditions related to CPP. Zoorob and colleagues[38] noted a greater than 50% improvement with reduced pelvic pain in patients receiving intravaginal manual treatment as well as patients receiving levator ani muscle trigger point injections. There was, however, a 0% dropout rate for those receiving the manual treatment compared with a 30% dropout rate for those receiving the trigger point injections. In 2012, FitzGerald and colleagues[39] noted an improvement in 59% of female participants with CPP receiving pelvic floor myofascial therapy as compared with only 26% of those receiving global massage for relaxation. In 2013, FitzGerald and colleagues[40] included men in a repeat study that showed similar results of 57% improvement in the myofascial pelvic floor physical therapy group compared with only 21% improvement in those receiving global massage. More specifically concerning coccydynia, a recent retrospective study noted a 62% mean improvement in average pain ratings with the addition of pelvic floor physical therapy to traditional medical interventions with treatment, including both internal and external myofascial release, biofeedback-guided pelvic floor muscle relaxation, perineal bulges, diaphragm breathing, posture corrections, and use of dilators and a therapy wand as a part of the home program of self-management.[41] More research, including additional prospective trials, is certainly needed to clarify the role of pelvic physical therapy for patients with pelvic pain.

SUMMARY

Skilled pelvic floor therapists possess a wide range of successful techniques to treat chronic pain. Working to normalize muscle activity for patients with pelvic floor pain is the key component of treatment. Tissue lengthening, muscle function restoration, and the ability to improve relaxation are required for successful reduction of overactivity symptoms and managing pain in the pelvic region. The physical therapist is an integral part of the chronic pain team of specialists who ensure effective treatment and restoration of function to the musculoskeletal and neuromuscular systems.[42]

REFERENCES

1. Bo D, Berghmans B, Morkved S, et al. Evidence-based physical therapy for the pelvic floor. Philadelphia: Churchill Livingstone; 2007.
2. Nygaard I, Barber MD, Burgio KL, et al. Prevalence of symptomatic pelvic floor disorders in US women. JAMA 2008;300(11):1311–6.
3. Krieger JN, Ross SO, Riley DE. Chronic prostatitis: epidemiology and role of infection. Urology 2002;60(Suppl 6):8–12.
4. Anothaisintawee T, Attia J, Nickel JC, et al. Management of chronic prostatitis/chronic pelvic pain syndrome: a systematic review and network meta-analysis. JAMA 2011;305(1):78–86.

5. Nee R, Butler D. Management of peripheral neuropathic pain: integrating neuro-biology, neurodynamics, and clinical evidence. Phys Ther Sport 2006;7:36–49.

6. Butler D, Moseley L. Explain pain. Adelaide (Australia): Noigroup Publications; 2003.

7. Vachon-Presseau E, Roy M, Martel MO, et al. The stress model of chronic pain: evidence from basal cortisol and hippocampal structure and function in humans. Brain 2013;136(Pt 3):815–27.

8. Bhattacherjee A, Karim Rumi MA, Staecker H, et al. Bone morphogenetic protein 4 mediates estrogen-regulated sensory axon plasticity in the adult female reproductive tract. J Neurosci 2013;33(3):1050–61.

9. Prendergast SA, Rummer EH. Pelvic pain explained: what everyone needs to know. Lanham (MD): Rowman & Littlefield; 2016.

10. Wijma AJ, van Wilgen CP, Meeus M, et al. Clinical biopsychosocial physiotherapy assessment of patients with chronic pain: the first step in pain neuroscience education. Physiother Theor Pract 2016;32(5):368–84.

11. Tu FF, As-Sanie S, Steege JF. Prevalence of pelvic musculoskeletal disorders in a female chronic pelvic pain clinic. J Reprod Med 2006;51:185–9.

12. Prather H, Camacho-Soto A. Musculoskeletal etiologies of pelvic pain. Obstet Gynecol Clin North Am 2014;41:433–42.

13. Mowers EL, Lim CS, Skinner B, et al. Prevalence of endometriosis during abdominal or laparoscopic hysterectomy for chronic pelvic pain. Obstet Gynecol 2016; 127(6):1045–53.

14. Section on Women's Health ATPA. Available at: http://www.womenshealthapta.org/about-us-sowh/. Accessed August 14, 2016.

15. Bi X, Zhao J, Zhao L, et al. Pelvic floor muscle exercise for chronic low back pain. J Int Med Res 2013;41(1):146–52.

16. Tuttle LJ, DeLozier ER, Harter KA, et al. The role of the obturator internus muscle in pelvic floor function. J Women's Health Phys Ther 2016;40(1):15–9.

17. Lee D. The pelvic girdle. 4th edition. Philadelphia: Churchill Livingstone; 2011.

18. Gordon AM, Huxley AF, Julian FJ. The variation in isometric tension with sarcomere length in vertebrate muscle fibres. J Physiol 1966;184:170–92.

19. Weiss JM. Pelvic floor myofascial trigger points: manual therapy for interstitial cystitis and the urgency-frequency syndrome. J Urol 2001;166(6):2226–31.

20. FitzGerald MP, Kotarinos R. Rehabilitation of the short pelvic floor. I: background and patient evaluation. Int Urogynecol J 2003;14:261–8.

21. Cozean N, Cozean J. The interstitial cystitis solution. Beverly (MA): Quarto Publishing Group; 2016.

22. Hilton S, Vandyken C. The puzzle of pelvic pain: a rehabilitation framework for balancing tissue dysfunction and central sensitization, I: pain physiology and evaluation for the physical therapist. J Women's Health Phys Ther 2011;35(3): 103–13.

23. DiNoto PM, Newman L, Wall S, et al. The homunculus: what is known about the representation of the female body in the brain? Cereb Cortex 2013;23:1005–13.

24. Van der Velde J, Everaerd W. The relationship between involuntary pelvic floor muscle activity, muscle awareness and experienced threat in women with and without vaginismus. Behav Res Ther 2001;39(4):395–408.

25. Guide to physical therapy practice. Phys Ther 2001;81:9–744.

26. Strauhal MJ, Frahm J, Morrison P, et al. Vulvar pain: a comprehensive review. J Women's Health Phys Ther 2007;31(3):7–26.

27. FitzGerald MP, Kotarinos R. Rehabilitation of the short pelvic floor. II: treatment of the patient with the short pelvic floor. Int Urogynecol J Pelvic Floor Dysfunct 2003; 14(4):269–75.

28. Schwartz G, Beatty J. Biofeedback: theory and research. New York: Academic Press; 1977.

29. Chiarioni G, Nardo A, Vantini I, et al. Biofeedback is superior to electrogalvanic stimulation and massage for treatment of levator ani syndrome. Gastroenterology 2010;138:1321–9.

30. Laycock J, Haslam J. Therapeutic management of incontinence and pelvic pain. New York: Springer-Verlag; 2002.

31. Moseley GL, Butler DS, Beames TB, et al. The graded motor imagery handbook. Adelaide (Australia): Noigroup Publications; 2012.

32. Zhao L, Wu H, Zhou X, et al. Effects of progressive muscular relaxation training on anxiety, depression and quality of life of endometriosis patients under gonadotrophin-releasing hormone agonist therapy. Eur J Obstet Gynecol Reprod Biol 2012;162:211–5.

33. Rosenbaum TY. Physiotherapy treatments of sexual pain disorder. J Sex Marital Ther 2005;31:329–40.

34. Oliveria CB, Pinto RA, Franco MR. Walking exercise for chronic musculoskeletal pain. Br J Sports Med 2016. http://dx.doi.org/10.1136/bjsports-2016-096245.

35. Oyama IA, Rejba A, Lukban JC, et al. Modified Thiele massage as intervention for female patients with interstitial cystitis and high tone pelvic floor dysfunction. Urology 2004;64(5):862–5.

36. Idama TO, Pring DW. Vaginal dilator therapy – an outpatient gynaecological option in the management of dyspareunia. J Obstet Gynaecol 2000;20(3):303–5.

37. Hilton L, Hempel S, Ewing BA, et al. Mindfulness medication for chronic pain: systematic review and meta-analysis. Ann Behav Med 2017;51(2):199–213.

38. Zoorob D, South M, Karram M, et al. A pilot randomized trial of levator injections versus physical therapy for treatment of pelvic floor myalgia and sexual pain. Int Urogynecol J 2015;26:845–52.

39. FitzGerald MP, Payne CK, Lukacz ES, et al. Randomized multicenter clinical trial of myofascial physical therapy in women with interstitial cystitis/painful bladder syndrome and pelvic floor tenderness. J Urol 2012;187:2113–8.

40. FitzGerald MP, Anderson RU, Potts J, et al. Randomized multicenter feasibility trial of myofascial physical therapy for the treatment of urological chronic pelvic pain syndromes. J Urol 2013;189:S75–85.

41. Scott KM, Fisher LW, Bernstein IH, et al. The treatment of chronic coccydynia and postcoccygectomy pain with pelvic floor physical therapy. Phys Med Rehabil 2016. http://dx.doi.org/10.1016/j.pmrj.2016.08.007.

42. Prendergast SA, Weiss JM. Screening for musculoskeletal causes of pelvic pain. Clin Obstet Gynecol 2003;46(6):773–82.

Iatrogenic Pelvic Pain

Surgical and Mesh Complications

Dominic Lee, MBBS, FRACS (Urology)[a], John Chang, MBBS[a],
Philippe E. Zimmern, MD[b],*

KEYWORDS

- Chronic pelvic pain • Vaginal mesh • Synthetic midurethral sling • Prolapse
- Stress urinary incontinence

KEY POINTS

- Chronic pelvic pain (CPP) from vaginal mesh is a diagnostic and management challenge that may require a multidisciplinary approach.
- CPP cannot always be cured, however a multimodal approach is required for optimal pain control and psychological support can be provided.
- The need for future large prospective cohort studies and national registries in assessing outcomes of patients following mesh/tape removal has never been more desirable.

INTRODUCTION

The increasing prevalence of stress urinary incontinence (SUI) and pelvic organ prolapse (POP) in our aging population has translated into an increased volume in surgical procedures among women afflicted with the condition. It is estimated that 1 in 8 women in the United States will require surgical management for SUI or POP by 80 years of age.[1]

In trying to offset the morbidity of more traditional reconstructive surgeries, such as the autologous pubovaginal sling for SUI or to lessen the recurrence rate of native tissue repair for POP, a range of synthetic mesh materials were gradually introduced in the market. Heavy promotion by the device companies offering various all inclusive "mesh-kits" have led to a significant uptake in surgeries by clinicians. In 210 alone, an estimated 210,000 women had placement of synthetic midurethral sling (MUS) for SUI treatment and 75,000 women had transvaginal mesh (TVM) placement for prolapse repair.[2,3]

The escalation of mesh-related complications, including mesh exposure, pain, dyspareunia, and revision surgeries, prompted the US Food and Drug Administration

The authors have nothing to disclose.
[a] Department of Urology, St George Hospital, Gray Street, Kogarah 2217, New South Wales, Australia; [b] Department of Urology, University of Texas Southwestern Medical Center, 5323 Harry Hines Boulevard, Dallas, TX 75390-9110, USA
* Corresponding author.
E-mail address: Philippe.zimmern@utsouthwestern.edu

(FDA) to issue safety communications for the use of TVM for POP in 2008,[2] and more recently in 2011.[3] The FDA safety notifications exempted MUS for SUI but these devices were not without complications either. Several issues were raised in the FDA report at the time including severity, incidence, and outcome results: "Serious complications associated with surgical mesh for transvaginal repair of POP are not rare." This is a change from what the FDA previously reported on October 20, 2008. Furthermore, it is not clear that transvaginal POP repair with mesh is more effective than traditional nonmesh repair in all patients with POP and it may expose patients to greater risk. Mesh-related complications seen in tertiary referral institutions have increased and their management has become more and more multifaceted and complicated; in fact it is now clear that the FDA warning "mesh erosion can require multiple surgeries to repair and can be debilitating for some women. In some cases, even multiple surgeries will not resolve the complication" was indeed accurate.

Furthermore, multidistrict litigations (MDLs) emerged against some of the device companies, reaching levels rarely seen before (approaching 100,000 in some reports). In March 27, 2013, the FDA updated the Urogynecologic Surgical Mesh Implant Web site to include more information for patients about SUI. At present, women electing to undergo a synthetic sling placement should have a thorough discussion with their surgeons on (1) the indication for using synthetic material, (2) how the surgeon trained to place such device, (3) which device specifically the surgeon was trained to place, (4) what might happen in terms of complications, and (5) who will deal with these complications should they happen. This detailed information has clearly changed the environment in caring for these patients.[4]

The incidence of requiring subsequent revision in patients with implanted mesh according to a recent Cochrane review was estimated at 7% to 18%.[5] Among these mesh-related complications, pelvic pain has proven to be extremely challenging to treat. Therefore, this review focuses on chronic pelvic pain (CPP) following synthetic mesh surgery.

VAGINAL AND URETHRAL NEURO-ANATOMY

The vagina is a highly vascular structure rich in nerve endings. Innervations to the vagina can be split into 2 parts: the upper third and the lower two-thirds. The upper two-thirds of the vagina is innervated in a visceral manner. The uterovaginal nerve plexus, which is derived from the inferior hypogastric plexus (IHP) and the pelvic splanchnic nerve (S2-S4) innervate the upper two-thirds of the vagina. The uterovaginal nerve plexus is found at the base of the broad ligament and forms a dense network on the lateral walls of the middle and proximal vagina. The uterovaginal nerve plexus carries sympathetic (T1-L2), parasympathetic (S2-S4), and visceral afferent fibers.[6,7] The lower third of the vagina is supplied by somatic innervations of the deep perineal nerve, which is a branch of the pudendal nerve (S2-S4). The deep perineal nerve carries sympathetic and visceral afferent fibers but lack any parasympathetic fibers. It fuses with autonomic nerves arising from the pelvic plexus (IHP) via the cavernous nerves of the clitoris and becomes the dorsal nerve of the clitoris (DNC) and runs on the medial aspect of the inferior pubic rami (IPR) to innervate the urethra and clitoris.[8]

Depending on the location of the mesh, either the deep perineal nerve, which carries the somatic sensation or the uterovaginal nerve plexus, which carries the vague autonomic mediated pain signals, may be injured, resulting in CPP.

Cadaveric studies by Achtari and colleagues[9] demonstrated the potential risks of 3 vaginal slings to the DNC in cadavers in which distances of a tension-free vaginal tape (TVT), in-out transobturator (TVT-O), and out-in transobturator (Monarc) varied from

19 mm to 40 mm, the TVT-O being the closest to the DNC. As the DNC courses along the medial side of the IPR, it could also potentially be damaged during obturator procedures, both outside in and inside out.

The obturator nerve and the pudendal nerve are particularly vulnerable to injury leading to neuralgia from pelvic prolapse or anti-incontinence sling surgeries, as these structures are in close proximity to the trocar passage of the device kits.

Obturator Nerve

The obturator nerve is a major lower limb nerve derived from the anterior division of L2-L4 nerve roots and enters the pelvis along the obturator foramen and exits into the thigh anterosuperiorly along a 2- to 3-cm oblique tunnel, the obturator canal, and splits into anterior and posterior divisions. It innervates the medial (adductor) compartment of the thigh and skin of the medial thigh. The obturator nerve can be damaged during surgery involving the pelvis or abdomen resulting in pain or numbness and paresthesia on the medial aspect of the thigh and/or posture and gait problems due to the loss of thigh adduction.

Pudendal Nerve

The pudendal nerve arises from the anterior division of ventral rami of S2-4 nerves of the sacral plexus. It exits from the pelvis via the greater sciatic foramen, below the piriformis muscle. It then turns forward around the sacrospinous ligament just medial to the ischial spine as it passes through the lesser sciatic foramen and runs along the pudendal canal and divides into the (1) inferior rectal nerve, (2) perineal nerve, and (3) DNC, which supplies the clitoris. Damage to the nerve most commonly from sacrospinous fixation or mesh kits for prolapse or trocar injury from MUS can result in pudendal neuralgia.[10–12] **Fig. 1** illustrate the large amount of synthetic mesh with multiple sling arms in a Prolift total mesh kit.

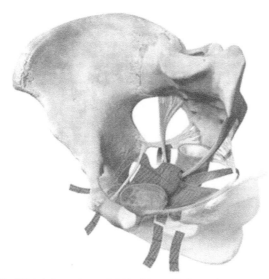

Fig. 1. Gynecare Prolift total repair mesh kit with multiple mesh arms and large surface area of mesh.

ETIOLOGY OF PAIN RELATED TO MESH PLACEMENT

The lack of consensus on the definition of CPP, apart from site and duration of symptoms, compromises the estimation of prevalence within the community. Most centers define CPP as persistent pain in the pelvis lasting more than 6 months.[13] The etiology is varied and can include gynecological, gastrointestinal, urologic, myofascial, musculoskeletal, and/or psychosomatic causes. **Box 1** provides a list of possible causes of CPP.

A large US population study survey on prevalence, economic burden, and health care utilization reported that 1 in 7 women aged between 18 and 50 years was affected by CPP within the past 3 months. Not surprisingly, those who reported CPP had significantly lower mean scores for general health than those who did not (70.5 vs 78.8, $P<.05$), and 61% of those with CPP had no known etiology. The estimated direct medical costs for outpatient visits for CPP was \$881.5 million per year; and among women

---

Box 1
Differential diagnoses of chronic pelvic pain

Gynecologic disease including the following:

- Endometriosis
- Adhesions (chronic pelvic inflammatory disease)
- Leiomyoma

Gastrointestinal disease including the following:

- Constipation
- Irritable bowel syndrome
- Diverticular disease
- Meckel diverticulum

Genitourinary disease including the following:

- Interstitial cystitis
- Vaginal mesh
- Chronic urethritis

Myofascial disease including the following:

- Fasciitis
- Nerve entrapment syndrome
- Herniae (inguinal, femoral, spigelian, umbilical, and incisional)

Skeletal disease including the following:

- Scoliosis
- Spondylolisthesis
- Osteitis pubis

Psychological disorders including the following:

- Somatization
- Psychosexual dysfunction (sexual abuse)
- Depression

in employment, 15% reported time lost from paid work and 45% reported reduced work productivity.[14]

CPP is not unique to transvaginal mesh repairs and is present after native tissue repairs as well. Recent systematic review and meta-analysis of native tissue repair reported a 4% rate of denovo dyspareunia[15] and a recent Cochrane review has shown no difference in dyspareunia with anterior mesh versus native tissue anterior repair.[5]

The incidence of chronic pelvic pain attributable to transvaginal mesh surgery is highly variable and is estimated to be between 0% and 30% based on case-series and small randomized control trials.[5,16] With regard to POP mesh complications, the FDA 2011 update stated that serious complications were "not rare,"[3] and mesh exposure rates after transvaginal mesh POP repairs were estimated at 10%.[5] A review by Daneshgari and colleagues[17] on synthetic sling complications reported adverse outcomes ranging from 4.3% to 75.1% for retropubic and 10.5% to 31.3% for transobturator MUS. The complications were wide ranging including viscus (bladder and bowel injury), vascular injury, vaginal extrusion, de novo urgency and urge incontinence, urinary tract infections (UTIs), dyspareunia/pelvic pain, and voiding dysfunction. A more recent review article by Shah and Badlani[18] over a 3-year period from 2008 to 2011 reported a composite MUS erosion/extrusion rate of 0% to 7.6%, dyspareunia 0% to 6.2%, and overall pelvic/groin pain 0% to 16.6%, respectively. Prevalent pain symptoms included dyspareunia; pelvic, vaginal, or buttock pain related to the distribution of the obturator or pudendal nerve; and most women were polysymptomatic reporting combinations of these symptoms.

Our understanding of the pathophysiology of iatrogenic CPP provoked by mesh placement either for incontinence or pelvic prolapse surgery is unclear. CPP may arise from trauma to any structure in or related to the pelvis, including the abdominal and pelvic walls,[19] and not uncommonly the cause of pain is multifactorial. **Box 2** outlines the potential mechanisms of mesh-induced pain.

Vaginal pain may be associated with changes that can occur with mesh contraction, retraction, or shrinkage, resulting in taut sections of mesh on the anchoring tissue, which is estimated at 11.7% based on large retrospective studies.[20] Due to the heterogeneity of studies published regarding iatrogenic mesh pain, it has not been possible to pinpoint the exact etiology of mesh contractures. Some would argue that the type of mesh used could be an important factor of iatrogenic pelvic pain. The prevalent mesh type used today is type 1 polypropylene, as it is a softer, lighter, monofilament in nature. But most importantly it is macroporous (pore size >75 μm). Theoretically, this important feature promotes a host–graft response that ultimately results in collagen in-growth and immune system–cell migration through the membrane to counter

---

Box 2
Etiology of chronic pelvic pain from mesh

1. Mesh contracture/shrinkage

2. Exposure and/or erosion

3. Mesh infection

4. Nerve entrapment (obturator/pudendal nerve)

5. Obstruction (sling)

6. Fistula

bacterial invasion and allows integration of the mesh material with the natural tissue.[21] However, no mesh is immune from the process of shrinkage or contracture.

It has been shown that the inorganic mesh materials commonly use cause a more intense inflammatory response than organic mesh (such as porcine dermis). Zheng and colleagues[22] in animal studies with rats have shown that Prolene meshes produce twice as much inflammation than the porcine dermis group. This inflammatory reaction (oxidative stress) causes free radical damage to the mesh and in turn causes more inflammation and results in mesh contraction and local fibrosis.[23] Perhaps it is the same inflammatory reaction that also gives the patient the side effect of pain as evident in abdominal wall or thoracic wall hernia mesh contractions.[24,25] To counter argue with the mesh contracture theory, some patients with clinically evident mesh contractures can be completely asymptomatic.[26]

If there are mesh erosions, the associated pain also could be from the ulceration of vaginal tissue or other complications to pelvic organs such as the bladder or rectum.[27] Pelvic organ fistula is another potential cause for iatrogenic pelvic pain following mesh repair surgeries. Other causes of pelvic pain after mesh placement include pelvic floor muscle spasms, nerve involvement (pudendal),[10] and infection.[28] Mesh infection has been contentious, as the rate of clinical sepsis following mesh implantation is low in the published literature with a reported incidence of 1%.[29,30] Vaginal epithelium is a clean contaminated field and thus mesh colonization on implantation is a genuine hazard. Recently Mellano and colleagues[31] evaluated their cohort of women undergoing synthetic MUS excision. Each patient's excised mesh was sent for microbiological culture and of the 107 cases reported, the positive culture rate was 82% (77 patients) and potential pathogens were isolated in 37% (40 patients). The presenting symptoms in this cohort were heterogeneous, including most commonly pelvic pain, mesh extrusion, voiding dysfunction, and recurrent UTIs and according to the investigators, persistent subclinical mesh infections were the raison d'être for the clinical presentation.[31]

A further confounding factor is the delayed onset of mesh related pain, which results in underreporting and thus make deciphering the cause even more difficult. Adding to this layer of complexity is the prevalence of psychological diagnoses apparent in up to 60% of women referred for CPP. They include depression (25%–50%), somatoform disorders (10%–20%), anxiety disorders (10%–20%), and multiple psychological diagnoses (20%–30%).[32] It is of note that although CPP is often associated with substantial psychosocial impact, the identification of psychosocial factors as cause or effect remains problematic.[33] Thus, each patient must be carefully assessed and managed accordingly.

EVALUATIONS/APPROACH TO DIAGNOSIS

Assessment of a woman presenting with CPP after mesh placement requires a multi-system approach. It is important to take a detailed pain history, including its nature, severity, quality, location, site of radiation, duration, and aggravating and relieving factors. In particular, its relation to the menstrual cycle; bowel, urinary, and sexual functions; and physical activity, and its impact on activities of daily living including work and personal relationships is vital.

The site of radiation of the pain can inform on the origin of the pain; for example, vaginal pathologies may refer pain to the low back or buttock, whereas nerve entrapment with pudendal or obturator neuralgia generally has pain localized to one side and refers to the buttock and/or medial aspect of the thigh. Associated symptoms particularly vaginal discharge, bleeding, dyspareunia, and recurrent urinary tract infections may indicate the presence of mesh exposure and/or erosion.

A thorough review of systems related to the possible causes of CPP (genitourinary, gynecologic, gastrointestinal, neurologic, and musculoskeletal) is required. Psychiatric causes for pain also should not be forgotten. Smoking status, advanced age, and early resumption of sex also should be noted, as they have been shown to be significant factors in mesh exposure.[27,34] These are all important questions that could provide insight to where the specific problems lie. Whether patients had pelvic pain or dyspareunia before mesh implantation also should be clarified, as the mesh implantation may exacerbate but not be the sole cause of pain.

It is then vital to perform a physical examination, in particular a detailed pelvic examination using a speculum to systematically examine all compartments of the vagina for any mesh exposure or signs of infection or fistula. Any areas of focal tenderness over the vaginal epithelium that could indicate mesh contraction, or excessive tension on the underlying mesh should be noted. Specific areas of trigger point pelvic floor muscle tenderness or increased muscle tone, especially of levator ani, bulbocavernous, obturator, and perineal body may suggest underlying pelvic floor muscle spasms. A periurethral band is often felt in an overtly tight transobturator midurethral sling.[20] The presence or absence of atrophic vaginitis, vaginal discharge, fluctuant masses, adnexal thickening, and fixation of any structures also should be noted. An office vaginoscopy, if tolerated, can be informative (**Fig. 2**). Concurrently, a rectal examination also should be undertaken to assess for rectal involvement with integrity of anal sphincter and evidence of mesh protrusion. Oftentimes the patient's pain may be so severe that a detailed pelvic examination is impossible, and this needs to be deferred and conducted under general anesthesia.

The investigations performed for women presenting with CPP is largely dictated by the history and physical examination findings. It is reasonable, however, to support the use of the following basic laboratory studies in most women presenting with CPP:

- Complete blood count
- Serum chemistry
- Urine microscopy, culture, and sensitivity
- Vaginal swab if discharge is present

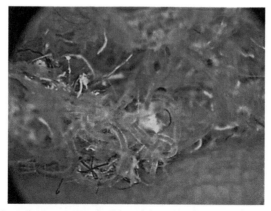

Fig. 2. Case 1. This patient presented with pelvic pain after mesh surgery but had severe pain on pelvic examination so that the vault of her vagina was overlooked. She was able to tolerate an office vaginoscopy, which revealed left-sided vaginal apical mesh erosion (magnified view with flexible scope). This case illustrates the utility of a simple office-based procedure that led to the missed diagnosis.

Other selected imaging studies may include the following:

- Ultrasound scan (USS) of the pelvis (in particular, translabial USS) to evaluate for mesh location
- Computed tomography (CT) to evaluate for abscess or visceral injury
- MRI to evaluate for soft tissue edema/abscess associated with pelvic mesh

Input from our radiology colleagues as part of a multidisciplinary approach is vital in the assessment of mesh burden and its associated complications. This bipartisan relationship as highlighted by Khatri and colleagues[35] facilitates the best possible evaluation before surgical exploration. For MUS, the mesh in the suburethral space is best visualized using an ultrasound. But for retropubic and transobturator sling arms and vaginal prolapse mesh kits in general, an MRI study is more helpful, as it can image the more peripheral aspects of the mesh[35] (**Fig. 3**).

Cystoscopy can be useful for patients with complaints of hematuria, recurrent UTI, or pelvic pain symptoms suggestive of fistula and/or mesh erosion through the urethral or bladder wall. Vaginoscopy can be done with a flexible scope after the completion of the cystoscopy to carefully examine the vaginal wall surface and each sulcus for mesh exposure, especially if there is a specific area of pain or the patient's partner has complained of hispareunia and has noted scratches on one side or another of the penis (**Fig. 4**). Urodynamics may be necessary if bladder outlet obstruction from sling is suspected. Other causes of pelvic pain should be investigated and excluded as necessary.

Patients may therefore require additional procedures to exclude other causes of pelvic pain including the following:

- Diagnostic laparoscopy for gynecologic pathology
- Sigmoidoscopy and/or colonoscopy to exclude bowel pathology

For that reason, several tertiary care centers dealing with CPP will have a dedicated multidisciplinary pelvic floor program that is ideal for the patient to have an easy access to various pelvic floor specialties and experts, and to know that these experts have an interest in evaluating and managing their CPP issues.

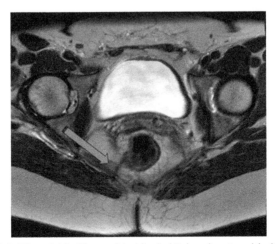

Fig. 3. MRI of pelvis. T2-weighted image-bladder (*white*) and rectum (*dark*). Arrow pointing to mesh remnant located alongside the right rectum wall.

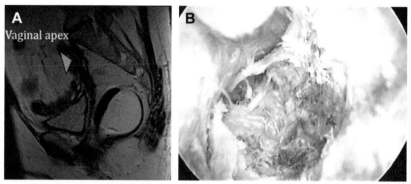

Fig. 4. Case 2. This woman presented with vaginal pain and discharge. Vaginal examination confirmed a very elongated vagina with no apparent abnormality. (*A*) MRI pelvis shows a stretched and elongated vagina with apex high up (rectum filled with gel). This patient proceeded to have an examination under anesthesia. (*B*) Intraoperative vaginoscopy reveals an exposed Ethibond suture beneath surrounding granulation tissues.

MANAGEMENT AND OUTCOMES

CPP from pelvic mesh surgeries are multifaceted problems with no consensus on management. Most outcome studies are from case series with varying treatment protocols and variable duration of follow-up. Specific identified causes of CPP should be treated according to medical guidelines. Conservative management include topical estrogen cream, topical antiseptic, and office-based trimmings of extruded mesh and optimization of pain with pain specialists with pelvic floor rehabilitation and trigger point injections, as appropriate.

The failure rate of conservative management for CPP secondary to mesh is significantly high. Success rates of conservative medical management for mesh extrusion is reported to be much lower. Only up to 42% of patients resolved with medical treatment alone[36] and most patients will proceed to have surgical intervention. The extent of mesh removal is not predictable depending on the individual but the ultimate goal is for maximal mesh excision within safety margins. Therefore, as outlined in the FDA mesh notifications of 2008/2011, mesh removal alone may not be curative and debilitating and life-altering changes may persist.[37]

Surgical Technique of Transvaginal Mesh Excision

The approach to mesh excision can be carried out either transabdominally or transvaginally. But there are obvious advantages to a transvaginal approach, as it carries less morbidity and can be performed safely and effectively.[38] There are multiple techniques that have been previously published.[38,39]

Success of mesh removal often depends on surgical experience in dealing with these complications and many patients travel great distances to tertiary referral centers for management.[40] Following lithotomy position, ureteral stents may be needed when the mesh is very close to the bladder wall or there is bladder base deformation noted on preoperative pelvic MRI. We routinely place a betadine-soaked rectal pack to help with identification of the lateral mesh arm dissection/excision, and detect small rectal wall tears. Our surgical technique is outlined in the next section. The vaginal incision can be an inverted U-shape for ease of access to the lateral pelvic sidewalls, or midline, or directed to one vaginal sulcus or another depending on the location of the pain or site of exposure and should allow for tissue interposition in case of intraoperative adjacent organ injury. Adequate thickness of the vaginal flaps must be maintained to prevent buttonhole or tearing of the flaps. The underlying mesh is grasped with an Ellis clamp and sharply dissected away from underlying tissue. Care is exercised to make sure the underlying viscus is not injured. Depending on whether an anterior mesh or posterior mesh is placed, it is vital to remember how the arms of the mesh will lie. For anterior mesh, the arms traverse the obturator foramen and the arcus tendineus fascia. Although in the posterior mesh, the arms will in addition travel through the ischiorectal fossa and terminate in the sacrospinous ligament.[18] It is important to excise as much mesh as possible when removing the mesh for the indication of pelvic pain.[19] Once maximal mesh excision is achieved, the bladder and rectum integrity is checked with repeat cystoscopy with dye to exclude ureteric injury and a rectal examination, respectively. The vagina is closed with absorbable sutures and a vaginal pack is inserted. Because of frequent lawsuits associated with mesh placement, it is best to document the procedure with intraoperative photographs whenever possible, and the extent and side of mesh removed at the conclusion of the procedure. All removed segments should be sent to pathology for documentation (**Figs. 5** and **6**).

Mesh erosions through the bladder and/or urethral wall can at times be treated with cystoscopy and Holmium laser ablation.[41] However, it is important to note that most mesh erosions are complicated and some may involve the bladder, urethra, or bowel. So because patients may require morbid procedures, such as laparotomies and temporary diversions, it is important to explain and clarify these risks during the consenting process.

Surgical Technique of Mid-urethral Sling Excision

Our technique has been previously described.[42] Following cystoscopy to exclude possible urethral erosion, a short transversal incision is made in the anterior vaginal wall following the natural vaginal wall ridges and over the course of the MUS. This exposure maximizes access to the lateral extensions of the MUS as compared with

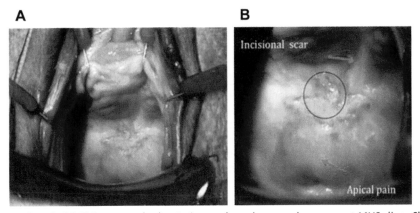

Fig. 5. Case 3. (*A*) This woman had anterior mesh prolapse and concurrent MUS sling. She reported pelvic pain, dyspareunia, and hispareunia. (*B*) On pelvic examination she had an incisional scar from MUS. Mesh exposure is visible in the midline (*circle*) explaining the hispareunia. Then, the apical pain prompted her request for complete mesh removal rather than just the exposed area.

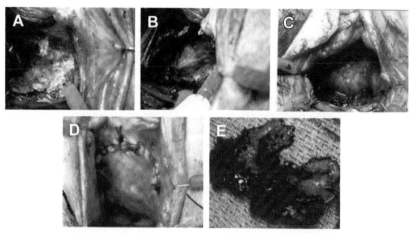

Fig. 6. Mesh excision surgery: this illustrates the steps of removal of anterior vaginal wall mesh kit from the previous case. (*A*) Mesh (*blue*) appears as dense, corrugated material following vaginal incision. (*B*) Mesh (superior right corner) dissected off the underlying bladder wall (*white*). (*C*) Complete mesh with free bladder wall. (*D*) Vaginal wall flap closure. (*E*) Excised large mesh fragments (*left* and *right*) from bladder base.

a vertical incision. Furthermore, this vaginal incision can be extended into an inverted U-shaped flap in case tissue interposition with a Martius fat pad graft and/or a fascial patch is needed should a urethral or bladder neck injury occur. Excision begins lateral to the urethra, at the 3 or 9 o'clock position, to minimize the risk of urethral injury directly at the undersurface of the urethra (6 o'clock). Once detached on one side of the urethra, the MUS is carefully dissected off the under surface of the urethra toward the contralateral side, staying close to the mesh. The lateral extensions of the MUS are removed as laterally (transobturator tape [TOT]) or superiorly (TVT) as possible toward the obturator fossa for a TOT or in the retropubic space for a TVT respectively. Urethro-cystoscopy is repeated to ensure that the urethral lumen is intact. The vaginal incision is closed in running absorbable layers.

MANAGEMENT AND OUTCOMES

The current literature is replete with single-center case study series with short-term follow-up in heterogeneous populations and a paucity of long-term outcomes after treatment of mesh complications.

In one of the earlier published series on contracted mesh removal, Feiner and Maher[43] reported that in 17 patients, 15 (88%) patients experienced a "substantial" reduction in vaginal pain, and 9 of 11 a substantial reduction in dyspareunia. But many women (22%–46%) had permanent quality-of-life–altering sequelae. Similar outcomes have been reported in other studies.[37,38,44] It is also not uncommon for patients to undergo repeated surgical procedures to rectify mesh complications.[45,46]

In a larger series with patients with TVM alone undergoing mesh excision, Crosby and colleagues reported an overall 51% (n = 43) resolution rate in 84 women with a median follow-up of 4 months (range 2.0–11.5). Of those presenting with mesh exposure, 95% were treated successfully in contrast to pain, which was only successfully treated in 51% of patients.[44] On a similar trend, Hokenstad and colleagues[47] reported a 54% success rate in a cohort of 68 women after mesh excision.

A larger mixed population case series by Hou and colleagues[48] on pain outcomes after mesh excision in 123 patients with prolapse mesh (69) and suburethral tape (54) reported pain-free status using an objective visual analogue scale (VAS) in 81% of tape and 67% of mesh cases, respectively. Similarly, Danford and colleagues[49] examined a larger cohort of 233 women who underwent vaginal mesh revision, excision or urethrolysis for pelvic pain (121 [65%] were sling alone and 66 [35%] had a concomitant prolapse procedure). They reported an overall improvement in 73%, whereas 19% reported no change in pain, and 18% reported worsened pain at a median follow-up of 12 months (range 1–120). Comparatively, those with mesh exposure (131 patients) were more likely to do better than those without (102 patients) (77% vs 67%) and were less likely to be worse after excision (5% vs 12%).[49] **Table 1** summarizes the outcomes of TVM excision.

With regard to MUS excision, **Table 2** summarizes the outcomes. Pain outcomes were variable and differed significantly from study to study. Hammett and colleagues recently reported on their series of 57 patients (26 slings, 23 transvaginal prolapse, 9 intraperitoneal prolapse) with mean follow-up of 6 weeks. Of those who had TVM excision, 95% had either complete or partial resolution of chronic pain but overall only 57.3% achieved complete symptom resolution, whereas 14.6% were improved.[50] From a multicenter retrospective study, Unger and colleagues[45] reported that 63% (19/30) improved, 30% (9/30) were worse, and 7% (2/30) reported no change in 30 of 101 patients who reported pelvic pain before intervention. Agnew and colleagues[51] reported on a 100% improvement in 8 of 47 women who underwent sling excision for pain alone. Mini-slings (SIMS) are not exempted from mesh complications. Misrai and colleagues[52] reported in one of the earlier series on sling excisions via a predominant laparoscopic approach and for those with CPP, there was 100% improvement. In a small series of 17 women in which 11 presented with pelvic pain alone, Coskun and colleagues[53] reported that 8 (73%) were cured or improved and 3 (27%) had persistent pain following sling excision. Of the 17 women, only 6 were considered "cured," with

Table 1
Outcomes following mesh excision for prolapse

Study	Symptoms	n	Intervention	Mean Follow-up, mo	Outcomes (Improved or Cured)/(%)
Danford et al,[49] 2015	Pelvic pain	233	Mesh excision/ revision	NR	73
Hou et al,[48] 2014	Pelvic pain	69	Mesh excision	22	67
Crosby et al,[44] 2014	Mesh extrusion	84	Mesh excision	4	95
	Pelvic pain	—		—	84
	Dyspareunia	—		—	84
Hammett et al,[50] 2014	Mesh extrusion	23	Mesh excision	1.5	100
	Pelvic pain	—		—	95
Lee et al,[37] 2013	Mesh extrusion	58	Mesh excision	13.3	100
	Pelvic pain	—		—	86
Tijdink et al,[27] 2011	Mesh extrusion	48	Mesh excision	6	92
	Pelvic pain	—		—	—
Feiner and Maher,[43] 2010	Pelvic pain	17	Mesh excision	6	88
	Dyspareunia	—		—	64

Abbreviation: NR, not reported.

Table 2
Outcomes following mid-urethral sling excision

Study	Symptoms	n	Intervention	Mean Follow-up, mo	Outcomes (Improved or Cured)/(%)
Coskun et al,[53] 2015	Pelvic pain	8	Sling excision	17	73
Hammett et al,[50] 2014	Chronic pain	22	Sling excision	1.5	95
	Dyspareunia/ hispareunia	—		—	42
	Urinary retention	—		—	100
	Urge incontinence	—		—	100
Agnew et al,[51] 2014	Mesh exposure/ extrusion	47	Sling excision	NR	100
	Vaginal/pelvic pain	—		—	100
	Mesh infection	—		—	100
Hou et al,[48] 2014	Chronic pain	55	Sling excision	35	81
Tijdink et al,[27] 2011	Mesh extrusion	15	Sling excision	6	92
	Pelvic pain	—		—	—
Misrai et al,[52] 2009	Mesh extrusion	75	Sling excision	38.4	100
	Mesh erosion	—	Transvaginal removal	—	100
	Urinary retention	—		—	82
	Chronic pain	—		—	100

Abbreviation: NR, not reported.

cure defined as continent, pain-free, and sexually active. Although suprapubic and groin pain are infrequent manifestations of MUS, some patients have requested total mesh removal at the time of surgery. The access to retropubic arms in a retropubic MUS can be challenging, and sometimes a combination transvaginal and retropubic approach is required. For this reason, many pelvic surgeons prefer a retropubic MUS, as complete removal of the MUS is achievable. On the contrary, removal of transobturator arms is more difficult and exacting and may even require a multidisciplinary surgical approach with the orthopedic team. Obturator foramen dissection for debilitating groin pain related to a transobturator mesh placement has been reported by Reynolds and colleagues.[54] In their series of 8 patients, obturator groin dissection was performed via a lateral groin incision over the inferior pubic ramus for women with intractable pain. In all cases, total excision was achieved and the mesh was noted to be deeply imbedded in the adductor longus muscle and tendon. Of these 8 patients, only 5 patients were cured of their pain.[54]

CONSERVATIVE MANAGEMENT OF CHRONIC PELVIC PAIN

If the previously described surgical excision has failed to rectify the patient's ongoing pain, then a multimodal therapy regimen may be considered. This consists of medications, pelvic floor muscle physiotherapy, and pudendal nerve blocks for patients with neuropathic-type pain. Gyang and colleagues[55] has provided a nice review and a management algorithm for mesh-related CPP.

No specific evidence is available to dictate which medication is most effective in the context of mesh complications. But it would be wise to start off with a stepwise approach, including paracetamol and nonsteroidal anti-inflammatory drugs, then possibly adding on[56] concurrent neuroleptics (Pregabalin, Gabapentin).

Pelvic floor muscle therapy also can be useful if there are components of pelvic floor muscle spasms as part of the CPP. If there are elements of nerve pain or pudendal nerve involvement, it can be effective to start the patient on oral neuroleptic or muscle relaxant, and concomitant pelvic floor muscle physiotherapy.[57] Failing that, a CT-guided Alcock canal pudendal nerve block with a local anesthetic can provide some relief[58] while confirming the diagnosis of pudendal neuralgia. Many tertiary centers benefit from the expertise of their physical medicine and rehabilitation and pelvic pain centers to administer these therapies.

COMPLICATIONS

Complications following removal of transvaginal mesh are related to the affected compartment. Other complications associated with mesh excision include large vaginal defects, possibly requiring skin grafting, residual pain that can be unremitting and life altering, and/or need for repeat surgery for secondary prolapse. In our TVM excision series of 58 women (mesh and tape) with a median of 13 months' follow-up, 17 (29%) required reexcision of residual mesh. Five women developed recurrent symptomatic POP (7%). The residual rate of dyspareunia and pelvic pain was 14% and 22%, respectively. Fourteen women (24%) were treated successfully, with complete resolution of all presenting symptoms.[37]

SUMMARY

The management of CPP from vaginal mesh is a challenge to patients and clinicians alike. Surgeries are often complicated and may require major reconstructive approaches. Unfortunately, cure is not always possible and women in these circumstances should be advised the pain can be managed and psychological support can be provided. For many women in these circumstances, a multidisciplinary approach to care and management produces the best results.

REFERENCES

1. Olsen AL, Smith VJ, Bergstrom JO, et al. Epidemiology of surgically managed pelvic organ prolapse and urinary incontinence. Obstet Gynecol 1997;89:501.
2. US Food and Drug Administration. FDA safety communication: update on serious complications associated with transvaginal placement of surgical mesh for pelvic organ prolapse. 2011. Available at: http://www.fda.gov/MedicalDevices/Safety/AlertsandNotices/ucm262435.htm. Accessed July 13, 2011.
3. FDA public health notification: serious complications associated with transvaginal placement of surgerical mesh in repair of pelvic organ prolase and stress urinary incontinence. 2008. Available at: http://www.fda.gov/MedicalDevices/Safety/AlertsandNotices/PublicHealthNotifications/ucm061976.htm. October 20, 2008.
4. Yanagisawa M, Rhodes M, Zimmern P. Mesh social networking: a patient-driven process. BJU Int 2011;108(10):1539–41.
5. Maher C, Feiner B, Baessler K, et al. Transvaginal mesh or grafts compared with native tissue repair for vaginal prolapse. Cochrane Database Syst Rev 2016;(2):CD012079.

6. Agur AM, Dalley AF. Grant's atlas of anatomy. Philadelphia: Lippincott Williams & Wilkins; 2009.

7. Zimmern PE, Chapple CC, Haab F, et al. Vaginal surgery for incontinence and prolapse. Berlin (Germany): Springer; 2006.

8. Bekker MD, Hogewoning CR, Wallner C, et al. The somatic and autonomic innervation of the clitoris; preliminary evidence of sexual dysfunction after minimally invasive slings. J Sex Med 2012;9(6):1566–78.

9. Achtari C, McKenzie BJ, Hiscock R, et al. Anatomical study of the obturator foramen and dorsal nerve of the clitoris and their relationship to minimally invasive slings. Int Urogynecol J Pelvic Floor Dysfunct 2006;17:330–4.

10. Sancak EB, Avci E, Erdogru T. Pudendal neuralgia after pelvic surgery using mesh: case reports and laparoscopic pudendal nerve decompression. Int J Urol 2016;23(9):797–800.

11. Maldonado PA, Chin K, Garcia AA, et al. Anatomic variations of pudendal nerve within pelvis and pudendal canal: clinical applications. Am J Obstet Gynecol 2015;213(5):727.

12. Fisher HW, Lotze PM. Nerve injury locations during retropubic sling procedures. Int Urogynecol J 2011;22(4):439–41.

13. Campbell F, Collett BJ. Chronic pelvic pain. Br J Anaesth 1994;73:571–3.

14. Mathias SD, Kuppermann M, Liberman RF, et al. Chronic pelvic pain: prevalence, health-related quality of life, and economic correlates. Obstet Gynecol 1996; 87(3):321–7.

15. Jha S, Gray T. A systematic review and meta-analysis of the impact of native tissue repair for pelvic organ prolapse on sexual function. Int Urogynecol J 2015;26:321–7.

16. Sentilhes L, Berthier A, Sergent F, et al. Sexual function in women before and after trans-vaginal mesh repair for pelvic organ prolapsed. Int Urogynecol J Pelvic Floor Dysfunct 2008;19:763–72.

17. Daneshgari F, Kong W, Swartz M. Complications of mid urethral slings: important outcomes for future clinical trials. J Urol 2008;180(5):1890–7.

18. Shah HN, Badlani GH. Mesh complications in female pelvic floor reconstructive surgery and their management: a systematic review. Indian J Urol 2012;28(2):129–53.

19. Moore J, Kennedy S. Causes of chronic pelvic pain. Best Pract Res Clin Obstet Gynaecol 2000;14:389–402.

20. Cholhan HJ, Hutchings TB, Rooney KE. Dyspareunia associated with paraurethral banding in the transobturator sling. Am J Obstet Gynecol 2010;202(5):481.

21. Silva WA, Karram MM. Scientific basis for use of grafts during vaginal reconstructive procedures. Curr Opin Obstet Gynecol 2005;17(5):519–29.

22. Zheng F, Lin Y, Verbeken E, et al. Host response after reconstruction of abdominal wall defects with porcine dermal collagen in a rat model. Am J Obstet Gynecol 2004;191(6):1961–70.

23. Costello CR, Bachman SL, Grant SA, et al. Characterization of heavyweight and lightweight polypropylene prosthetic mesh explants from a single patient. Surg Innov 2007;14(3):168–76.

24. Klosterhalfen B, Junge K, Klinge U. The lightweight and large porous mesh concept for hernia repair. Expert Rev Med Devices 2005;2(1):103–17.

25. Cappelletti M, Attolini G, Cangioni G, et al. The use of mesh in abdominal wall defects. Minerva Chir 1997;52(10):1169–76 [in Italian].

26. Hinoul P, Ombelet WU, Burger MP, et al. A prospective study to evaluate the anatomic and functional outcome of a transobturator mesh kit (prolift anterior) for symptomatic cystocele repair. J Minim Invasive Gynecol 2008;15(5):615–20.

27. Tijdink MM, Vierhout ME, Heesakkers JP, et al. Surgical management of mesh-related complications after prior pelvic floor reconstructive surgery with mesh. Int Urogynecol J 2011;22(11):1395–404.

28. de Tayrac R, Letouzey V. Basic science and clinical aspects of mesh infection in pelvic floor reconstructive surgery. Int Urogynecol J 2011;22(7):775–80.

29. Vollebregt A, Troelstra A, van der Vaart CH. Bacterial colonisation of collagen-coated polypropylene vaginal mesh: are additional intraoperative sterility procedures useful? Int Urogynecol J Pelvic Floor Dysfunct 2009;20:1345–51.

30. Falagas ME, Velakoulis S, Iavazzo C, et al. Mesh-related infections after pelvic organ prolapse repair surgery. Eur J Obstet Gynecol Reprod Biol 2007;134:147–56.

31. Mellano EM, Nakamura LY, Choi JM, et al. The role of chronic mesh infection in delayed-onset vaginal mesh complications or recurrent urinary tract infections: results from explanted mesh cultures. Female Pelvic Med Reconstr Surg 2016; 22(3):166–71.

32. Reiter RC. Evidence based management of chronic pelvic pain. Clin Obstet Gynecol 1998;41:422–35.

33. Stones RW, Selfe SA, Fransman S, et al. Psychosocial and economic impact of chronic pelvic pain. Best Pract Res Clin Obstet Gynaecol 2000;14:415–31.

34. Kaufman Y, Singh SS, Alturki H, et al. Age and sexual activity are risk factors for mesh exposure following transvaginal mesh repair. Int Urogynecol J 2011;22(3): 307–13.

35. Khatri G, Carmel ME, Bailey AA, et al. Postoperative imaging after surgical repair for pelvic floor dysfunction. Radiographics 2016;36(4):1233–56.

36. Caquant F, Collinet P, Debodinance P, et al. Safety of Trans Vaginal Mesh procedure: retrospective study of 684 patients. J Obstet Gynaecol Res 2008;34(4): 449–56.

37. Lee D, Dillon B, Lemack G, et al. Transvaginal mesh kits–how "serious" are the complications and are they reversible? Urology 2013;81(1):43–8.

38. Firoozi F, Ingber MS, Moore CK, et al. Purely transvaginal/perineal management of complications from commercial prolapse kits using a new prostheses/grafts complication classification system. J Urol 2012;187(5):1674–9.

39. Rane A, Iyer J. Pearls and pitfalls of mesh surgery. J Obstet Gynaecol India 2012; 62(6):626–9.

40. Isom-Batz G, Zimmern PE. Vaginal mesh for incontinence and/or prolapse: caution required! Expert Rev Med Devices 2007;4(5):675–9.

41. Frenkl TL, Rackley RR, Vasavada SP, et al. Management of iatrogenic foreign bodies of the bladder and urethra following pelvic floor surgery. Neurourol Urodyn 2008;27(6):491–5.

42. Dillon B, Gurbuz C, Zimmern P. Long term results after complication of "prophylactic" suburethral tape placement. Can J Urol 2012;19:6424–30.

43. Feiner B, Maher C. Vaginal mesh contraction: definition, clinical presentation, and management. Obstet Gynecol 2010;115(2 Pt 1):325–30.

44. Crosby EC, Abernethy M, Berger MB, et al. Symptom resolution after operative management of complications from transvaginal mesh. Obstet Gynecol 2014; 123(1):134–9.

45. Unger CA, Abbott S, Evans JM, et al. Outcomes following treatment for pelvic floor mesh complications. Int Urogynecol J 2014;25(6):745–9.

46. Abbott S, Unger CA, Evans JM, et al. Evaluation and management of complications from synthetic mesh after pelvic reconstructive surgery: a multicenter study. Am J Obstet Gynecol 2014;210(2):163.

47. Hokenstad ED, El-Nashar SA, Blandon RE, et al. Health-related quality of life and outcomes after surgical treatment of complications from vaginally placed mesh. Female Pelvic Med Reconstr Surg 2015;21(3):176–80.
48. Hou JC, Alhalabi F, Lemack GE, et al. Outcome of transvaginal mesh and tape removed for pain only. J Urol 2014;192(3):856–60.
49. Danford JM, Osborn DJ, Reynolds WS, et al. Postoperative pain outcomes after transvaginal mesh revision. Int Urogynecol J 2015;26(1):65–9.
50. Hammett J, Peters A, Trowbridge E, et al. Short-term surgical outcomes and characteristics of patients with mesh complications from pelvic organ prolapse and stress urinary incontinence surgery. Int Urogynecol J 2014;25(4):465–70.
51. Agnew G, Dwyer PL, Rosamilia A, et al. Functional outcomes following surgical management of pain, exposure or extrusion following a suburethral tape insertion for urinary stress incontinence. Int Urogynecol J 2014;25(2):235–9.
52. Misrai V, Roupret M, Xylinas E, et al. Surgical resection for suburethral sling complications after treatment for stress urinary incontinence. J Urol 2009;181(5):2198–202.
53. Coskun B, Lavelle RS, Alhalabi F, et al. Mini-slings can cause complications. Int Urogynecol J 2015;26(4):557–62.
54. Reynolds WS, Kit LC, Kaufman MR, et al. Obturator foramen dissection for excision of symptomatic transobturator mesh. J Urol 2012;187(5):1680–4.
55. Gyang AN, Feranec JB, Patel RC, et al. Managing chronic pelvic pain following reconstructive pelvic surgery with transvaginal mesh. Int Urogynecol J 2014;25(3):313–8.
56. Vargas-Schaffer G. Is the WHO analgesic ladder still valid? Twenty-four years of experience. Can Fam Physician 2010;56(6):514–7.
57. Hibner M, Desai N, Robertson LJ, et al. Pudendal neuralgia. J Minim Invasive Gynecol 2010;17(2):148–53.
58. Robert R, Prat-Pradal D, Labat JJ, et al. Anatomic basis of chronic perineal pain: role of the pudendal nerve. Surg Radiol Anat 1998;20(2):93–8.

Interventional Management for Pelvic Pain

Ameet S. Nagpal, MD, MS, MEd*, Erika L. Moody, MD, MBS

KEYWORDS

- Pelvic pain • Interventional pain management • Pelvic injections • Nerve block
- Hypogastric plexus • Ganglion impar

KEY POINTS

- Depending on the etiology of pelvic pain, various interventions may be used to aid in diagnosis and treatment.
- Multiple imaging modalities are increasingly being used with these procedures, with the goal of enhancing efficacy and safety.
- Interventional procedures can be applied for diagnostic evaluation and treatment, often once more conservative measures have failed to provide relief.

INTRODUCTION

A multimodal approach to treatment is often necessary in the patient with pelvic pain. Interventional procedures can be applied for both diagnostic evaluation and treatment, often once more conservative measures have failed to provide relief. This article reviews interventional management strategies for pelvic pain. Such interventions are recommended to be performed by an appropriately trained pain medicine specialist.

SUPERIOR HYPOGASTRIC PLEXUS BLOCK

Superior hypogastric plexus (SHP) blocks provide targeted intervention to sympathetic-mediated pain pathways. The SHP is part of the abdominopelvic autonomic nervous system, a complex network of fibers surrounding the anterior and lateral aspects of the abdominal aorta. These fibers divide just below the aorta to course in the endopelvic fascia of the pelvic basin to form a separate, inferior hypogastric plexus (IHP).[1] The SHP provides visceral innervation to most pelvic structures, the descending colon, rectum, and internal genitalia, except the ovaries and fallopian

The authors have nothing to disclose.
UT Health San Antonio, 7703 Floyd Curl Drive MC 7838, San Antonio, TX 78229, USA
* Corresponding author.
E-mail address: NagpalA@uthscsa.edu

Phys Med Rehabil Clin N Am 28 (2017) 621–646
http://dx.doi.org/10.1016/j.pmr.2017.03.011
1047-9651/17/© 2017 Elsevier Inc. All rights reserved.

tubes.[2] Given the complexity of the IHP, the SHP is targeted, in essence, to block the innervation of both the SHP and IHP. The SHP is retroperitoneal at the level of the lower one-third of the fifth lumbar vertebral body and upper one-third of the first sacral vertebral body at the sacral promontory, and in proximity to the bifurcation of the common iliac vessels. SHP blocks are performed for pelvic pain secondary to endometriosis, inflammatory disease, postoperative adhesions, and cancer unresponsive to more conservative measures.[3] There are also reports of the blocks providing post-prostatectomy penile and urethral pain relief.[4,5]

The traditional posterior approach using fluoroscopic guidance is described using bilateral 6- or 7-inch, 22-gauge beveled needles oriented 30° caudad and 45° medial, to direct the needle to the anterolateral aspect of the L5 vertebral body (**Fig. 1**). Fluoroscopic anteroposterior views should demonstrate the needle tip at the junction of the L5 and S1 vertebral bodies (**Fig. 2**). This imaging is important to avoid potential spread of the injected agent toward the L5 roots. Lateral views should confirm placement of the needle tip about 1 cm past the vertebral body. Contrast spread should be confined to the midline region on anteroposterior view and a smooth posterior continuous spread corresponding with the anterior psoas fascia should be seen in the lateral view. The block should be performed with 6 to 8 mL of 0.25% bupivacaine on each side for diagnostic or prognostic blockade and 6 to 8 mL of 10% aqueous phenol for therapeutic neurolysis.[6] De Leon-Casasola and colleagues[7] reported a 69% success rate with neurolytic SHP blocks in patients with severe pelvic cancer pain. There was a mean oral opioid therapy decrease of 67% in the 2 weeks after the procedure. Potential complications include accidental dislodgement of atherosclerotic plaques from iliac vessels, intraarterial injection of iliac vessels, retroperitoneal hematomas, and ureter and bladder puncture.[7]

Alternate methods include a fluoroscopically guided anterior approach. This method avoids contact of the needle with the lumbar nerve roots. Although technically easier to perform, this approach carries an increased risk of inadvertent perforation of

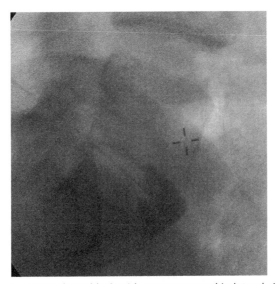

Fig. 1. Superior hypogastric plexus block with contrast spread in lateral view. The needle is visualized at the L5 vertebral body.

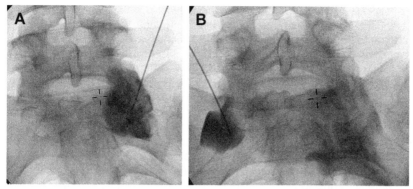

Fig. 2. (*A, B*) Superior hypogastric plexus block with contrast spread in an anteroposterior view. The needle is visualized at the junction of L5 and S1 vertebral bodies.

structures overlying the plexus, including the bowel, bladder, and vasculature.[2] In addition, a posterior paramedian transdiscal approach through the L5 to S1 transdiscal space has been described. Some authors find this technique to be easier, faster, and more effective than the traditional posterior approach described by Plancarte and associates.[6] Potential complications secondary to puncture of the intervertebral disc include discitis, disc rupture, and herniation.[8] It is also difficult to perform in patients with osteophytes of the lumbosacral spine.[5] For either approach, antibiotic prophylaxis is recommended given the potential risks of bowel perforation with the anterior approach and discitis with the transdiscal approach.[2,8]

Alternatives to fluoroscopic guidance include axial computed tomography (CT) scans and ultrasound imaging. CT scanning assists in the visualization of vascular and soft tissue structures, although it increases the radiation dose. The major disadvantage of this technique is the potential for small intestine perforation and significantly increased radiation exposure. Avoidance of large intestine injury is important to prevent bacterial flora from entering the abdominal cavity, leading to peritonitis or retroperitoneal infection.[5] Advantages of ultrasound guidance include avoidance of radiation associated with CT and fluoroscopic guided blocks and improved visualization of medication spread in real time. A recent trial of an anterior ultrasound-guided approach was described in 22 patients with pelvic cancer pain and demonstrated a marked decrease in pain scores and morphine consumption with similar efficacy as the traditional posterior fluoroscopic-guided approach.[9] Disadvantages of this technique are the same as other anterior approaches.

INFERIOR HYPOGASTRIC PLEXUS BLOCK

The IHP is presacral, located on either side of the rectum ventral to the S2, S3, and S4 spinal segments. It is formed by efferent sympathetic fibers from the hypogastric and pelvic splanchnic nerves, preganglionic parasympathetic fibers from pelvic splanchnic nerves, and visceral afferent fibers from the pelvic viscera. IHP blocks are described in the literature as useful for the diagnosis and treatment of chronic pain conditions involving the lower pelvic viscera, specifically pain involving the bladder, penis, vagina, rectum, anus, and perineum. They are not commonly performed in clinical practice.[10]

Schultz[10] was the first to describe fluoroscopically guided transsacral IHP blocks on 11 female patients with chronic pelvic pain involving the lower pelvic viscera (not further defined). He reported a 73% success rate (11 of 15 procedures performed with statistically significant reduction in pain scores, p<0.05) with no complications. This technique involves the use of a 3.5-inch, 25-gauge spinal needle entering 1 to 2 cm lateral to the lateral edge of the S2 or S3 sacral foramen unilateral to the target. The block can be performed through the S1, S2, S3, or S4 levels, with the recommendation to choose the foramen most easily visible. The needle should be advanced slowly under fluoroscopic guidance through the dorsal sacral foramen toward the medial inferior edge of the ventral sacral foramen until contact is made with the medial bony edge of the ventral sacral foramen. If sacral paresthesia occurs, the needle should be retracted and rotated slightly to move past the sacral nerve root. Small doses of 1% or 2% lidocaine (0.1–0.3 mL) during needle advancement should improve patient comfort without blockade of the sacral nerve roots. The needle should be advanced to exit the ventral sacral foramen as medially as possible. Contrast spread should appear cephalad and caudad along the presacral plane conforming to the midline, ventral surface of the sacrum. The author recommends the use of 10 to 15 mL of a local anesthetic/steroid combination. Transient paresthesia is reported as the most common adverse effect, occurring in 5% of IHP blocks (reported by Schultz).[10] In our experience, the paresthesia experienced by the patient is severe and this discomfort has limited our ability to continue performing this procedure in our clinic.

Mohamed and colleagues[11] were the first to describe neurolytic IHP blocks in 20 patients with pelvic cancer pain using 6 to 8 mL of 10% phenol bilaterally using the approach described by Schultz. Pain levels were reduced by 43.8% at 1 week with no complications reported.[11] In addition to paresthesia, other possible complications include rectal puncture if the needle is advanced too deep into the presacral tissues. This complication can be avoided by careful visualization of the needle depth on lateral fluoroscopy, because the rectum is separated by the ventral sacrum by more than 1 mm. Additional risks include vascular penetration of pelvic vessels, hematoma, and infection.[10,11]

GANGLION IMPAR BLOCK

The bilateral paravertebral sympathetic chain terminates anteriorly as a midline single fused ganglion impar (also known as the Ganglion of Walther). The ganglion impar is traditionally described as being found anterior to the anterior sacrococcygeal ligament. It may be found at variable positions in the precoccygeal space, located anywhere from the anterior surface of the sacrococcygeal junction to the lower coccygeal vertebral bodies. The ganglion impar is thought to supply nociceptive and sympathetic fibers to the perineum, distal rectum, perianal region, distal urethra, vulva/scrotum, and distal one-third of the vagina, as well as sympathetic innervation to the pelvic viscera.[3,12]

Ganglion impar blocks were originally described for sympathetically mediated cancer pain involving the perineum. They are now used to treat visceral and sympathetic pelvic and perineal pain, both malignant and benign.[12] One common indication is coccydynia after trauma, infection, degenerative change, or subluxation.[3] Although most cases of coccydynia are considered to be caused by sacrococcygeal or intercoccygeal joint instability, approximately one-third of cases are idiopathic. The coccygeal plexus or its branches may be involved in such cases, because affected patients often respond to injections of local anesthetic or corticosteroids. The coccygeal plexus is formed from the ventral rami of S4, S5, and coccygeal nerves and is found within the ischiococcygeus muscle at the level of first intercoccygeal joint. The plexus gives off 1 to 3 anococcygeal nerves that penetrate posteriorly through the distal fibers of the ischiococcygeus muscle and the sacrospinous ligament to enter the subcutaneous fat of the post anal region, before passing inferiorly to the distal border of the sacrotuberous ligament (**Fig. 3**). Injection to the ganglion impar could diffuse to affect nearby somatic nerves of the coccygeal plexus.[13]

Ganglion impar blocks were initially described using fluoroscopic guidance using a 22-gauge, 8-cm spinal needle bent 5 to 7 cm from the tip to facilitate positioning near the ganglion. After traversing the anococcygeal ligament, the needle is directed cephalad toward the ganglion. Simultaneously, the operator performs a continuous rectal examination using the nondominant index finger to prevent accidental perforation of the rectum by the needle. The disadvantages of this technique are numerous. It is technically challenging, risks injury to the patient's rectum and vasculature, and places

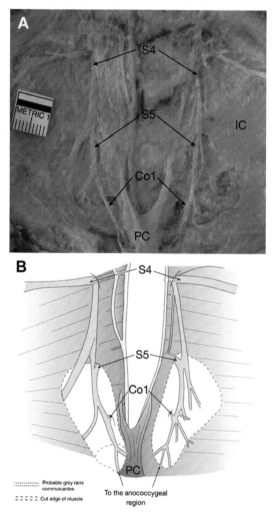

Fig. 3. (*A*) Anterior view of coccygeal plexus in cadaver. (*B*) Schematic representation of dissection with the ischiococcygeus (IC) incised to expose sacral and coccygeal nerves and sacral sympathetic trunk. Co1, coccygeal nerve; PC, pubococcygeus. (*From* Woon JT, Stringer MD. Redefining the coccygeal plexus. Clin Anat 2014;27:255; with permission.)

the operator at high risk of needle stick. Additional disadvantages include tissue trauma along the plane of angulation, risk of needle breakage, failure of injection spread to the ganglion impar with local tumor spread, and periosteal injection with failure to confirm posteroanterior orientation of the needle.[14] Also, a failure rate of up to 30% has been reported.[12,15]

To improve technical feasibility and overcome the risks of rectal perforation with the conventional approach, a modified transsacrococcygeal approach is most commonly used. Here, the patient is placed in a prone position and a 22-gauge 3.5-inch needle is placed in the retroperitoneal space through the sacrococcygeal disc/junction using fluoroscopic guidance.[16] One obstacle to this approach is that there may be difficulty with needle placement because the sacrococcygeal disc is made up of glycoproteins, which ossify with age. One method of overcoming this problem is using a "needle inside a needle" technique. This can be accomplished using an 18-gauge needle to facilitate penetration of a 22-gauge or 25-gauge needle through ossified discs without complication.[15] Also described is the use of a 22-gauge, 1.5-inch spinal needle to guide a 25-gauge, 2-inch spinal needle through the sacrococcygeal disc. It is advanced until the tip is anterior to the ventral sacrococcygeal ligament, felt as a loss of resistance. Needle position is confirmed by injecting 1 mL of contrast into the retroperitoneal space. A "reverse comma" dye spread appearance is seen on the lateral view (**Fig. 4**). In cases of nonmalignant pain, 5 to 10 mL of 0.5% bupivacaine are injected for diagnostic block. Steroid may be added to the injectate if the provider feels that this will improve the patient's outcome. In cases of cancer pain, a neurolytic block may be performed using 4 to 6 mL of at least 6% aqueous phenol.[15] Potential complications of chemical neurolysis include motor, sexual, bowel, or bladder dysfunction as a result of inadvertent spread of the neurolytic agent. Neuritis or neuralgia is a potential risk after any chemical neuroablation.[3,17,18] Several other approaches using various imaging modalities have been described in the literature, including CT- and ultrasound-guided approaches, but these have not been widely adopted.

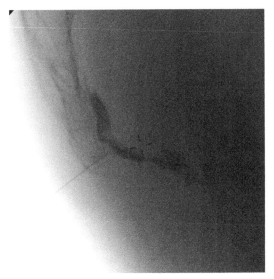

Fig. 4. Ganglion impar block with contrast spread in lateral view. "Reverse comma" dye spread.

After diagnostic local anesthetic injection, cryoablation or radiofrequency ablation of the ganglion may be performed in place of chemical neurolysis. Reig and colleagues[17] report using a 2-needle conventional radiofrequency ablation technique at 80°C for 80 seconds to the ganglion impar in 13 patients with nonmalignant perineal pain. One needle is placed at the sacrococcygeal ligament and the other needle is placed through the coccygeal disc. This allows coverage of a larger area, increasing the likelihood that the ganglion will be reached. Advantages of radiofrequency ablation over chemical neurolysis are increased selectivity and fewer complications.[17] Cryoablation involves a cryoprobe with N_2O or CO_2 gas used to cool the probe tip to −60°C. This causes the probe tip to extract heat from the surrounding tissue and form an ice ball, resulting in axonal degeneration and neural disruption. Cryoablation is most appropriate for painful conditions amenable to small, well-localized lesions because the ice ball is typically 3.5 to 5.5 mm in diameter. The amount of tissue destruction depends on the size of the cryoprobe, freezing time, tissue permeability to water, and presence of vascular structures. Cryoablation has a lower incidence of neuritis and neuroma formation compared with chemical neurolysis. After cryoablation, the perineurium and epineurium remain intact, ensuring that neural regeneration occurs and that there is less of a risk of neuroma formation. Potential major complications of cryoablation include trauma to pelvic structures.[18]

TRANSVERSUS ABDOMINIS PLANE BLOCK

The transversus abdominis plane (TAP) block delivers local anesthetic into the fascial plane superficial to the transversus abdominis muscle and deep to the internal oblique muscle (**Fig. 5**). Above the iliac crest, spinal nerves T7 to T11 emerge from the intercostal space and run along the neurovascular plane between the internal oblique and transversus abdominis muscles. Below the iliac crest, the subcostal nerve (T12) and the ilioinguinal (II) and iliohypogastric (IH) nerves (L1) also travel in the plane between the transversus abdominis and internal oblique muscles. Targeting these nerves with

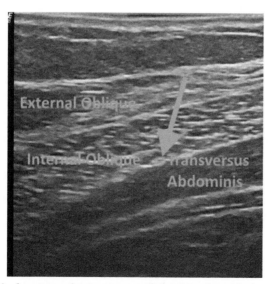

Fig. 5. Ultrasound of anatomy for transversus abdominis plane block. Arrow depicts the target site for injection between transversus abdominis and internal oblique muscles.

local anesthetics allows blockade of pain signals both above and below the umbilicus.[19] TAP blocks have traditionally been used for analgesia after abdominal surgeries, including laparoscopic cholecystectomy, gynecologic surgery, colorectal surgeries, appendectomy, renal transplant, inguinal hernia repair, and cesarean section.[3,19,20] Women who underwent TAP blocks after total abdominal hysterectomy had significant shorter hospital durations of stay and lower opioid use.[21] Schaeffer and colleagues[22] report successful TAP blockade using a continuous ropivicaine infusion via TAP catheter placement under ultrasound guidance in patients with traumatic pelvic ring fractures.

In 2001, Rafi[23] described the TAP block using superficial landmarks and a "double pop" loss of resistance technique to find the plane between the internal oblique and transversus abdominis muscles. This blind approach involves identification of the lumbar triangle of Petit, created by the boundaries of the iliac crest inferiorly, the external oblique muscle anteriorly, and the latissimus dorsi muscle posteriorly. In most people, this triangle is situated just behind the highest point of the iliac crest. As the examiner's finger moves posteriorly, a gap is felt in the musculature of the lateral abdominal wall. Here, a 22- or 24-gauge, 5-cm blunt needle is inserted perpendicular to the skin, approximately 1 to 2 cm above the iliac crest and posterior to the midaxillary line, toward the apex of the triangle. The needle is inserted until 2 "pops" (loss of resistance) are felt. The first "pop" indicates penetration through the external oblique muscle and the second "pop" indicates penetration through the internal oblique muscle.[19] After negative aspiration, 15 to 20 mL of local anesthetic are injected.[3,20,23]

Ultrasound imaging allows direct visualization of external oblique, internal oblique, and transverse abdominal musculature, allowing better visualization of the targeted plane (see **Fig. 5**). This technique potentially reduces complications and improves effectiveness. This block is performed between the iliac crest and subcostal margin via an in-plane approach with needle insertion from anterior to posterior with an endpoint in the plane between the internal oblique and the transversus abdominis in the midaxillary line.[24,25] Variations of this traditional lateral ultrasound-guided approach are described elsewhere in the literature, including an oblique subcostal and posterior approach.[25]

Potential complications of TAP blocks include visceral organ injuries, because the peritoneal cavity is located deep to the TAP. Also, the concern for local anesthetic systemic toxicity has been raised given the high local anesthetic volumes used in bilateral blocks.[25] Femoral nerve palsy after TAP block has been reported in the literature. The femoral nerve lies in the same tissue plane as the space deep to the transversus abdominis. If the needle is advanced into the wrong tissue plane, between the transversus abdominis muscle and the transversus fascia, the injectate can travel along the transversus fascia and accumulate along the femoral nerve.[26] Ultimately, this is an extremely safe procedure when performed with ultrasonographic guidance.

ILIOINGUINAL, ILIOHYPOGASTRIC, AND GENITOFEMORAL NERVE BLOCK

The II and IH nerves arise from T12 and L1 roots of the lumbar plexus, supplying sensory innervation to the suprapubic and inguinal regions. At the lateral border of the quadratus lumborum, both the II and IH nerves pass through the fascia lumborum and extend to the area between the internal oblique and transversus abdominis muscles. The IH nerve perforates the transversus abdominis to lie between it and the external oblique muscle before dividing into anterior and lateral branches. The lateral branch supplies sensory innervation to the posterolateral gluteal region. The anterior branch pierces the external oblique just past the anterior superior iliac spine (ASIS), providing sensory innervation to the abdominal skin above the pubis. The II nerve perforates the transversus abdominis at the level of the ASIS. It may interconnect with the IH nerve as it continues medially and inferiorly, where it accompanies the spermatic cord in men or round ligament of the uterus in women, through the inguinal ring and into the inguinal canal.[3,27] The II nerve provides sensory innervation to the upper inner thigh, root of the penis, and upper scrotum in men and the mons pubis and lateral labia in women, although the sensory innervation is variable.

The genitofemoral (GF) nerve is mainly a sensory nerve arising from the L1 and L2 roots. It descends through the psoas major muscle, emerging at the abdominal surface opposite L3 and L4. It then divides into genital and femoral branches above the inguinal ligament. The genital branch enters the inguinal canal though the deep inguinal ring and supplies and to the fibers to the cremaster muscle and sensory fibers to the scrotal skin in men and mons pubis and labia majora in women. The femoral branch descends lateral to the external iliac artery, passing behind the inguinal ligament. The nerve enters the femoral sheath lateral to the femoral artery and supplies sensory innervation to the skin over the femoral triangle.[3]

II, IH, and GF blocks have historically been used as perioperative anesthesia techniques during inguinal herniorrhaphy, orchidopexy, and hydrocelectomy. Unlike IH and II blocks, the GF block has more limitations on analgesic distribution, primarily limiting pain related to traction on the hernia sac. These nerve blocks may be helpful in the evaluation and management of groin pain and have been recommended in patients with persistent pain and paresthesia after inguinal herniorrhaphy, appendectomy, cesarean section, and hysterectomy.[3]

GF blocks can be helpful diagnostically in the evaluation of groin pain to differentiate peripheral nerve entrapment from lumbar radiculopathy. The II and GF nerves have been known to become adhered after laparoscopy for endometriosis.[28] Successful pain relief after a diagnostic nerve block may indicate nerve entrapment.[1,3]

Historically, landmark-based approaches have been used for these blocks. The IH block has an insertion point 1 inch medial and 1 inch inferior to the ASIS, advancing the needle at an oblique angle toward the pubic symphysis (**Fig. 6**). The II block has an insertion point 2 inches medial and 2 inches inferior to the ASIS, advancing the needle at an oblique angle toward the pubic symphysis (see **Fig. 6**). The GF block involves identification of the ASIS, femoral artery, inguinal crease, and pubic tubercle by palpation. The needle is inserted at the lateral border of the femoral artery in the inguinal crease, if targeting the femoral branch of the GF nerve. Alternatively, to block the genital branch, the pubic tubercle and inguinal ligament are identified and the needle is advanced through the skin and subcutaneous tissue at an insertion point just lateral to the pubic tubercle, just below the inguinal ligament (see **Fig. 6**). For all approaches, a 25-gauge, 1.5-inch needle is recommended. For both IL and IH blocks, 2 to 5 mL of local anesthetic are injected in a fanlike manner as the needle pierces the fascia of the external oblique (loss of resistance may be felt as the aponeurosis of the external oblique muscle is pierced).[29] Potential complications include placing the needle too deep and entering the peritoneal cavity, piercing the abdominal viscera, hematoma formation (especially if the patient is taking anticoagulants), and block of adjacent nerves such as the femoral nerve. If the pain has an inflammatory component, local anesthetic can be combined with steroid.[30–32]

Landmark-based approaches can be inaccurate with failure rates reported to be as high as 30%. The use of high-frequency, high-resolution ultrasound imaging decreases complications and improves quality of blocks. Willschke and colleagues[29] compared the use of ultrasound imaging with the landmark-based approaches for II and IH nerve blocks and found that the amount of local anesthetic used in the

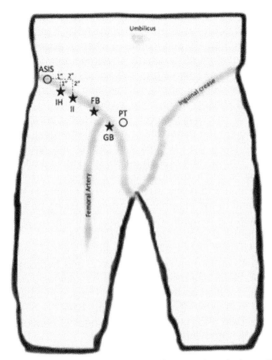

Fig. 6. Iliohypogastric (IH) block anatomically based target site 1 inch medial and 1 inch inferior to the anterior superior iliac spine (ASIS). Ilioinguinal (II) block anatomically based target site 2 inches medial and 2 inches inferior to the ASIS. Femoral branch of the genitofemoral nerve (FB) target site at the lateral border of the femoral artery in the inguinal crease. Genital branch of the genitofemoral nerve (GB) target site just lateral to the pubic tubercle (PT) and just inferior to the inguinal crease.

ultrasound group was significantly lower than the conventional landmark-based group. During the intraoperative period, only 4% of the children in the ultrasound group received additional analgesics compared with 26% in the landmark-based group.[29] Recommended local anesthetic doses with the ultrasound approach are 0.075 mL/kg in children and 0.2 mL/kg in adults.[3]

Ultrasound examination should be performed with a high-frequency linear transducer. The II nerve is best visualized immediately medial to the ASIS, whereas the IH nerve is found less than 1 cm from the II nerve. It is standard to block both of these nerves simultaneously. Using an out-of-plane approach, the needle is inserted between the internal oblique and the transversus abdominis muscles. It is important to realize that the external oblique muscle is often present only as an aponeurosis when ultrasound imaging is performed in the lower abdominal region below the ASIS. Thus, instead of the 3 muscles typically seen in the abdominal wall, there might only be 2 at this location (**Fig. 7**).[33] An alternative ultrasound approach was described by Eichenberger and colleagues[32] with an injection point 5 cm cranial and posterior to the ASIS, with a success rate of 95%. At this point, all 3 muscle layers of the abdominal wall were easily identified on ultrasound imaging. Of the 37 cadavers studied, all 37 had the IH and II nerves lying between the internal oblique and transverse abdominis muscles, which may explain the high incidence of failure reported in the literature with the conventional landmark-based approach.[32]

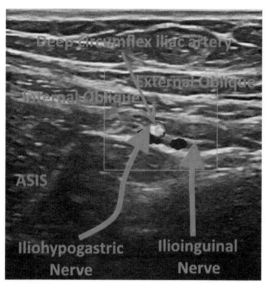

Fig. 7. Ultrasound of anatomy for ilioinguinal and iliohypogastric nerve blocks. ASIS, anterior superior iliac spine.

The ultrasound-guided approach to the GF block involves placement of the transducer in long axis over the femoral artery. The transducer is advanced in a cephalad direction following the femoral artery until it begins to descend beneath the inguinal ligament into the abdominal cavity as it becomes the external iliac artery. At this transition, the inguinal canal should be visible just above the external iliac artery, appearing as an ovoid structure containing tubular structures (the spermatic cord in males and round ligament in women) **(Fig. 8)**. In the out-of-plane approach, the needle is

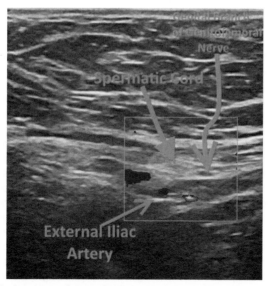

Fig. 8. Ultrasound of anatomy for genital branch of genitofemoral nerve block.

advanced to the inguinal canal and solution is injected around the spermatic cord in men and around the round ligament in women.[34] Other image-guided approaches have been reported in the literature, including a transpsoas method using CT guidance.[35]

PUDENDAL BLOCK

The pudendal nerve originates from ventral rami of S2 to S4. It passes around the sacrospinous ligament and attaches to the medial aspect of the ischial tuberosity (pudendal or Alcock's canal) then terminates by passing through the urogenital diaphragm to reach the external genitalia.[1] The pudendal nerve innervates the penis, clitoris, bulbospongiosus muscle, ischiocavernosus muscles, perineum, and anus. The pudendal nerve may become entrapped or irritated along several points in its course leading to intractable pelvic and perineal pain, hyperalgesia, genital numbness, sexual dysfunction, and even abnormal urinary frequency. Patients with pudendal neuralgia typically present with burning pain in the distribution of the pudendal nerve or a small region involving only a particular branch. Pain is localized to the vulva, vagina, clitoris, perineum, and rectum in females and to the glans penis, scrotum, perineum, and rectum in males. The classic presentation is unilateral pain in this distribution, worsened throughout the day and with sitting, although there are reports of bilateral involvement.[36–38]

Blind pudendal nerve blocks have traditionally been used for diagnosis and treatment. Essentially, the pudendal nerve is blocked where it rotates around the ischial spines, using a transvaginal approach.[39] The patient is placed in the lithotomy position. The transvaginal approach is used primarily in obstetric anesthesia as an adjunct to pain relief in the second stage of labor. Also, it has historically been used to provide surgical anesthesia for surgery on the labia, including lesion removal and laceration repair.[40] In the female, the ischial spine is palpated through the vaginal wall. A needle guider is placed between the index and middle fingers against the vaginal mucosa and just in front of the ischial spine. A 20-gauge, 6-inch needle can then be placed into the needle guider, advanced through the sacrospinous ligament, just beyond the ischial spine.[40] In the male, the ischial spine is palpated through the rectum, and the needle is inserted transperineally.[38] Waldman[30] recommends using 10 mL of 1% lidocaine with 3 to 4 mL of additional local anesthetic used during needle withdrawal to ensure blockade of the inferior rectal nerve.[40] Major risks of this procedure include perforation of the bowel, bladder, and vasculature (close proximity of pudendal artery and vein) as well as an increased risk of needle puncture to the examiner as they are directing the needle through landmark palpation.[38] There is a potential increased risk of infection or fistula formation in patients who are immunocompromised or have a history of radiation therapy to the perineum.[40]

Several image-guided approaches to pudendal nerve blocks have been described in the literature and are preferable to the blind approaches when treating chronic pain. The fluoroscopic approach involves placing the patient in a prone position and obtaining an optimal ischial spine view. Using a 25-gauge, 3.5-inch needle, the entrance point is just above the tip of the ischial spine. The needle is advanced to the base of the ischial spine. The correct position of the needle is confirmed in lateral view and after contrast injection demonstrating dye spread directly above the ischial spine and the absence of vascularity (**Fig. 9**). A solution of long-acting local anesthetic (ie, 0.75% ropivacaine or 0.5% bupivacaine) with or without 4 to 10 mg dexamethasone can be administered.[41] Hibner and colleagues[37] report using a series of 3 CT-guided injections into the pudendal nerve canal, each 6 weeks apart. Ultrasound guidance

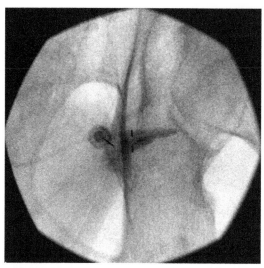

Fig. 9. Pudendal block. Needle advancing to base of ischial spine.

has been described with the patient in the prone position, using a 2- to 5-MHz curvilinear transducer placed at the ischial spine in transverse view. Here, the ischial spine, sacrospinous and sacrotuberous ligaments, internal pudendal artery, and the pudendal nerve can be visualized. The location of the pudendal nerve can be targeted between the 2 ligaments.[42] The pudendal nerve is predominantly located medial to the internal pudendal artery (76%–100%; **Fig. 10**).[43] Direct ultrasound guidance of a 25- or 22-gauge, 3.5- or 6-inch needle should be visualized until the tip of the needle lies next to the pudendal nerve. In the final position, a mixture of 2 mL of long-acting local anesthetic with or without dexamethasone is injected.[42] We advise against the use of particulate steroids in this procedure owing to the proximity of the pudendal nerve to the internal pudendal artery and the possibility of particle embolization and infarction in this artery.

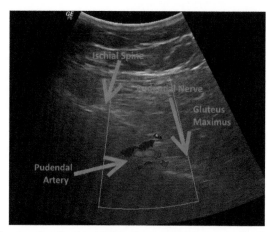

Fig. 10. Pudendal nerve visualized medial to the pudendal artery with ultrasound guidance.

Bellingham and colleagues[44] performed a randomized, controlled trial comparing the effectiveness and safety between ultrasound and fluoroscopically guided pudendal nerve blocks. They found no difference in the degree of neural blockage or adverse effects between the 2 techniques. The time to complete the procedure was longer using the ultrasound guided approach (428 seconds) compared with fluoroscopy (219 seconds).

SELECTIVE NERVE ROOT BLOCK

Selective nerve root blocks involve placing the needle adjacent to the nerve root sleeve as it emerges from the intervertebral foramen. This is typically performed under fluoroscopic guidance, although ultrasound and CT guidance have also been used. A selective nerve root block serves to identify a specific level where the pain generator arises. Pain relief after a selective nerve root block implicates a specific nerve as the source, because pain referral patterns from the lumbar and sacral nerve roots can be an etiology of pelvic pain.[45]

For injection of the lumbar spine, vertebral bodies are squared, with their endplates paralleled under fluoroscopy. The target is beneath the pedicle of the vertebrae or "eye of the Scotty dog" and is in the region of the safe triangle as described by Bogduk and colleagues. This region is above the exiting nerve root. A 25-gauge, 3.5-inch spinal needle is inserted in a paramedian direction through the muscle, immediately below the pedicle, and along the superior border of the foramen. The needle is not advanced more medial than the lateral one-fourth of the pedicle. The needle is aspirated to avoid blood or cerebrospinal fluid (**Fig. 11**).[45]

For injection of the sacral spine, the foramina are directly posterior and are aligned so that the anterior and posterior foramina overlap. The spinal needle is inserted into

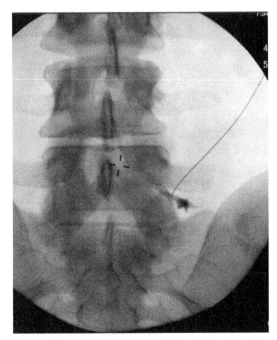

Fig. 11. Fluoroscopic guided selective nerve root block of the right L5 nerve root.

the foramen perpendicular to the dorsal surface of the sacrum. The needle is advanced through the epidural space and then viewed in lateral projection. The needle is seen approaching the anterior foramen and presacral space. Contrast is injected to view the outline of the sacral nerve. Anesthetic solution and corticosteroid medications are injected around the nerve root sleeve.[45]

Potential complications include infection, bleeding, and allergic reaction to contrast media or anesthetic. Direct procedural complications include leakage of cerebrospinal fluid from a tear along the nerve root sleeve, direct nerve puncture, and injection of material directly into the nerve root. Bowel or visceral perforation is possible if the needle is advanced too far. Vascular or ischemic injury can occur if spinal arteries are lacerated or directly injected. Direct injection can cause embolization of the spinal artery and devascularize the cord. Another unintended complication is the possibility of epidural spread of medication, leading to the procedure being a transforaminal epidural steroid injection rather than a selective nerve root block. This could lead to a spurious false-positive diagnostic block. Care should be taken to ensure that the contrast spread is lateral to the epidural space.[45]

TRIGGER POINT INJECTION

A myofascial trigger point (MTrP) is a hyperirritable spot in skeletal muscle that is associated with a hypersensitive palpable nodule in a taut band. The spot is painful on compression and can give rise to characteristic referred pain and tenderness, motor dysfunction, and autonomic phenomena.[46] MTrPs display a "local twitch response," defined as a transient visible or palpable contraction or dimpling of the muscle or skin as the taut band of the trigger point contracts as pressure is applied. This response is caused by a sudden change of pressure on the trigger point by needle penetration into the trigger point or by transverse snapping palpation of the trigger point across the direction of the tense band of muscle fibers.[47]

MTrPs in the low back, abdominal wall, lower extremities, and pelvic girdle can be the primary referral sources of pelvic pain.[28] Although the cause of pelvic myofascial pain is not completely understood, the involved muscles are shortened and often weak, and therefore more likely to develop MTrPs. Theories of etiology include metabolic imbalance at the peripheral tissue, centralized pain phenomenon, and neuromuscular microtrauma secondary to sustained positions and impaired movements in the lumbopelvic region.[48] Common muscular causes of pelvic pain include MTrPs involving the levator ani, obturator internus, piriformis, gluteal muscles, and quadratus lumborum. Spasms of the levator ani can lead to chronic vaginal discomfort, dyspareunia, perineal pain with sitting, painful bowel movements, and tailbone, hip, and back pain.[49,50] Sites of pain can often be reproduced digitally using either a transvaginal or transrectal approach (**Fig. 12**).[51] MTrPs in the obturator internus may refer pain to the vagina, anococcygeal region, and posterior thigh. Symptoms may be reported as rectal fullness and posterior thigh pain. Piriformis MTrPs may refer pain to the low back, buttock, and pelvic floor. Symptoms include worsening of pain with sitting, standing, walking, or "sciatica"-type complaints. Gluteus maximus MTrPs refer pain to the buttock region and pain may be exacerbated with prolonged sitting or walking uphill. Gluteus medius MTrPs refer pain to the posterior crest of the ilium, sacrum, and posterior and lateral buttock, and symptoms can be aggravated with walking, lying on one's side, and sitting. Quadratus lumborum MTrPs can refer pain to the sacroiliac (SI) joint and buttock, anterior ilium, lower abdomen, groin, and greater trochanter. The patient may complain of pain in the low back exacerbated by walking, coughing, or sneezing.

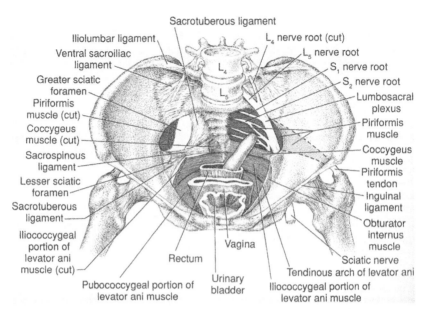

Fig. 12. Internal palpation of the levator ani, obturator internus, and piriformis muscles via the rectum, viewed from in front and above. The sacrospinous ligament is the major transverse landmark, attaching mainly to the coccyx, which is typically easily palpated and mobile. (*From* Simons DG, Travell JG, Simons LS. Myofascial pain and dysfunction. In: Johnson EP, editor. Myofascial pain and dysfunction, vol. 2. 2nd edition. Baltimore (MD): Williams and Wilkins; 1999. p. 200; with permission.)

A shortened quadratus lumborum may create an apparent leg length discrepancy and secondary pelvic obliquity. This could then lead to SI joint dysfunction and pelvic floor muscle imbalance and pain.[28]

Trigger point injection is a treatment option and involves injection into the involved muscle with various agents, typically local anesthetics.[51] Injection of local anesthetic versus local anesthetic with corticosteroid was shown to be as effective as dry needling (penetrating the most painful area of the muscle with a fine needle, using rapid in-and-out maneuvers), thus emphasizing the importance of mechanically rupturing the trigger point, irrespective of the substance administered.[52] Hong[53] found dry needling to be as effective as injecting 0.5% lidocaine; however, postinjection soreness was of significantly greater intensity and duration than those treated with lidocaine injection. In a controlled, double-blind study of 28 patients receiving trigger point injections with either 0.5% mepivicaine or equivalent volume saline, 68% of patients treated with saline reported improvement in symptoms versus 74% of patients treated with mepivicaine.[54]

Lewit[55] described that when the most painful spot was touched by the needle, immediate analgesia without hypesthesia was observed in the majority of cases, termed the "needle effect." Needling may cause postneedle soreness, hematoma, hemorrhage at the needling site, and syncopal episodes.[28] Corticosteroid injection may be associated with local changes to musculature and connective tissue with prolonged use.[52] Contraindications to MTrP injections include local or systemic infection, anticoagulation therapy, bleeding disorders, allergy to the injected agent, and acute muscle trauma.[28]

Although the mechanism of action of trigger point injections is not completely understood, inactivation of the trigger point likely occurs through multiple mechanisms. This may include mechanical disruption of abnormal contractile elements, dilution of nociceptive substances by the infiltrated anesthetic, and inducing muscle fiber trauma subsequently releasing intracellular potassium, which then depolarizes and blocks nerve fibers.[49] Additional theories include interruption of the positive feedback loop that perpetuates pain and a vasodilatory effect of anesthetic to remove excess metabolites.[56]

Levator ani trigger point injection involves placement of the patient in the dorsal lithotomy position. Using a sweeping technique, manual transvaginal palpation from the posterior portion to the anterior portion of the levator ani muscles is used to identify the trigger points. The obturator internus and piriformis can be palpated laterally from this position as well (see **Fig. 12**). Langford and colleagues[49] reported using a mixture of 10 mL of 0.25% bupivacaine, 10 mL of 2% lidocaine, and 1 mL (40 mg) of triamcinolone injected in 5-mL increments into the trigger points using a 23-gauge spinal needle through a 5.5-inch needle guider. At the follow-up period at 3 months, 13 of the 18 patient's studied (72.2%) improved after their first trigger point injection and 6 of the 18 (33%) were completely pain free. No adverse effects were reported. Complications of this procedure include worsening of localized pain at sites of injection, bleeding, infection, and allergic reaction to the injected solution. Care should be taken to aspirate before injection, because injection within a blood vessel may cause systemic and cardiac effects.[49]

Various piriformis injection techniques have been described using needle electromyography, peripheral nerve stimulation, and fluoroscopic, ultrasound, and CT guidance.[57,58] Effective and near immediate pain relief after injection of local anesthetic with or without corticosteroid is considered a diagnostic aid for piriformis syndrome.[57] One validated method involves injecting one-fourth to one-third of the way along an imaginary line drawn from the acetabulum to the SI joint. The needle is inserted to the level of the ischium and retracted until maximum motor unit action potential activity is appreciated on electromyography while the leg is externally rotated. If motor unit action potentials are generated when the leg is extended, the needle is likely in the gluteus maximus and the needle is advanced further. Another common method involves injection halfway along the line connecting the sciatic notch and greater trochanter using fluoroscopy. Contrast is then injected and successful placement is confirmed with medial to lateral spread of contrast along the piriformis distribution.[58] Fishman and colleagues[59] reported that patients receiving injection with 200 units of botulinum toxin A (BoNT) to the piriformis muscle experienced more pain relief than in patients receiving lidocaine with steroid or normal saline (placebo).

BoNT injection is being increasingly used in the treatment of myofascial pain and has shown benefit in refractory myofascial pelvic pain.[51,58] BoNT is a potent neurotoxin that binds to peripheral nerve terminals, preventing the release of acetylcholine into the synaptic cleft, leading to muscle paralysis. BoNT has been shown to act at the level of the muscle spindle by inhibiting gamma motor neurons and blocking type 1A afferent signals, thereby affecting both motor and sensory pathways. BoNT may also have additional analgesic properties by inhibiting the release of substance P by the nerve terminals.[58] The clinical effect of the toxin is dose related and decreases as presynaptic molecules turn over and neural sprouts develop from the toxin-affected axonal terminal to create a new functional synapse, eventually with muscle cells returning to normal contractility.[51]

Various concentrations of BoNT injections have been reported in the literature with variable results. Jarvis and colleagues[60] reported the use of BoNT in 12 women with chronic pelvic pain for more than 2 years with objective evidence of pelvic muscle spasm by vaginal manometry. These women were treated with 40 units of BoNT injected into the puborectalis and pubococccygeus muscles identified by digital vaginal palpation. The study reported a significant reduction in dyspareunia and dysmenorrhea scores at 2, 4, 8, and 12 weeks after injection. There was not significant improvement in dyschezia or nonmenstrual pelvic pain.[60] Ghazizadeh and Nikzad[61] reported using 150 to 400 units of BoNT into the puborectalis muscles in 3 sites bilaterally in 24 women with moderate to severe vaginismus refractory to other treatment. Twenty-three patients (95.8%) had little or no vaginismus on vaginal examination 1 week after injection and 18 patients (75%) achieved satisfactory intercourse after the first injection.[61] Similarly, Adelowo and colleagues[62] reported a 79.3% improvement in pain scores in their study cohort receiving 100 to 300 units of BoNT for refractory myofascial pelvic pain. Targeted muscles included the coccygeus, iliococcygeus, pubococcygeus, puborectalis, obturator, and piriformis, with injection locations individualized to findings on physical examination and patient-reported tenderness at each site.[62] A double-blinded, randomized, placebo-controlled trial in women with chronic pelvic pain of more than 2 years' duration with evidence of pelvic floor spasm received either 80 units of BoNT to the pelvic floor muscles or saline injection. There was significant reduction in pelvic floor pressures in both groups, with greater reduction in the BoNT group. There was significant reduction in some types of pelvic pain (dyspareunia and nonmenstrual pelvic pain) in the BoNT group compared with placebo. There were no differences in pain compared with the control group who had physical therapy as an intervention. The main complication reported was bleeding from the injection sites, which was controlled by digital pressure followed by insertion of a medium dilator.[63] Other potential complications of BoNT include toxin reactions, typically a dose-related effect when more than 200 units are used. Also, loss of pelvic sphincter control is reported, particularly in women with a history of stress urinary continence, in addition to the possibility of temporary fecal incontinence and inability to control flatus. Repeated injections may lead to the development of secondary treatment failure as a result of antibody production, although this is reported to be low at 4%.[64] BoNT is a category C drug; thus, women should be advised against pregnancy after treatment anywhere in the body.[65]

Investigators have used a variety of techniques to aide placement of BoNT for gynecologic indications, including electromyography and ultrasound imaging. Injection into the most painful areas on palpation during clinical examination seems to produce appropriate clinical outcomes. Transrectal ultrasound imaging may be helpful in localization of deeper structures, such as the puborectalis.[65]

SACROILIAC JOINT INJECTION

The SI joint is a diarthroidal joint with variable and extensive innervation. During an injection, the needle is directed at the inferior portion of the joint, because this is the synovial part. The upper portion is amphiarthrodial or fibrous and does not constitute a true joint. The innervation of the SI joint is complex and controversial. Roberts and colleagues[66] concluded that the posterior aspect of the SI joint is innervated by the posterior sacral network, formed by the lateral branches of S1 to S3 in most specimens, after evaluation of 25 cadaveric hemipelvices. S4 contributions were highly variable and contributions from the dorsal ramus of L5 was inconsistent. Although the number of lateral branches varied at each level, they were found to emerge from the superolateral and inferolateral quadrants of the posterior sacral foramina.[66]

Local anesthetic with or without a corticosteroid can be injected into the SI joint into the intraarticular space or into the periarticular space, in particular into the posterior ligamentous structures for the treatment of SI joint pain. Unfortunately, the origin of SI joint pain is often unclear and has been reported to originate from both the intraarticular space as well as periarticular structures. Murakami and colleagues[67] reported that injection into the middle periarticular area was more effective for SI joint pain, with an improvement rate of 96% after periarticular injection versus 62% improvement after intraarticular injection.

SI joint injections are traditionally performed with fluoroscopic and, less commonly, with CT guidance. The patient is placed in a prone position with a pillow under the abdomen to flex the spine. Under a straight anteroposterior view, the SI joint presents several lines that course caudocranially. The lateral line represents the ventral or anterior margin of the joint, and the medial line represents the dorsal or posterior margin of the joint. The inferior-most portion of the SI joint demonstrates overlap of the anterior and posterior components. The C-arm is rotated approximately 30° caudal to the axial plane to better visualize the area underneath the posterior superior iliac spine and iliac crest. The C-arm is then angled obliquely to the contralateral side until the inferior joint space is clearly demarcated. The target point for intraarticular injection is along the inferoposterior aspect of the joint, in the area 1 to 2 cm cephalad from its most caudal end. A 22-gauge, 3.5-inch spinal needle is advanced into the lower one-third of the SI joint with intermittent images obtained every 2- to 4-mm advancement of the needle to confirm trajectory. When the posterior surface of the SI joint is contacted, the needle is advanced to just penetrate the joint capsule. A change in resistance is commonly felt as the needle passes through the capsular tissue, and the needle tip is often deflected slightly as it traces the surface of the ilium. Lateral imaging should be performed to confirm proper needle placement. Once the needle is within the joint, contrast is injected to demonstrate intraarticular spread followed by injection of a solution of steroid and local anesthetic (**Fig. 13**). The capacity of the SI joint is small and distension may exacerbate pain, thus a volume of 2 to 2.5 mL has been recommended.[3,68] Periarticular injection as described by Murakami and associates[67] involves placing the patient is placed in the same position as the intraarticular injection, except that the fluoroscope is slanted cranially to detect the whole SI joint line. The posterior margin of the SI joint line is then visually divided into 3 equal sections (upper, middle, and lower). An additional section is the cranial portion of the SI joint over the ilium. The spinal needle is then inserted at the center of each section, with 0.5 to 1.0 mL of 2% lidocaine and contrast mixture injected.[67]

SI joint injection under ultrasonographic guidance was described by Pekkafali and colleagues.[69] Patients received injections under ultrasound guidance with fluoroscopic spot images obtained to assess accuracy of the sonographically guided technique with a success rate reported of 46 out of the 60 injections performed (76.7%; ie, intraarticular). Various techniques have been described in the literature, typically using a low-frequency curvilinear or linear transducer placed perpendicular to the distal sacrum to identify the sacral hiatus. The probe is then moved laterally until the lateral edge of the sacrum comes into view, then moved cephalad to find the medial aspect of the iliac bone. The SI joint appears as a hypoechoic cleft area between 2 echogenic lines of the sacrum and the iliac bone (**Fig. 14**). The entrance point of the needle is approximately 2 cm medial to the perpendicular line of the SI joint's opening, making the needle route and the joint's axis parallel. As the tip of the needle touches the posterior ligament and encounters resistance, an abrupt decrease in resistance is felt as a "pop" as the needle enters the joint space. Limitations of ultrasound-guided SI joint injections include the difficulty distinguishing anatomic structures clearly, especially in obese patients. Sufficient training is required to optimize the accuracy of intraarticular needle placement in this complexly configured joint.[3,69,70]

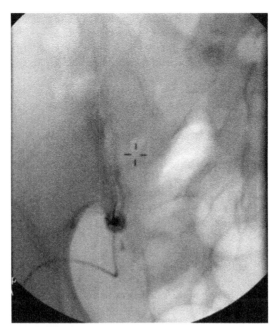

Fig. 13. Fluoroscopic-guided sacroiliac joint injection demonstrating intraarticular contrast spread.

NEUROMODULATION

Spinal cord stimulation (SCS) is an invasive, interventional surgical procedure that is useful in refractory chronic pain syndromes. It has been used as a method for controlling complex, intractable pain syndromes for decades. An SCS system is made up of 3 parts including the electrodes or leads, the implantable pulse generators or battery, and the charging and programming systems. Placement of the electrodes into the

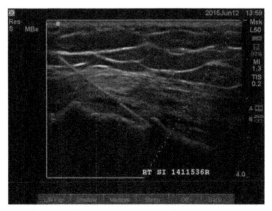

Fig. 14. Ultrasound-guided sacroiliac joint injection demonstrating target hypoechoic cleft between sacrum and ileum. (*From* Perry JM, Colberg RE, Dault SL, et al. A cadaveric study assessing the accuracy of ultrasound-guided sacroiliac joint injections. PM R 2016;8(12):1170; with permission.)

epidural space is technically challenging (**Fig. 15**). A careful trial period, typically 3 to 10 days in duration, is essential to avoid a failed implant. Patient selection is thought to be the most challenging and important step in the decision to offer neurostimulation.[3]

SCS has demonstrated limited ability to alleviate malignant and nociceptive pain, but its efficacy in treating neuropathic and sympathetically associated pain is well documented.[71,72] Although the mechanism of action for SCS is not completely understood, the Gate Control Theory proposed by Melzack and Wall is a proposed mechanism.[73] Stimulation of either the dorsal horn or the dorsal nerve roots at an intensity and frequency to selectively activate large Aβ fibers reduces the spontaneous firing of wide dynamic range neurons in animals with neuropathic injuries.[72] SCS likely influences multiple components and levels within the central nervous system by both interneuron and neurochemical mechanisms.[3] Additional mechanisms of action of SCS include facilitation of physiologic inhibitory mechanisms, changes in the activity of a number of neurotransmitters, especially gamma-aminobutyric acid, and also glutamate, adenosine, acetylcholine, substance P, calcitonin gene-related peptide, brain-derived neurotrophic factor, bradykinin, and others. Orthodromic activation of dorsal column fibers may activate descending serotonergic pathways from brainstem centers, as well as alter pain processing in the cerebrum.[72] Multicontact, multiprogram systems have demonstrated improved outcomes and reduced the incidence of surgical revisions.[3] The most common complications are lead breakage or migration and wound infections, although more serious complications like paralysis, nerve injury, or death are possible.

Stimulation parameters with a wide range of frequencies (30–120 Hz) have been studied and are used in commercially available SCS to optimize pain therapy.[72,74] There is a more recent focus on new frequencies and waveforms such as

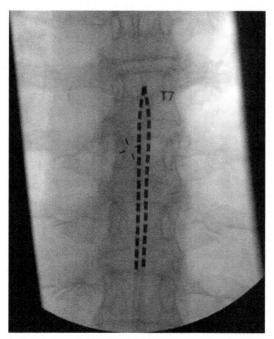

Fig. 15. Spinal cord stimulator trial under fluoroscopic guidance. Leads are placed in the epidural space over T7, T8, and T9 vertebral levels.

high-frequency (10 kHz) and "burst" stimulation. One model currently being used is 10-kHz frequency with a pulse width of 10 μs and amplitude of 1 to 5 mA. Hypotheses of the mechanism of action of this high-frequency waveform have varied to include temporal summation (multiple impulses build on each other to achieve neuronal activation), depolarization blockade (propagating action potentials are blocked by high-frequency stimulation), and desynchronization (kilohertz stimulation results in pseudospontaneous neuronal activity).[72] The Senza system (Nevro Corp, Menlo Park, CA) allows high frequency stimulation (up to 10 kHz) to be delivered to the spinal cord without inducing paresthesia. Preclinical data reports that high-frequency stimulation of wide dynamic range neurons, which are hyperactive in chronic pain states, results in decreased output of these cells (desensitization), and brings them closer to preinjury states. Van Buyten and colleagues[75] reported that at the 6-month follow-up, 74% of patients experienced at least 50% pain reduction, significantly improved disability scores and sleep as well as high satisfaction rates, in a prospective, multicenter study in patients receiving high-frequency waveform SCS for chronic, intractable back pain. Clinical trials for this system for pelvic pain are ongoing.

The "burst" pattern waveform is a series of five, 1000-μs pulses at a pulse frequency of 500 Hz followed by a single repolarization pulse, with each train repeated at 40 Hz. This is proposed to provide a signal that is more similar and relevant to endogenous activation patterns in the nervous system. Neurons responsible for encoding aspects of pain signaling from peripheral neurons and the thalamus have been reported to fire in bursting patterns. It is not clear how "burst" pattern SCS alters ongoing burst activity in pain pathways.[72] De Vos and colleagues[74] reported that "burst" stimulation caused a 25% further reduction in pain compared with tonic stimulation, which resulted in a 52% average reduction in pain scores compared with baseline. Clinical trials for this system for pelvic pain are ongoing.

Kapural and colleagues reported on a T11 to L1 placement of leads in 6 patients with chronic pelvic pain who experienced significant improvements in pain and reductions of opioid requirements.[76] Stimulation as cephalad as T11 can provide appropriate coverage for the treatment of chronic pelvic pain, most likely by stimulation of the sacrally exiting fibers of the dorsal columns. Hunter and colleagues[71] report a case series of successful sacral coverage even more cephalad, with lead placement at T6 and T7. Placement of SCS at the conus level of L1 and L2 theoretically is ideal for chronic pelvic pain given the convergence of information via the cauda equina. There has yet to be reported successes at this level as well as several drawbacks associated with lead placement at this level. First, its mobility within the spinal column makes it difficult to provide consistent paresthesia. Additionally, there is an increased volume of cerebrospinal fluid between the epidural space and neural tissue at the conus. Thus, higher voltages may be required to access the dorsal columns, leading to inadvertent stimulation of segmental roots and associated patient discomfort and inability to tolerate neuromodulation.[71]

Peripheral nerve stimulation was first developed in the 1960s and has since been applied to treat refractory pelvic pain syndromes. The mechanism of action for peripheral nerve stimulation might be different than SCS. The voltage level for peripheral nerve stimulation likely activates only large, myelinated fibers. Constant peripheral stimulation might provide a constant blockade of afferent peripheral input; therefore, allowing central processing to return to normal. Additionally, afferent impulses might block abnormal nociceptive impulses at the spinal cord level in a gate control manner.[77] Sacral nerve stimulation is an effective treatment for some chronic pelvic pain conditions, including interstitial cystitis, coccygodynia, vulvodynia, anorectal pain, and pelvic pain from general pelvic floor dysfunction and spinal cord infarction.[71,78]

SUMMARY

Depending on the etiology of pelvic pain, various interventions may be used to aid in diagnosis and treatment. Multiple imaging modalities are increasing being used with these procedures, with the goal of enhancing efficacy and safety.

REFERENCES

1. Willard FH, Schuenke MD. The neuroanatomy of female pelvic pain. In: Bailey A, Bernstein C, editors. Pain in women: a clinical guide. New York: Springer Science + Business Media; 2013. p. 17–55.
2. Kanazi GE, Perkins FM, Thakur R, et al. New technique for superior hypogastric plexus block. Reg Anesth Pain Med 1999;24(5):473–6.
3. Benzon HT, Rathmell JP, Wu CL, et al. Practical management of pain. 5th edition. Philadelphia: Elsevier Mosby; 2014. p. 683–800.
4. Rosenberg SK, Tewari R, Boswell MV, et al. Superior hypogastric plexus block successfully treats severe penile pain after transurethral resection of the prostate. Reg Anesth Pain Med 1998;23(6):618–20.
5. Michalek P, Dutka J. Computed-tomography guided anterior approach to the superior hypogastric plexus for noncancer pelvic pain: a report of two cases. Clin J Pain 2005;21:553–6.
6. Plancarte R, Amescua C, Patt RB, et al. Superior hypogastric plexus block for pelvic cancer pain. Anesthesiology 1990;73:236–9.
7. de Leon-Casasola OA, Kent E, Lema MJ. Neurolytic superior hypogastric plexus block for chronic pelvic pain associated with cancer. Pain 1993;54:145–51.
8. Gamal G, Helaly M, Labib YM. Superior hypogastric block: transdiscal versus classic posterior approach in pelvic cancer pain. Clin J Pain 2006;22:544–7.
9. Mishra S, Bhatnagar S, Rana SPS, et al. Efficacy of the anterior ultrasound-guided superior hypogastric plexus neurolysis in pelvic cancer pain in advanced gynecological cancer patients. Pain Med 2013;14:837–41.
10. Schultz DM. Inferior hypogastric plexus blockade: a transsacral approach. Pain Physician 2007;10:757–63.
11. Mohamed SAE, Ahmed DG, Mohamed MF. Chemical neurolysis of the inferior hypogastric plexus for the treatment of cancer-related pelvic and perineal pain. Pain Res Manag 2013;18(5):249–52.
12. Scott-Warren JT, Hill V, Rojasekaram A. Ganglion impar blockade: a review. Curr Pain Headache Rep 2013;17:306–12.
13. Woon JT, Stringer MD. Redefining the coccygeal plexus. Clin Anat 2014;27:254–60.
14. Munir MA, Zhang J, Ahmad M. A modified needle-inside-needle technique for the ganglion impar block. Can J Anaesth 2004;51(9):915–7.
15. Toshniwal GR, Dureja GP, Prashanth SM. Transsacrococcygeal approach: to ganglion impar block for management of chronic perineal pain: a prospective observational study. Pain Physician 2007;10:661–6.
16. Wemm K, Saberski L. Modified approach to block the ganglion impar (ganglion of Walther). Reg Anesth 1995;20(6):544–5.
17. Reig E, Abejón D, del Pozo C, et al. Thermocoagulation of the ganglion impar or ganglion of Walther: description of a modified approach. Preliminary results in chronic nononcological pain. Pain Pract 2005;5(2):103–10.
18. Loev MA, Varklet VL, Wilsey BL, et al. Cryoablation: A novel approach to neurolysis of the ganglion impar. Anesthesiology 1998;88(5):1391–3.

19. Taylor R, Pergolizzi JV, Sinclair A, et al. Transversus abdominis block: clinical uses, side effects, and future perspectives. Pain Pract 2013;13(4):332–4.
20. McDonnell JG, O'Donnell B, Curley G, et al. The analgesic efficacy of transversus abdominis plane block after abdominal surgery: a prospective randomized controlled trial. Anesth Analg 2007;104:193–7.
21. Pather S, Loadsman JA, Gopalan PD. The role of transversus abdominis plane blocks in women undergoing total laparoscopic hysterectomy: a retrospective review. Aust N Z J Obstet Gynaecol 2011;51:544–7.
22. Schaeffer E, Millot I, Landy C, et al. Another use of continuous transversus abdominis plane (TAP) block in trauma patient: pelvic ring fractures. Pain Med 2014;15:166–70.
23. Rafi A. Abdominal field block: a new approach via the lumbar triangle. Anaesthesia 2001;56:1003–29.
24. Hebbard P, Fujiwara Y, Shibata Y. Ultrasound-guided transversus abdominis plane (TAP) block. Anaesth Intensive Care 2007;35(4):616–7.
25. Lissauer J, Mancuso K, Merritt C. Evolution of the transversus abdominis plane block and its role in postoperative analgesia. Best Pract Res Clin Anaesthesiol 2014;28:117–26.
26. Manatakis DK, Stamos N, Agalianos C, et al. Transient femoral nerve palsy complicating "blind" transversus abdominus plane block. Case Rep Anesthesiol 2013;2013:874215.
27. Kowalska B, Sudot-Szopinska I. Normal and sonographic anatomy of selected peripheral nerves. Part III: peripheral nerves of the lower limb. J Ultrason 2012; 12:148–63.
28. Prendergast SA, Weiss JM. Screening for musculoskeletal causes of pelvic pain. Clin Obstet Gynecol 2003;46(4):773–82.
29. Willschke H, Marhofer P, Bösenberg A, et al. Ultrasonography for ilioinguinal/iliohypogastric nerve blocks in children. Br J Anaesth 2005;95(2):226–30.
30. Waldman SD. Iliohypogastric nerve block. In: Waldman, editor. Atlas of interventional pain management. 4th edition. Philadelphia: Elsevier Saunders; 2015. p. 435–40.
31. Waldman SD. Ilioinguinal nerve block. In: Waldman, editor. Atlas of interventional pain management. 4th edition. Philadelphia: Elsevier Saunders; 2015. p. 432–5.
32. Eichenberger U, Greher M, Kirchmair L, et al. Ultrasound-guided blocks of the ilioinguinal and iliohypogastric nerve: accuracy of a selective new technique confirmed by anatomical dissection. Br J Anaesth 2006;97(2):238–43.
33. Gucev G, Yasui GM, Chang TY, et al. Bilateral ultrasound-guided continuous ilioinguinal-iliohypogastric block for pain relief after cesarean delivery. Anesth Analg 2008;106:1220–2.
34. Waldman SD. Genitofemoral nerve block. In: Waldman, editor. Atlas of interventional pain management. 4th edition. Philadelphia: Elsevier Saunders; 2015. p. 441–6.
35. Parris D, Fischbein N, Mackey S. A novel CT-guided transpsoas approach to diagnostic genitofemoral nerve block and ablation. Pain Med 2010;11(5):785–9.
36. Khoder W, Hale D. Pudendal neuralgia. Obstet Gynecol Clin North Am 2014;41: 443–52.
37. Hibner M, Desai N, Robertson LJ, et al. Pudendal neuralgia. J Minim Invasive Gynecol 2010;17:148–53.
38. Hong MJ, Kim YD, Park JK, et al. Management of pudendal neuralgia using ultrasound-guided pulsed radiofrequency: a reports of two cases and discussion of pudendal nerve block techniques. J Anesth 2016;30:356–9.
39. Cok OY, Eker HE, Cok T, et al. Transsacral S2-S4 nerve block for vaginal pain due to pudendal neuralgia. J Minim Invasive Gynecol 2011;18:401–4.

40. Waldman SD. Pudendal nerve block. In: Waldman, editor. Atlas of interventional pain management. 4th edition. Philadelphia: Elsevier Saunders; 2015. p. 638–40.

41. Choi SS, Lee PB, Kim YC, et al. C-arm guided pudendal nerve block: a new technique. Int J Clin Pract 2006;60(5):553–6.

42. Rofaeel A, Peng P, Louis I, et al. Feasibility of real-time ultrasound for pudendal nerve block in patients with chronic perineal pain. Reg Anesth Pain Med 2008;33:139–45.

43. Peng PWH, Tumber PS. Ultrasound guided interventional procedures for patients with chronic pelvic pain - a description of techniques and review of literature. Pain Physician 2008;11:215–24.

44. Bellingham GA, Bhatia A, Chan C, et al. Randomized controlled trial comparing pudendal nerve block under ultrasound and fluoroscopic guidance. Reg Anesth Pain Med 2012;37:262–6.

45. Dean LM. Chapter 163: Selective nerve root block. In: Matthew AM, Kieran PJ, editors. Image-guided interventions. 2nd edition. Philadelphia: Elsevier Saunders; 2014. p. 1217–32.

46. Simons DG, Travell JG, Simons LS. Myofascial pain and dysfunction. In: Johnson EP, editor. Myofascial pain and dysfunction, vol. 1, 2nd edition. Baltimore (MD): Williams and Wilkins; 1999. p. 5.

47. Alvarez DJ, Rockwell PG. Trigger points: diagnosis and management. Am Fam Physician 2002;65:653–60.

48. Spitznagle TM, Robinson CM. Myofascial pelvic pain. Obstet Gynecol Clin North Am 2014;41:409–32.

49. Langford CF, Nagy SU, Ghoniem GM. Levator ani trigger point injections: an underutilized treatment for chronic pelvic pain. Neurourol Urodyn 2007;26:59–62.

50. Nicosia JF, Abcarian H. Levator syndrome: a treatment that works. Dis Colon Rectum 1985;28:406–8.

51. Zoorob D, South M, Karram M, et al. A pilot randomized trial of levator injections versus physical therapy for treatment of pelvic floor myalgia and sexual pain. Int Urogynecol J 2015;26:845–52.

52. Venancio RD, Alencar FG, Zamperini C. Different substances and dry needling injections in patients with myofascial pain and headaches. J Craniomandibular Pract 2008;26(2):96–103.

53. Hong CZ. Lidocaine injection versus dry needling to myofascial trigger point. The importance of the local twitch response. Am J Phys Med 1994;73(4):256–63.

54. Frost FA, Jessen B, Siggaard-Andersen A. A control, double-blind comparison of mepivicaine injection versus saline injection for myofascial pain. Lancet 1980; 1(8167):499–500.

55. Lewit K. The needle effect in the relief of myofascial pain. Pain 1979;6:83–90.

56. Moldwin RM, Fariello JY. Myofascial trigger points of the pelvic floor: associations with urological pain syndromes and treatment strategies including injection therapy. Curr Urol Rep 2013;14:409–17.

57. Misirlioglu TO, Akgun K, Palamar D, et al. Piriformis syndrome: comparison of the effectiveness of local anesthetic and corticosteroid injections: a double-blinded, randomized controlled study. Pain Physician 2015;18:163–71.

58. Kirschner JS, Foye PM, Cole JL. Piriformis syndrome, diagnosis and treatment. Muscle Nerve 2009;40:10–8.

59. Fishman M, Anderson C, Rosner B. BOTOX and physical therapy in the treatment of piriformis syndrome. Am J Phys Med Rehabil 2002;81(12):936–42.

60. Jarvis SK, Abbott JA, Lenart MB, et al. Pilot study of botulinum toxin type A in the treatment of chronic pelvic pain associated with spasm of the levator ani muscles. Aust N Z J Obstet Gynaecol 2004;44:46–50.

61. Ghazizadeh S, Nikzad M. Botulinum toxin in the treatment of refractory vaginismus. Obstet Gynecol 2004;104:922–5.
62. Adelowo A, Hacker MR, Shapiro A, et al. Botulinum toxin type A (BOTOX) for refractory myofascial pelvic pain. Female Pelvic Med Reconstr Surg 2013;19:288–92.
63. Abbott J, Jarvis SK, Lyons SD. Botulinum toxin type A for chronic pain and pelvic floor spasm in women: a randomized controlled trial. Obstet Gynecol 2006;108(4):915–23.
64. Abbott J. The use of botulinum toxin in the pelvic floor for women with chronic pelvic pain - a new answer to old problems? J Minim Invasive Gynecol 2009;16:130–5.
65. Abbott J. Gynecologic indications for the use of botulinum toxin in women with chronic pelvic pain. Toxicon 2009;54:647–53.
66. Roberts SL, Burnham RS, Ravichandiran K, et al. Cadaveric study of sacroiliac joint innervation: implications for diagnostic blocks and radiofrequency ablation. Reg Anesth Pain Med 2014;39:456–64.
67. Murakami E, Tanaka Y, Aizawa T, et al. Effect of periarticular and intraarticular lidocaine injections for sacroiliac joint pain: prospective comparative study. J Orthop Sci 2007;12:274–80.
68. Maldjian C, Mesgarzadeh M, Tehranzadeh J. Diagnostic and therapeutic features of facet and sacroiliac joint injection. Radiol Clin North Am 1998;36(3):497–508.
69. Pekkafali MZ, Kiralp MZ, Başekim CC. Sacroiliac joint injections performed with sonographic guidance. J Ultrasound Med 2003;22:553–9.
70. Harmon D, O'Sullivan M. Ultrasound guided sacroiliac joint injection technique. Pain Physician 2008;11:543–7.
71. Hunter C, Davé N, Diwan S, et al. Neuromodulation of pelvic visceral pain: review of the literature and case series of potential novel targets for treatment. Pain Pract 2013;13(1):3–17.
72. Miller JP, Eldabe S, Busher E, et al. Parameters of spinal cord stimulation and their role in electrical charge delivery: a review. Neuromodulation 2016;19:373–84.
73. Valovska A, Peccora CD, Philip CN, et al. Sacral neuromodulation as a treatment for pudendal neuralgia. Pain Physician 2014;17:E645–50.
74. de Vos CC, Born MJ, Vanneste S, et al. Burst spinal cord stimulation evaluated in patients with failed back surgery syndrome and painful diabetic neuropathy. Neuromodulation 2014;17:152–9.
75. Van Buyten SP, Al-Kaisey A, Smet I, et al. High frequency spinal cord stimulation for the treatment of chronic back pain patients: results of a prospective multicenter European clinical study. Neuromodulation 2013;16:59–66.
76. Kapural L, Narouze SM, Janicki TI, et al. Spinal cord stimulation is an effective treatment for chronic intractable visceral pelvic pain. Pain Med 2006;7(5):440–3.
77. Hassenbusch SJ, Stanton-Hicks M, Shoppa D, et al. Long-term results of peripheral nerve stimulation for reflex sympathetic dystrophy. J Neurosurg 1996;84:415–23.
78. Datir A, Connell D. CT guided injection for ganglion impar blockade: a radiological approach to the management of coccydynia. Clin Radiol 2010;65:21–5.

Index

Note: Page numbers of article titles are in **boldface** type.

Phys Med Rehabil Clin N Am 28 (2017) 647–657
http://dx.doi.org/10.1016/S1047-9651(17)30044-X
1047-9651/17

pmr.theclinics.com

Moving?

Make sure your subscription moves with you!

To notify us of your new address, find your **Clinics Account Number** (located on your mailing label above your name), and contact customer service at:

Email: journalscustomerservice-usa@elsevier.com

800-654-2452 (subscribers in the U.S. & Canada)
314-447-8871 (subscribers outside of the U.S. & Canada)

Fax number: 314-447-8029

Elsevier Health Sciences Division
Subscription Customer Service
3251 Riverport Lane
Maryland Heights, MO 63043

*To ensure uninterrupted delivery of your subscription, please notify us at least 4 weeks in advance of move.

ELSEVIER

Printed and bound by CPI Group (UK) Ltd, Croydon, CR0 4YY

03/10/2024

01040388-0001